ANESTHESIA
REVIEW
Blasting the Boards

Acquisitions Editor: Keith Donnellan
Product Development Editor: Nicole Dernoski
Editorial Assistant: Kathryn Leyendecker
Marketing Manager: Dan Dressler
Production Project Manager: Priscilla Crater
Design Coordinator: Stephen Druding
Manufacturing Coordinator: Beth Welsh
Prepress Vendor: S4Carlisle Publishing Services

Library of Congress Cataloging-in-Publication Data

Names: Berg, Sheri M., author. | Bittner, Edward A., 1967- , author. | Zhao,
    Kevin H., author.
Title: Anesthesia review : blasting the boards / Sheri M. Berg, Edward A.
    Bittner, Kevin H. Zhao.
Description: Philadelphia : Wolters Kluwer Health, [2016]
Identifiers: LCCN 2015048903 | ISBN 9781496317957
Subjects: | MESH: Anesthesia | Examination Questions
Classification: LCC RD82.3 | NLM WO 218.2 | DDC 617.9/60076—dc23 LC record available at
    http://lccn.loc.gov/2015048903

ANESTHES

REVIE

Blasting the Bo

Sheri M. Be

Instructor
Harvard M
Massachusetts Ge
Boston, N

Edward A. Bittner, M

Assistant Professor
Harvard M
Program Director, Critical Ca
Associate Director, Surgical Inten
Massachusetts Ge
Boston, N

Kevin H. Zh

Anesthesiologist a
Anesthesiology Associates
Ann Ar

Revie

Archit Shar

Clinical Fellow, Critical C
Department of Anesthesia, C
F
Massachusetts Ge
Boston, N

🔷. Wolters Kluwer

Philadelphia • Baltimore • New York • London
Buenos Aires • Hong Kong • Sydney • Tokyo

This book is dedicated to all of the trainees that
demand the best teaching, challenge us to
be paramount in our field, and continue to provide
excellent care to all of the patients.

Preface

As each of us approached board certification and recertification exams in anesthesiology, we realized the need for a resource that was evidence-based, succinct, and composed of high-yield examination topics. This book is the compilation of hundreds of pages of handwritten notes from us (the three authors) that we took while we were studying for (and passed) our board exams. The content reflects topics that we thought were important, covered inadequately in other resources, or appeared in prior board certification exams.

Over the course of one year, we compiled, sorted, and fact-checked our notes into this book. We then added the most commonly encountered anesthesiology keywords (which are in bold face for easy recognition) to ensure that we covered the exams for certification and recertification to the fullest extent.

Our goal was to create a resource that was comprehensive, yet quick to read, and, most importantly, would enable you to understand and remember the information, with its bullet-point style. Furthermore, "In-training" scores are used for securing competitive fellowship positions. While there are a number of question and review books on the market, there are few that combine core content and questions in an easy-to-use format. The questions were designed to reinforce key concepts and simulate actual test questions. *Blasting the Boards* is intended to fill that unmet need and help you to succeed in "blasting" your board exam.

We hope this book can improve your knowledge base in anesthesiology, prepare you for examinations, and serve as a reference in the future.

SMB
EAB
KHZ

Acknowledgment

We would like to thank Dr. Archit Sharma for his brilliant editing skills.

Contents

Preface   vii
Acknowledgment   ix

Chapter 1   Equipment 1
Chapter 2   Monitors and Labs 17
Chapter 3   Induction Drugs 29
Chapter 4   Inhaled Anesthetics 45
Chapter 5   Perioperative Management 53
Chapter 6   Cardiovascular System 79
Chapter 7   Respiratory System 117
Chapter 8   Neurologic System 129
Chapter 9   HEENT System 149
Chapter 10   General/Genitourinary System 157
Chapter 11   Renal 169
Chapter 12   Hematologic System 181
Chapter 13   Endocrine System 199
Chapter 14   Neuromuscular and Musculoskeletal System 209
Chapter 15   Pediatric Anesthesia 215
Chapter 16   Obstetrics 237
Chapter 17   Pain 257
Chapter 18   Regional 271
Chapter 19   Intensive Care Medicine 283
Chapter 20   Toxins and Drugs of Abuse 295
Chapter 21   Statistics and Data 301
Chapter 22   Ethics and Practice Management 307

Answer Key   313

Index   337

CHAPTER 1

Equipment

ANESTHETIC BREATHING CIRCUITS

- Definition: an anesthetic breathing circuit must deliver gas and eliminate carbon dioxide (CO_2)
  - Circuits vary in components and organization
  - Rebreathing can be used to assess circuit efficiency by affecting the amount of fresh gas required and the amount of waste produced
- Circuit classification
  - On the basis of the rebreathing of CO_2, circuits can further be classified as
    - Open: no rebreathing
    - Semi-open: partial rebreathing
    - Closed: complete rebreathing
  - **Rebreathing** is dependent on
    - Circuit design
    - Fresh gas flow
    - Mode of ventilation
    - Mechanics of respiration including tidal volume, respiratory rate, inspiratory-to-expiratory ratio, and inspiratory flow rate
- **Mapleson breathing circuits** (Fig. 1.1)
  - Semi-open breathing circuits that are composed of a facemask, pop-off valve, reservoir tubing, fresh gas inflow tubing, and a reservoir bag
  - Designated by the letters A through F based on circuits construction
    - Mapleson A
      - Fresh gas flow (FGF) is opposite from the patient while the pop-off valve is adjacent to the patient
      - Best at eliminating CO_2 → most efficient for spontaneous breathing
        - FGF equal to minute ventilation prevents rebreathing during spontaneous breathing
        - FGF may need to be as high as 20 L/min to prevent rebreathing during controlled ventilation
      - Expiratory valve must be tightened to assist ventilation → least efficient for controlled ventilation
    - Mapleson B and C
      - Both the FGF and pop-off valve are adjacent to the patient
    - Mapleson D, E, and F
      - Fresh gas flow is adjacent to the patient while the pop-off valve is opposite the patient
      - Mapleson D is the most efficient for controlled ventilation, but least efficient for spontaneous ventilation
  - Bain circuit
    - Modification of a Mapleson D where FGF enters through a narrow tube within the corrugated expiratory limb of the circuit
- **Circle breathing system** (Fig. 1.2)
  - A closed breathing circuit composed of an FGF inlet, reservoir bag, pop-off valve, two unidirectional valves, tubing, and a CO_2 absorber
    - FGF should enter proximal to the inspiratory unidirectional valve
    - The pop-off valve should be distal to the expiratory unidirectional valve

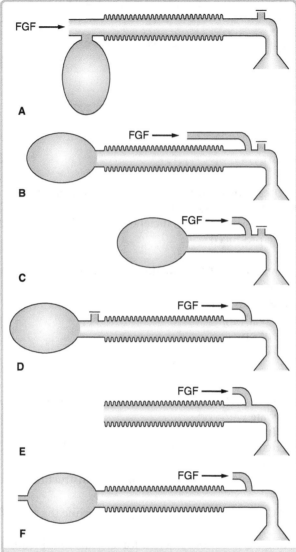

FIGURE 1.1 Mapleson Circuits. Mapleson circuits are semi-open circuits that vary by design. The Mapleson A circuit is the most efficient for spontaneous breathing and the Mapleson D circuit is the most efficient for controlled breathing. FGF, Fresh gas flow. (Reproduced from Riutort KT, Eisenkraft JB. The anesthesia workstation and delivery systems for inhaled anesthetics. In: Barash PG, Cullen BF, Stoelting RK, et al., eds. *Clinical Anesthesia.* 7th ed. Philadelphia, PA: Wolters Kluwer Health; 2013:663.)

- Benefits of a closed system
  - ◆ Reduced use of FGF
  - ◆ Decreased anesthetic pollution
  - ◆ Decreased heat loss
  - ◆ Humidification of gases
- ■ **Bag valve mask**
  - Self-inflating bag often used in emergency settings to provide positive pressure ventilation
  - Composed of an FGF inlet, a reservoir bag, inflatable bag, and facemask
  - Function
    - ◆ Squeezing of the bag forces gas through a one-way valve to the patient
    - ◆ Release of the bag draws ambient air or gas from a wall source

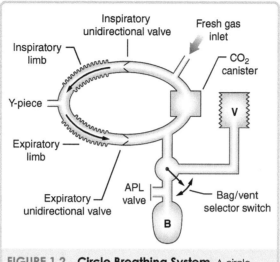

FIGURE 1.2 **Circle Breathing System.** A circle breathing system differs from open circuits through carbon dioxide removal. (Reproduced from Riutort KT, Eisenkraft JB. The anesthesia workstation and delivery systems for inhaled anesthetics. In: Barash PG, Cullen BF, Stoelting RK, et al., eds. *Clinical Anesthesia.* 7th ed. Philadelphia, PA: Wolters Kluwer Health; 2013:649.)

- Used primarily for resuscitation
  - Cannot be connected to anesthetic vaporizers
  - Self-inflating property distinguishes a bag valve mask from a Mapleson circuit

ANESTHESIA MACHINE

- Basic components for fresh gas delivery
  - **Inspiratory and expiratory limbs**
    - Each limb contains a one-way valve to control gas flow
    - Each limb is connected to a Y-piece adjacent to the patient
      - **Dead space ventilation** occurs distal to the Y-piece
      - Dead space includes bronchial tree, endotracheal tube or airway device, and tubing distal to the Y-piece
  - Access to oxygen, air, and nitrous oxide via **gas cylinders** or a **pipeline source** (Fig. 1.3)
    - Gas E-cylinders are attached to the anesthesia machine via a Pin Index Safety System
    - Pipeline source are attached to the anesthesia machine via Diameter Index Safety System
  - **Pressure regulators** and pressure-reduction valves
    - Pressures of up to 2,200 pounds per square inch (PSI) must be decreased prior to reaching the patient
    - Oxygen
      - First stage regulators reduce oxygen pressure to 45 PSI
      - Second stage regulators reduce pressure to about 14 to 16 PSI
      - Oxygen flush exists between the 1st and 2nd stage regulator
        - Does not require anesthesia machine to be turned on
        - Capable of flow rates up to 75 L/min
    - Nitrous
      - Nitrous pressure regulator reduces pressure of up to 745 to 45 PSI
  - **Pressure relief valves**
    - Ventilator pressure relief valve
      - During positive pressure ventilation, removes gas at a pressure greater than the setting of the relief valve to the scavenging system

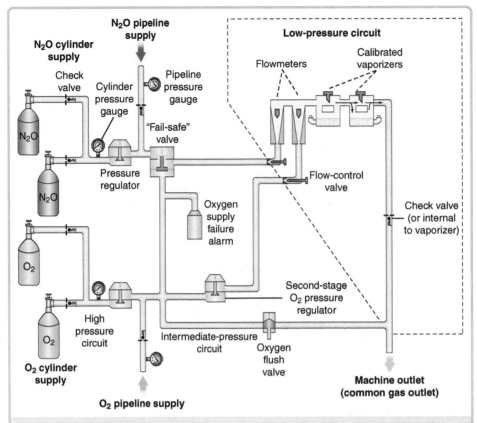

FIGURE 1.3 **Anesthesia Machine Pipeline.** Circuitry of wall gases connections to an anesthesia machine. (Reproduced from Riutort KT, Eisenkraft JB. The anesthesia workstation and delivery systems for inhaled anesthetics. In: Barash PG, Cullen BF, Stoelting RK, et al., eds. *Clinical Anesthesia.* 7th ed. Philadelphia, PA: Wolters Kluwer Health; 2013:647.)

- ◆ **Adjustable pressure limiting valve**
  - ➤ During spontaneous ventilation, removes gas at a pressure greater than the pressure setting
- ● **Gas analyzers**
  - ◆ Two types of oxygen analyzers
    - ➤ Clark electrode
      - ❖ Increased oxygen tension generates increased current across two electrodes in a gel
      - ❖ Clark electrodes require calibration and eventual replacement when electrodes are consumed
    - ➤ Paramagnetic device
      - ❖ Increased oxygen tension generates increased magnetic attraction
      - ❖ Paramagnetic devices have a faster response time, are self-calibrating, and have no consumable parts
- ● **Flow meters**
  - ◆ Measures gas flow to the common gas outlet
    - ➤ Upward force provided through gas flow
    - ➤ Downward force provided by gravity
  - ◆ Oxygen flowmeter is downstream of other flow meters to prevent a hypoxic mixture from reaching the patient
- ● Power source and bellows
  - ◆ Ventilators can be powered by electricity or compressed gas
    - ➤ Piston ventilators are driven by an electric motor
    - ➤ Pneumatic ventilators are driven by compressed gas

- ◆ Bellows
  - ➤ Descending bellows (descend during expiration)
    - ❖ During inspiration, driving gas pressurizes the bellows → bellows rise and delivers gas to patient
  - ➤ Ascending bellows (ascend during expiration)
    - ❖ During exhalation, depressurization of the bellows allows exhaled gas to fill the bellows
    - ❖ Considered safer because during a disconnect, the ascending bellows will fail to fill
  - ◆ Tidal volume measurements
    - ➤ Some older mechanical ventilators will deliver additional tidal volume based on FGF
      - ❖ (FGF × percentage of inspiratory time)/respiratory rate = additional volume delivered per breath
    - ➤ Compression volume
      - ❖ Compression volume is the volume absorbed by the circuit
      - ❖ Compression volume = (respiratory rate × set tidal volume) − minute ventilation
- ● **Reservoir bag**
  - ◆ Used to collect gases and squeezed to assist ventilation
  - ◆ Bag size should be selected based on the expected tidal volume of the patient
- ■ **CO^2 elimination**
  - ● Absorber collects exhaled CO_2 through soda lime or Baralyme
    - ◆ Soda lime: 75% $Ca(OH)_2$, 3% NaOH, 1% KOH, 20% H_2O
    - ◆ Baralyme: 80% $Ca(OH)_2$ + $Ba(OH)_2$
  - ● Exhausted soda changes color from white to purple, which can revert to white with time
  - ● Absorbent can create **carbon monoxide (CO)**
    - ◆ Factors associated with CO production
      - ➤ Degree of absorbent dryness
        - ❖ Absorbents not used for several days (over the weekend) commonly implicated in CO case reports
        - ❖ Low FGF rates can dry absorbent
      - ➤ High concentrations of volatile
      - ➤ Higher temperatures
      - ➤ Volatile used (desflurane > enflurane > isoflurane > halothane and sevoflurane)
      - ➤ Use of Baralyme over soda lime
  - ● Absorbent can create **compound A**
    - ◆ Sevoflurane + CO_2 absorbents → vinyl ether (compound A)
      - ➤ Nephrotoxic to rats at high concentrations
      - ➤ Implications on humans is less clear
    - ◆ Gas flows at >2 L/min prevents rebreathing of compound A, but not its formation
    - ◆ Factors increasing compound A
      - ➤ Low FGF
      - ➤ High absorbent temperatures
      - ➤ Fresh absorbent
      - ➤ Higher concentrates of sevoflurane
      - ➤ Use of Baralyme over soda lime
        - ❖ Dehydration of Baralyme increases compound A
        - ❖ Dehydration of soda lime decreases compound A
- ■ **Heat and moisture exchangers**
  - ● Used in ventilators to prevent drying of the respiratory tract
    - ◆ Minimal clinical effect because only 10% of heat loss is through respiratory tract
  - ● Heat and moisture exchangers are hydrophobic or hygroscopic
    - ◆ Hydrophobic
      - ➤ Better at filtering infectious agents
      - ➤ Long-term use associated with tube occlusion due to inadequate humidity to break secretions
    - ◆ Hygroscopic
      - ➤ Better at providing humidity
      - ➤ Increases circuit resistance

VAPORIZERS AND GAS CYLINDERS

- Vaporizers
  - Volatile anesthetics exist in a liquid state
    - The amount of liquid vaporized is dependent on the saturated vapor pressure of the volatile and the temperature
  - Contemporary vaporizers are variable-bypass (Fig. 1.4)
    - Gas enters through a common inlet
    - Concentration control dial alters the ratio of flow between the bypass chamber and vaporizing chamber
    - Gas from both chambers merge at a common outlet
  - Factors affecting vaporizer output
    - Flow rate
    - Gas concentration
    - Temperature
  - Altitude
    - Higher altitude → greater vaporizer output
    - Vapors are at constant potency at constant temperature irrespective of altitude
      - Except desflurane, which has decreased anesthetic potency with increased altitude because of its partial pressure
  - Problems that may occur with vaporizers
    - Vaporizer tipped
      - Anesthetic liquid in vaporizing chamber may enter the bypass chamber and increase the concentration of delivered anesthetic gas
        - The transport dial prevents this bypass
      - If tipped, the vaporizer should be flushed at high flows with the vaporizer set to low concentrations for 30 minutes
    - Wrong volatile is filled into the vaporizer
      - If a volatile of higher saturated vapor pressure is used → higher concentration of gas administered to patient

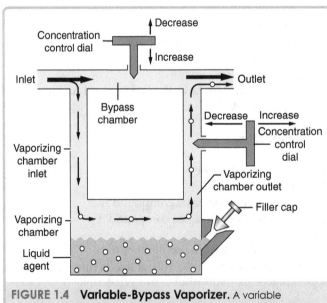

FIGURE 1.4 Variable-Bypass Vaporizer. A variable bypass vaporizer splits fresh gas flow between the mixing and bypass chamber to deliver a specific volatile gas concentration. (Reproduced from Riutort KT, Eisenkraft JB. The anesthesia workstation and delivery systems for inhaled anesthetics. In: Barash PG, Cullen BF, Stoelting RK, et al., eds. *Clinical Anesthesia*. 7th ed. Philadelphia, PA: Wolters Kluwer Health; 2013:663.)

> ➤ If a volatile of lower saturated pressure vapor is used → lower concentration of gas administered to patient
- ◆ Overfilling vaporizer
  - ➤ Volatile liquid can enter the bypass chamber → an elevated concentration of gas is delivered to the patient
  - ➤ Side-fill design of modern vaporizers minimizes the likelihood of overfilling
- ◆ Pumping effect and back pressure
  - ➤ Pumping effect
    - ❖ Intermittent back pressure from circuit prevents outflow of gases from vaporizing chamber and bypass
    - ❖ More anesthetic is vaporized
  - ➤ Back pressure effect
    - ❖ Back pressure may decrease concentration of gas
    - ❖ Compresses the carrier gas, but the anesthetic agent in chamber is unchanged because the amount of agent vaporized depends on saturated vapor pressure of the drug and not the drug in the chamber
- ■ **Anesthetic gas vapor pressures**
  - ● Methoxyflurane: 23 mm Hg
  - ● Sevoflurane: 160 mm Hg
  - ● Enflurane: 172 mm Hg
  - ● Isoflurane: 240 mm Hg
  - ● Halothane: 243 mm Hg
  - ● Desflurane: 669 mm Hg
- ■ **Calculating anesthetic gas output**
  - ● Vapor output (mL) = (carrier gas flow × saturated vapor pressure of gas)/(barometric pressure − saturated vapor pressure of gas)
    - ◆ At low flow rates (<250 cc/min), insufficient pressure to advance molecules of volatile upward
    - ◆ At high flow rates (>15 L/min), insufficient mixing in vaporizing chamber
  - ● Volatile uptake
    - ◆ Amount of uptake in the first minute is equal to the amount taken up between the squares of any two consecutive minutes
    - ◆ Example: between the 16th and 25th minute, the amount taken up is equal to the 1st minute
- ■ Gas cylinders
  - ● **Oxygen**
    - ◆ Green canister
    - ◆ Compressed gas cylinder holds 625 L at 2,000 PSI
  - ● Air
    - ◆ Yellow canister
    - ◆ Compressed gas cylinder holds 625 L at 2,000 PSI
  - ● **Nitrous oxide**
    - ◆ Blue canister
    - ◆ Compressed gas cylinder holds 1,590 L at 750 PSI
      - ➤ When pressure drops from 750 PSI, only 400 L of nitrous oxide remain
  - ● Helium
    - ◆ Brown canister
    - ◆ Helium has a lower density than nitrogen and oxygen, so it can decrease the density of a gas mixture by as much as a 3×
      - ➤ In laminar flow, gas flow is dependent on viscosity
      - ➤ In turbulent flow, gas flow is dependent on density
      - ➤ Reynolds number = 2 × radius × velocity × density/viscosity
        - ❖ Reynolds <2,000 = laminar flow
        - ❖ Reynolds >4,000 = turbulent flow
        - ❖ Reynolds between 2,000 and 4,000 = both flows
    - ◆ Helium–oxygen combination (heliox) can be used to decrease the work of breathing and improve gas flow through a stenotic lesion
  - ● Carbon dioxide

- ◆ Gray canister
- Nitrogen
  - ◆ Black canister

ANESTHESIA MACHINE SAFETY DEVICES

- **Fail-safe device**
  - Shuts off nitrous oxide if there is a loss of oxygen supply pressure
  - Does not allow oxygen concentration to fall below 19%
    - ◆ Fail-safe device checks only pressure and not flow
    - ◆ A hypoxic mixture can still be delivered if low flows are used
- Positive pressure and negative pressure relief valves
  - Exist in the scavenging system to prevent positive or negative pressure from being transmitted to the breathing circuit
  - The positive pressure valve opens if positive pressure accumulates in the scavenging system
  - The negative pressure valve opens and entrains room air if a vacuum develops in the scavenging system
- Common gas outlet check valve
  - Prevents expired gas from transmitting back to the vaporizers or flowmeters
- Interlock device
  - Prevents two vaporizers from working simultaneously
  - Two volatiles being administered together is referred to as an azeotrope

ANESTHETIC GAS POLLUTION

- **Anesthetic pollution**
  - Volatiles are allowed at 0.5 parts per million
  - Nitrous is allowed at 25 parts per million
    - ◆ Dental facilities permit up to 50 parts per million
- Anesthesia machine sterilization
  - Methods for anesthesia machines to kill bacteria
    - ◆ Shifts in humidity
    - ◆ Shifts in temperature
    - ◆ High oxygen concentration
    - ◆ Metallic ions in machine
  - Bacterial filter on breathing circuit is not effective at preventing cross-infection
- **Environmental risk**
  - Historical reports suggested that anesthesiologists and those working in the operating room had increased risks of liver disease, memory deficits, and miscarriages
    - ◆ Reports were done before effective scavenging systems
    - ◆ Studies were poor qualities (retrospective surveys)
  - Recent investigations into historical reports suggest that the fears are exaggerated and largely unfounded

ULTRASOUND

- Ultrasound imaging utilizes a sound wave at a frequency greater than the upper limit of human hearing
  - Ultrasound frequencies are >20 kHz
  - Ultrasound imaging is done at 2.5 to 10 MHz
- Frequency and image quality (Fig. 1.5)
  - Relationships
    - ◆ Wavelength and frequency are inversely related
      - ➤ Increased frequency → lower wavelength
    - ◆ Resolution is 2× wavelength
      - ➤ Lower resolution → improved image quality

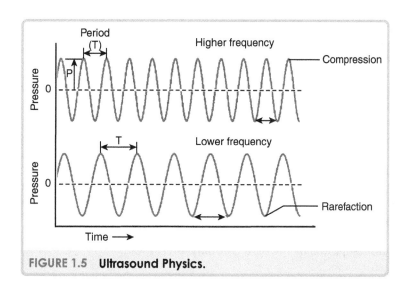

FIGURE 1.5   **Ultrasound Physics.**

- ◆ Penetration is 200× to 400× wavelength
  - ➤ Increased frequency → lower penetration, improved resolution
- ■ Image acquisition
  - ● A sound wave is emitted from a piezoelectric transducer and received after bouncing off an object
    - ◆ Time and strength of sound wave return determines image formation
  - ● Water based–gel improves coupling between transducer and patient
    - ◆ Air–tissue interface loses 99% of ultrasound beam
    - ◆ Gel has similar acoustic impedance between transducer and the patient
  - ● Speed of propagation
    - ◆ Fastest in bone, slowest in air (denser = faster)
    - ◆ Very rapid
      - ➤ 1,540 m/sec in soft tissue
- ■ Application
  - ● Ultrasound is used for vascular access, regional anesthesia, echocardiography, and focused assessment with sonography for trauma (FAST) exams
  - ● Probe selection
    - ◆ Linear
      - ➤ Used in **line placement** and regional anesthesia
    - ◆ Phased array (cardiac)
      - ➤ Used for transthoracic echocardiography
    - ◆ Curvilinear (abdominal)
      - ➤ Used for abdominal and obstetric exams
    - ◆ Transesophageal (matrix array)
      - ➤ Used for transesophageal echocardiography
  - ● **Doppler**
    - ◆ Uses the Doppler effect to assess blood flow
      - ➤ Doppler effect: a wave changes in frequency based on whether the wave is moving away or toward a focal point
    - ◆ Color interpretation during ultrasonography (BART = Blue Away, Red Toward)
      - ➤ Red color = flow toward the probe
      - ➤ Blue color = flow away from the probe
  - ● **Transthoracic echocardiogram**
    - ◆ Parasternal long-axis views
      - ➤ Offers views of the left atrium, mitral valve, left ventricle, right ventricular outflow tract, aortic valve, and descending aorta
    - ◆ Parasternal short-axis views
      - ➤ Offers five cross-sectional levels that include the pulmonary artery, aortic valve, mitral valve, mid-papillary, and apex

- Apical views
  - Offers a four- or five-chamber view of the heart
- Subcostal views
  - Provides a four-chamber view of the heart as well as clear views of the pericardium and inferior vena cava
- **Transesophageal echocardiogram**
  - Mid-esophageal views
    - The mid-esophagus offers numerous views through the left atrium including the four-chamber view, two-chamber view (left atrium and left ventricle), bicaval view, and views of the left ventricular outflow tract and aortic valve
    - The four-chamber view displays the anterolateral (supplied by the left anterior descending and circumflex) and inferoseptal (supplied by the left anterior descending and right coronary artery) walls
    - The two-chamber view displays the anterior (supplied by the left anterior descending) and inferior (supplied by the right coronary artery) walls
  - Transgastric views
    - The transgastric and deep transgastric views transmit through the stomach to offer important information about left and right ventricular function as well as valvular function
    - Offers views of all three major coronary arteries
  - High esophageal views
    - Offers views of the great vessels, coronary vessels, and aorta
- **Transesophageal echocardiogram contraindications**
  - Patient refusal
  - Esophageal obstruction or tracheoesophageal fistula
  - History of an esophagectomy
  - Perforated viscus
  - Active gastrointestinal bleed
  - Coagulopathy and varices are relative contraindications

ELECTRICITY

- Pacemakers
  - Types
    - **Transcutaneous**
      - Two pacing pads and ECG leads are placed on the chest or back
      - Used for temporary stabilization of hemodynamically unstable bradycardias before a more permanent modality is established
    - **Transvenous**
      - Pacing wires are placed into the right atrium or ventricle through an introducer in a central vein
    - **Epicardial**
      - Pacing wires are placed during open heart surgery in the epicardium
    - **Permanent**
      - Pacing wires are placed in the right atrium and/or right ventricle and an electronic pacemaker is implanted under the skin
      - Electrodes require an implantation time of up to 4 weeks to avoid dislodgement
  - **Nomenclature**
    - First letter: chamber paced
    - Second letter: chamber sensed
    - Third letter: response to sensing
    - Fourth letter: programmability
      - Example: rate modulation
        - An increase in vibration, motion, or minute ventilation is sensed → pacing rate increases
    - Fifth letter: multistate pacing
  - **Interrogation**
    - Recommended 30 days prior to surgery

- Routine follow-up recommended every 3 to 4 months
- **Preoperative considerations**
  - Determine pacer type
  - Determine setup (e.g., DDD, VOO)
  - Determine what happens when a magnet is applied
  - Discontinue rate modulation, if applicable
  - Consider programming to an asynchronous mode
- **Intraoperative considerations**
  - Disable artifact filter on monitor
  - Avoid **R on T phenomenon**
    - R on T occurs if a pacemaker paces during the heart's refractory period
- Risk exists if the native HR exceeds the programmed rate in an asynchronous mode → the native sinus node and the pacemaker will both fire
  - If the native rate is faster than the pacemaker, consider administering β-blockade to allow the pacemaker to lead
  - Encourage the use of bipolar, not monopolar, cautery
    - Bipolar transmits across only the distance between the two leads
    - Monopolar transmits to the grounding pad and can go a longer direction
    - Use short bursts of cautery at low settings
  - Consider whether magnet should be used
- **Postoperative considerations**
  - Re-interrogate pacemaker
  - Reprogram if needed
- Defibrillators
  - Function
    - Treatment for life-threatening dysrhythmias such as ventricular fibrillation and tachycardia
      - Depolarizes heart muscle and allows normal sinus rhythm to take over pacing function
    - Can be monophasic or biphasic
      - Monophasic delivers current in one direction
      - Biphasic delivers current in two directions and allows a measure of impedance
        - Higher efficacy at terminating ventricular fibrillation
        - Less postresuscitation myocardial dysfunction
        - Fewer skin burns
  - Types
    - **External**
      - Deliver a shock through paddles or pads placed on a patient's chest
      - **Paddle placement**
        - One below the right clavicle in the midclavicular line
        - One over the left lower ribs in the mid/anterior axillary line
      - **Energy**
        - Biphasic 200 J or monophasic 360 J should be used
      - Automated external defibrillators (AEDs) utilize a computer to read the patient's heart rhythm to determine if a shock is warranted
        - Delay for AED to read the heart rhythm can delay chest compressions and defibrillation
        - If trained health-care providers are available, the monitor should be read by the providers to expedite decision making
    - **Internal**
      - An internal cardiac defibrillator monitors a patient's heart rhythm and shocks during life-threatening dysrhythmias
        - Can remodel the left ventricle over time and increase cardiac output
      - Lead placement
        - One at right atrium, one at right ventricle, and one at the coronary sinus
      - Indications
        - Ejection fraction <35% or New York Heart Association class II or III
      - Nomenclature
        - First letter: chamber shocked

- ❖ Second letter: chamber stimulated for overdrive packing
- ❖ Third letter: chamber where rhythm is sensed
  - ➤ Magnet inhibits the cardioverter-defibrillator, but does not reprogram the pacer to an asynchronous mode
- **Cardioversion**
  - ❖ Used to convert an arrhythmia with a pulse into a sinus rhythm
  - ❖ Example: atrial fibrillation or ventricular tachycardia with a pulse

OPERATING ROOM ELECTRICITY AND FIRES

- ■ Operating room electricity
  - ● A **transformer** connects the **grounded** hospital to ungrounded electricity in the operating room
  - ● Operating rooms use an isolation transformer to convert grounded power to an ungrounded or isolated power system to avoid macroshocks
- ■ **Line-isolation monitor**
  - ● Measures total amount of current leakage in an isolated power system by monitoring the integrity of the isolated power system
    - ❖ Intact equipment ground wires key to function
    - ❖ Detects 2 to 5 mA
      - ➤ Prevents macroshocks, not microshocks
      - ➤ Understanding shocks
        - ❖ 1 mA = perceived
        - ❖ 10 to 2 mA = muscle contractions
        - ❖ 100 mA to 4 A = ventricular fibrillation
    - ❖ Does not suggest current is actively leaking, but suggests the potential for leaking
  - ● If line isolation monitor alarm goes off → unplug unneeded equipment or the last piece of equipment plugged in
- ■ Electrocautery
  - ● A metal probe is heated by an electric current
    - ❖ Used to stop bleeding or cut through tissue
  - ● Monopolar vs. bipolar
    - ❖ Monopolar: a small electrode contacts the tissue → current exits through grounding pad
    - ❖ Bipolar: circuit established between two tips of forceps → does not require a grounding pad
  - ● Grounding pads should have large surface area and be placed away from the heart
- ■ **Lasers**
  - ● Frequently used in otolaryngology, urological, and gynecological surgery
  - ● Greatest safety concern with laser usage is corneal and retinal damage
    - ❖ Milliseconds of exposure can cause permanent damage
  - ● Types of lasers
    - ❖ KTP-Nd: YAG (potassium, titanyl, phosphate-neodymium: ytrium, aluminum, garnet)
      - ➤ Light passes through cornea without causing damage → absorbed by pigment tissue → burns retina
    - ❖ Ruby lasers
      - ➤ Higher frequency light penetrates corneas → risk to retina
    - ❖ CO_2 lasers
      - ➤ Highest wavelength in the infrared range
      - ➤ Energy absorbed at water and tissue → increases corneal damage risk
      - ➤ Any clear glass or plastic is opaque to CO_2 energy, making this protective
        - ❖ Contact lenses fail due to high moisture
        - ❖ Patients can have water/saline soaked gauzes or metal shields at eyes
- ■ Operating room and airway fires
  - ● **National Fire Protection Association (NFPA)** governs and regulates operating room fire safety
  - ● **Triad for fire**
    - ❖ Ignition
    - ❖ Fuel
    - ❖ Oxidizer

- Skin antiseptic solutions contain flammable isopropyl alcohol
  - Must be allowed to dry prior to surgical draping
- Airway fires
  - Airway fires typically begin on the outside of tube, but it can have a devastating blowtorch effect if it reaches the inside of the tube
  - Immediate interventions in the event of an airway fire
    - Remove the endotracheal tube
    - Stop flow of all gases, especially oxygen
    - Remove burning material from the patient
    - Pour saline on airway
    - Mask ventilate with minimal inspired oxygen
    - Examine endotracheal tube for fragments
    - Perform a bronchoscopy to assess for debris, fragments, and degree of injury

RADIATION

- Radiation exposure
  - Radiation use is increasing in the medical field and in anesthetic locations
    - Locations and methods include interventional radiology, vascular operating rooms, cardiac catheterization suits, computerized tomography, and x-rays
  - Radiation exposure is permanent and cumulative
    - Radiation impart energy that can dislodge electrons and result in free radicals → adverse biological effects
- Radiation doses and safety
  - Maximum recommended annual accumulation is 50 mSv
  - Non–blood-forming agents, gonads, and lens should have maximum annual accumulation of 150 mSv
    - Cover eyes to prevent cataract formation
  - Total recommended dose of pregnancy should be <5 mSv
- Examples of radiation from typical medical equipment
  - Single x-ray
    - Chest x-ray: 0.1 mSv
    - Hip x-ray: 5 to 6 mSv
    - Fluoroscopy: 12 to 40 mSv/min
  - CT = 5 to 10 mSV
  - Interventional radiology or catheterization lab = 20 to 80 mSv
- Strategies to avoid radiation exposure
  - Minimize time near radiation source
  - Maintain distance from radiation source
    - Relationship of radiation and distance is the inverse of distance squared
      - Doubling distance → one-quarter of radiation
    - 1 m distance = 0.1% of patient's dose
    - 5 m distance = background radiation levels
  - Shielding
    - Lead aprons that contain 0.5-mm thick lead reduce 75% of radiation dose
    - Use barriers, such as a leaded glass, when possible
  - Be perpendicular to beam

MAGNETIC RESONANCE IMAGING (MRI)

- MRI mechanism
  - A magnetic field aligns nuclei in a patient
  - Radiofrequency pulses are emitted by the MRI machine and absorbed by the patient's cells
    - Different tissues emit a different response to radiofrequency
    - The various signals are compiled to form an image
- Equipment selection

- All equipment used in an MRI suite must not interfere with the magnetic field
- All equipment must function properly in the setting of a strong magnet
- Positioning
  - Careful attention must be made to avoid any metal objects being on, in, or near the patient
  - Prevent burns by avoiding loops in leads and cables
- Monitoring
  - ST-segment and T wave interpretation may not be possible during MRI acquisition
    - If a patient is at high risk of a cardiac event, a 12-lead ECG before and after the MRI may be advisable
  - Temperature
    - Body temperature can increase from heat created by the radiofrequency pulses
    - Body temperature can decrease due to the cold temperature in the scanner
- Quench
  - Termination of magnet operation
    - Can be done intentionally for a life-threatening emergency
  - Magnet turns resistive and all stored energy is released
    - Coolant evaporates → oxygen supply in the room can drop rapidly if venting does not occur
  - Procedures
    - Remove patient from scanner immediately
    - Oxygen should be administered to the patient
    - Oxygen should be available for all personnel in the room

MEDICAL INFORMATICS

- Computer hardware and software
  - **Central processing unit**
    - Receives input from various sources, integrates information, and responds with output
    - Conduit for information transmission
  - **Operating system**
    - Coordinates activity between hardware and software programs
    - Sets up the framework for software to operate (e.g., Apple, Windows)
    - Responsible for management of storage, memory, and user interfacing
- **Anesthesia information management system (AIMS)**
  - Electronic version of the anesthesia record
    - Captures information from monitors and laboratory services
    - Integrates record into hospital system for documentation and billing
    - Largely replaced paper charting
      - Up to 40% of operating room time can be spent charting
  - Benefits
    - Increased accuracy of data from monitoring
    - Increased legibility
    - Allowing the anesthesiologist to focus more on patient care than documentation
      - Patients that require the most charting are usually also the most unstable
    - Ability to program reminders such as antibiotic dosing and missing documentation
    - Data can be collected for research and quality improvement

QUESTIONS

1. Which of the following statements regarding the sensitivity setting of a temporary pacemaker is most correct?

    A. Increasing the sensitivity setting will reduce the occurrence of "R on T" phenomenon
    B. Increasing the sensitivity setting will result in an asynchronous pacing
    C. Decreasing the sensitivity setting will make the pacemaker more sensitive is to intracardiac signals
    D. Once the sensitivity threshold is determined, the sensitivity setting should be set 1–2 times higher

2. During an MRI scan for a patient, an unintentional shutdown of the magnet (quench) occurs. Which of the following statements regarding emergency management is most correct?

    A. Emergency personnel can safely enter the scanner
    B. Oxygen can safely be administered in the scanner
    C. The patient should be cared for in Zone IV if possible
    D. Ferromagnetic materials can safely enter the scanner

3. The annual whole-body effective dose limit for an occupational worker is 50 mSv. The average effective dose of radiation from a CT scan is:

    A. 0.05–0.25 mSv
    B. 0.5–1 mSv
    C. 2–20 mSv
    D. 5–70 mSv

4. Which of the following factors reduces the production of CO during the degradation of volatile anesthetics and CO_2 absorbers?

    A. Use of Baralyme instead of soda lime
    B. Increasing FGF
    C. Use of sevoflurane instead of desflurane
    D. Flushing the breathing circuit with fresh gas before use

5. Which of the following circuits is most efficient for spontaneous respiration?

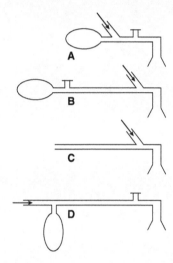

ASA STANDARD MONITORS

- Circulation
  - Continuous ECG monitoring
  - Blood pressure (BP) at least every 5 minutes
- Oxygenation
  - Inspired oxygen analyzer with a low-oxygen-concentration alarm
  - Blood oxygenation via pulse oximetry with pitch tone and a low-saturation alarm
- Ventilation
  - Capnography with alarm to indicate low end-tidal CO_2 for inadequate ventilation or circuit disconnect
- Temperature

ECG MONITORING (FIG. 2.1)

- Unipolar vs. bipolar
  - Unipolar leads measure the electrical activity at one location
  - Bipolar leads measure difference in electrical activity between two locations
    - Example: I, II, III
- Types of ECG monitoring
  - 3-lead
    - Right atrium (RA), left atrium (LA), and left leg (LL) leads
      - Allows calculation of leads I, II, and III
    - Adequate for assessing sinus rhythm and detection of dangerous arrhythmias
    - Inadequate for ST-segment monitoring due to lack of precordial leads and ability to detect a right bundle branch block, left bundle branch block, or more complex arrhythmias
  - 5-lead
    - LA, RA, LL, RL (right leg), and V5
    - Allows calculation of I, II, III, aVR, aVL, and aVF
    - Superior monitoring for patients with suspected ischemia
  - 12-lead
    - Most comprehensive electrocardiogram
    - Used for preoperative risk assessment and to further assess intraoperative arrhythmias

BLOOD PRESSURE MONITORING

- Noninvasive
  - BP cuff should have a width equal to 40% of the arm circumference
    - If width is too narrow or cuff is too loose → more pressure is needed to occlude artery → falsely elevated BP
    - If width is too wide → less pressure is needed to occlude artery → falsely low BP
  - Devices
    - **Auscultation**
      - Use a stethoscope over the brachial artery
      - Inflate the cuff to 180 mm Hg, and slowly release the cuff

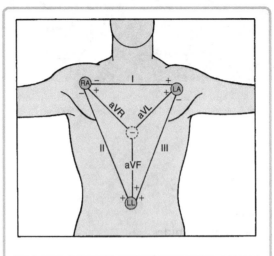

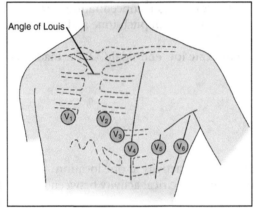

FIGURE 2.1   ECG Lead Placement. Placement of precordial and limb ECG leads for cardiac monitoring. (Reproduced from Badescu GC, Sherman B, Zaidan JR, et al. Atlas of electrocardiography. In: Barash PG, Cullen BF, Stoelting RK, eds. *Clinical Anesthesia*. 7th ed. Philadelphia, PA: Wolters Kluwer Health; 2013:1701.)

> ➤ The first sound (**Korotkoff**) is heard at the systolic pressure
> ➤ The sound disappears at the diastolic pressure
- ◆ **Oscillometry**
  > ➤ An electronic pressure sensor monitors cuff pressure oscillations
  > ➤ Inflate the cuff to 180 mm Hg, and slowly release the cuff
  > ➤ Blood flow returns and causes oscillations from expansion and contraction of the artery
  >   ❖ An algorithm determines systolic, mean, and diastolic pressure
- ◆ **Doppler**
  > ➤ Place a Doppler probe on an artery distal to the BP cuff
  > ➤ Inflate the cuff until the pulse is no longer audible, and slowly deflate the cuff
  > ➤ The first Doppler sound is the systolic BP
  > ➤ The point where the Doppler sound disappears is the diastolic BP
- • Complications
  - ◆ Frequent cuff inflations can cause distal edema, nerve paresthesias (particularly ulnar), compartment syndrome, drip failure, or friction blisters
- ■ Invasive
  - • **Arterial line**
    - ◆ Commonly inserted into the radial artery, but can also be inserted into the brachial, ulnar, femoral, or dorsalis pedis artery

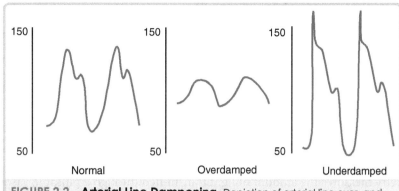

FIGURE 2.2 Arterial Line Dampening. Depiction of arterial line over- and underdampening. Systolic and diastolic pressures vary, but the mean arterial pressure is unchanged.

- ◆ Connected to a **pressure transducer** that transmits BPs in real time
- ● Level of transducer should align with the phlebostatic axis
  - ◆ Phlebostatic axis is at the 4th intercostal space along the midaxillary line
    - ➤ Not the level of the arterial catheter
  - ◆ If the transducer is not leveled properly, BP readings can be falsely high or low
    - ➤ Conversion: 10 cm H_2O = 7.5 mm Hg
    - ➤ Example: a transducer that is 10 cm below the patient will have a BP reading that is falsely elevated by 7.5 mm Hg
  - ◆ Transducer should be zeroed to eliminate the effects of atmospheric pressure
- ● Dampening (Fig. 2.2)
  - ◆ Can be tested using the square test
    - ➤ Evaluation of the waveform immediately following a flush of the catheter from the transducer
  - ◆ Underdamped
    - ➤ Exaggerated oscillations
      - ❖ Overestimates systolic pressure, underestimates diastolic pressure
      - ❖ Widened pulse pressures
    - ➤ Causes
      - ❖ Catheter whip, noncompliant tubing
  - ◆ Overdamped
    - ➤ Diminished oscillations
      - ❖ Underestimates systolic pressure, overestimates diastolic pressure
      - ❖ Narrow pulse pressures
    - ➤ Causes
      - ❖ Narrow tubing, increased tubing length, kinks, air bubbles, loose tubing connections
  - ◆ Mean BP is often accurate in both over- and underdamping

OXYGEN ANALYZER

- ■ Inspired oxygen
  - ● Oxygen analyzers on anesthesia machines indicate inspired oxygen concentration (FIO_2)
    - ◆ Types
      - ➤ Clark electrode uses oxygen to generate a current
      - ➤ Paramagnetic analyzers use the magnetic properties of oxygen to distinguish oxygen from other gases
  - ● FIO_2 from supplemental oxygen sources
    - ◆ Room air: 21% O_2
    - ◆ Oxygen by nasal cannula
      - ➤ 4% increase per liter of oxygen
      - ➤ FIO_2 concentration is no longer reliable beyond 6 L O_2

- ❖ Example: 6 L oxygen by nasal cannula
  - › 4% × 6 L = 24%
  - › 24% + 21% = 45% FIO_2
- ❖ Oxygen by non-rebreather
  - ➤ Can deliver 100% oxygen
  - ➤ FIO_2 may not be 100%, depending on flow rate, minute ventilation, and respiratory pattern
    - ❖ Example: minute ventilation > flow rate
- ■ **Pulse oximetry**
  - ● Properties of oxygen
    - ❖ Oxyhemoglobin absorbs light poorly at 660 nm, but well at 940 nm
    - ❖ Deoxyhemoglobin absorbs light well at 660 nm, but poorly at 940 nm
  - ● Pulse oximetry measures the amount of light transmitted through a pulsatile vascular bed
    - ❖ Measures the difference between background absorption during diastole and peak absorption with systole
    - ❖ Divides alternating current at 660 and 940 nm, direct current at 660 and 940 nm
    - ❖ (AC660/DC660)/(AC940/DC940)
  - ● Causes of inaccurate readings
    - ❖ Fixed reading
      - ➤ **Methemoglobin**: 85% regardless of saturation
      - ➤ **Prilocaine** can cause methemoglobin
    - ❖ Falsely low readings
      - ➤ Blue nail polish absorbs at 660 nm
      - ➤ Hypothermia
        - ❖ Due to peripheral vasoconstriction
      - ➤ Severe anemia (Hb <5 g/dL)
      - ➤ Sulfhemoglobin
        - ❖ Caused by medications such as dapsone, metoclopramide, phenacetin, and sulfonamides
      - ➤ Dyes
        - ❖ Indigo carmine, indocyanine green, methylene blue
      - ➤ Significant venous pulsations
        - ❖ Caused by severe tricuspid regurgitation, intra-aortic balloon pump, or high airway pressures
    - ❖ Falsely high readings
      - ➤ Carboxyhemoglobin absorbs at same frequency as oxyhemoglobin
        - ❖ Requires the use of a co-oximeter to distinguish the difference
      - ➤ Fluorescent light

CAPNOGRAPHY

- ■ Monitors the partial pressure of carbon dioxide of exhaled gas
  - ● A beam of infrared light is passed through the gas sample
    - ❖ CO_2 absorbs infrared light
  - ● A reduced amount of infrared light reaches the sensor for analysis
- ■ Capnography phases (Fig. 2.3)
  - ● 0: inspiratory downstroke
  - ● I: inspiratory phase
  - ● II: expiratory upstroke
  - ● III: alveolar plateau
- ■ Shape and level of the curve can be diagnostic
  - ● Height, frequency, shape, and baseline value can give information about the ventilator, connections, and underlying pulmonary disease
  - ● Increased $ETCO_2$ causes
    - ❖ Increased metabolic rate or cardiac output (malignant hyperthermia)
    - ❖ Tourniquet release
    - ❖ Hypoventilation
    - ❖ Rebreathing

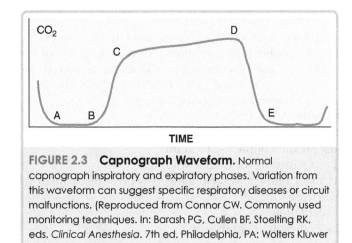

FIGURE 2.3 Capnograph Waveform. Normal capnograph inspiratory and expiratory phases. Variation from this waveform can suggest specific respiratory diseases or circuit malfunctions. (Reproduced from Connor CW. Commonly used monitoring techniques. In: Barash PG, Cullen BF, Stoelting RK, eds. *Clinical Anesthesia.* 7th ed. Philadelphia, PA: Wolters Kluwer Health; 2013:704.)

- ◆ Exhausted CO_2 absorber (bicarbonate infusion)
- ● Decreased ETCO$_2$ causes
  - ◆ Reduced metabolic rate or cardiac output
  - ◆ Hypotension or hypovolemia
  - ◆ Embolism
  - ◆ Hyperventilation
  - ◆ Bronchospasm
- ● Zero ETCO$_2$
  - ◆ Circuit disconnect/extubation
  - ◆ Kinked endotracheal tube
- ● Specific patterns
  - ◆ Prolonged upward slope at alveolar plateau may indicate obstructive lung disease
  - ◆ Steeple sign may be due to a leak at the sampling tube
  - ◆ Prolonged downstroke may be due to an incompetent inspiratory valve
  - ◆ Failure to return to zero during the inspiratory phase may be due to rebreathing or an incompetent expiratory valve
- ■ Esophageal detector device
  - ● Bulb used to detect esophageal intubations (inflates when in trachea)
  - ● Poor sensitivity and specificity for intubations

TEMPERATURE

- ■ Temperature should be monitored during general anesthetics to avoid hypothermia/hyperthermia and monitor for malignant hyperthermia
- ■ Body temperature is not homogenous, and the site of monitoring is important
  - ● Core temperature monitoring sites
    - ◆ Tympanic membrane, pulmonary artery, distal esophagus, and nasopharynx
    - ◆ Sites remain valid during cardiopulmonary bypass
  - ● Near-core sites
    - ◆ Axilla, mouth, bladder, rectum, and skin surface

CENTRAL VENOUS AND PULMONARY ARTERY CATHETERIZATION

- ■ **Central venous catheterization**
  - ● Sites
    - ◆ Central venous cannulation can be done at the internal jugular, subclavian, or femoral vein
      - ➢ Risk of infection

✧ Femoral > internal jugular > subclavian
  ➤ Left subclavian most likely to cause thoracic duct injury
  ➤ Left pleural apex is higher than the right and has a higher risk of causing a pneumothorax
✧ Ultrasound is commonly used for internal jugular and femoral vein cannulation
  ➤ The internal jugular vein is lateral to the common carotid artery
  ➤ The femoral vein is medial to the femoral artery
- **Central venous pressure (CVP)** (Fig. 2.4)
  - ✧ CVP is measured at the junction of the vena cava and right atrium
    - ➤ Reflects filling pressure of the right atrium
    - ➤ CVP is used as a surrogate for cardiac volume
  - ✧ Normal value is 1 to 7 mm Hg in a spontaneously breathing patient
  - ✧ Causes of CVP increase
    - ➤ Mechanical ventilation
    - ➤ High positive end-expiratory pressure
    - ➤ Valsalva
    - ➤ Abdominal muscle contraction
    - ➤ Venous constriction
    - ➤ Cardiogenic shock or heart failure
    - ➤ Tricuspid regurgitation
    - ➤ Volume overload
- CVP trace
  - ✧ *a* Peak: atrial contraction
  - ✧ *c* Peak: ventricular contraction
  - ✧ *x* Descent: atrial relaxation
  - ✧ *v* Peak: venous filling of atrium
  - ✧ *y* Descent: tricuspid valve opening
- **Pulmonary artery (PA) catheterization** (Fig. 2.5)
  - Placement
    - ✧ Placed through an introducer at any central venous cannulation site
      - ➤ Right internal jugular provides the most linear path to the heart
    - ✧ "Floated" through the right side of the heart with the distal balloon inflated
      - ➤ Passage is monitored by the tracings from the distal port
      - ➤ In the vena cava and right atrium: CVP trace
      - ➤ In the right ventricle: rapid systolic upstroke and beats

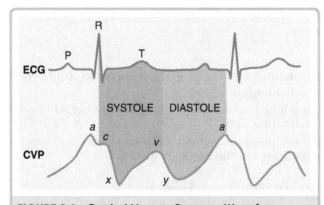

FIGURE 2.4   Central Venous Pressure Waveform.
Central venous pressure waveform with atrial contraction
(a peak), ventricular contraction (c peak), venous atrial
filling (v peak), atrial relaxation (x descent), and tricuspid
valve opening (y descent). (Reproduced from Connor CW.
Commonly used monitoring techniques. In: Barash PG, Cullen
BF, Stoelting RK, eds. *Clinical Anesthesia*. 7th ed. Philadelphia,
PA: Wolters Kluwer Health; 2013:711.)

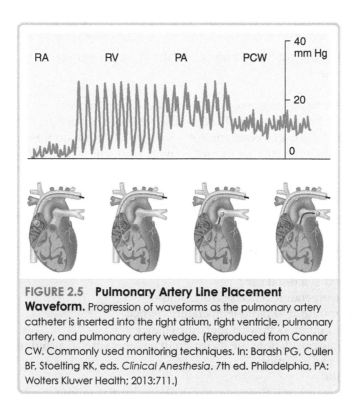

FIGURE 2.5 Pulmonary Artery Line Placement Waveform. Progression of waveforms as the pulmonary artery catheter is inserted into the right atrium, right ventricle, pulmonary artery, and pulmonary artery wedge. (Reproduced from Connor CW. Commonly used monitoring techniques. In: Barash PG, Cullen BF, Stoelting RK, eds. *Clinical Anesthesia*. 7th ed. Philadelphia, PA: Wolters Kluwer Health; 2013:711.)

➤ In the pulmonary artery: similar systolic pressure, but increased diastolic pressure
➤ In the pulmonary artery wedge: decreased systolic pressure and *a, c, v* trace, reflecting the left heart
◆ PA placement distances
   ➤ Distance from entry at the right internal jugular vein
      ❖ Right atrium is at 20 cm
      ❖ Right ventricle is at 30 to 35 cm
      ❖ PA is at 40 to 45 cm
      ❖ Wedge is at 45 to 55 cm
   ➤ Distance from entry at the left internal jugular vein
      ❖ Add 10 cm to all right internal jugular distances
   ➤ Distance from entry at the femoral vein
      ❖ Add 15 cm to all right internal jugular distances
   ➤ Distance from entry at an antecubital vein
      ❖ Add 30 cm from all right internal jugular distances
◆ Complications
   ➤ Bundle branch block
      ❖ If a patient has a preexisting left bundle branch block, a PA catheter could cause a right bundle branch block, leading to complete heart block
   ➤ Pulmonary artery rupture
      ❖ Risk increased with age, hypothermia, pulmonary hypertension, anticoagulation, and catheter migration
      ❖ Presents with hemoptysis
      ❖ Requires endobronchial intubation and emergent surgical management
● Measurements
◆ **Pulmonary artery pressure**: monitored at the distal port with the balloon down
◆ **Pulmonary artery occlusion pressure** (wedge pressure): monitored at the distal port with the balloon inflated
   ➤ The wedge pressure provides an indirect measurement of left atrial pressure
   ➤ **Left atrial pressure** is a surrogate for **left ventricular end-diastolic pressure**
◆ **Mixed venous saturation** can be collected from the distal PA port
◆ **The normal Svo$_2$ is 65% to 75%,** which denotes tissue oxygen extraction to be 25% to 35%

CARDIAC OUTPUT ASSESSMENT AND CALCULATION

- Cardiac output is the volume of blood pumped by the heart per minute
- Methods for measurement
  - **Fick principle**
    - Calculated by knowing oxygen consumption and oxygen content
      - Values can be found or extrapolated from an anesthesia machine
    - Assumes that rate of oxygen consumption relates to rate of blood flow and oxygen uptake
    - Oxygen consumption = (cardiac output × oxygen content of arterial blood) − (cardiac output × oxygen content of venous blood)
  - **Dye dilution**
    - Calculated by sampling blood distal to a site of injection
    - Cardiac output = dye injected/concentration in arterial blood at a downstream sampling site
  - **Thermodilution**
    - Calculated by measuring temperature change from a pulmonary artery catheter
    - Cold or room temperature fluid is injected into the proximal port, and the temperature of blood is assessed at a distal site
      - Change in temperature reflects cardiac output
      - High cardiac output → rapid temperature change
      - Low cardiac output → slow temperature change
    - Risk of inaccurate calculations are increased in patients with tricuspid regurgitation, intracardiac shunts, and atrial fibrillation
  - **Doppler ultrasound**
    - Uses flow seen on echocardiography to calculate a cardiac output
      - Both transthoracic and transesophageal echocardiography can be used
    - Cardiac output = heart rate × (velocity time integral over the left ventricular outflow tract × valve cross-sectional area)
  - **Pulse wave analysis**
    - Uses an algorithm to calculate cardiac output using the arterial BP tracing
  - **Impedance**
    - Uses an algorithm that measures current transmitted through the chest to calculate cardiac output
      - Current uses the path of least resistance to transverse the body
      - The aorta offers the least resistance
    - Uses the velocity and volume changes in the aorta per heartbeat to calculate a cardiac output

ANESTHETIC DEPTH MONITORING

- Expired gas analysis
  - **Mass spectrometry**
    - Concentrations of gas are determined by the volatile's mass to charge ratio
    - Procedure
      - A gas sample is passed through an ionizer → particles become positively charged → particles separated by mass
      - A detector converts the number of ions at each mass into a concentration
    - Largely phased out of clinical use due to inconvenience
  - **Infrared absorption**
    - Concentrations of gas are determined based on intensity of transmission after being passed through an infrared light
  - **Raman Scatter analysis**
    - Concentrations of gas are determined by energy scatter patterns
      - Light strikes gas molecules → energy scatters
      - Gases produce unique patterns
- **Bispectral index**
  - Uses electroencephalography (EEG) to evaluate the **depth of anesthesia** and sedation
    - EEG is monitored at multiple locations along the scalp

- EEG is converted into a number using an algorithm that indicates anesthetic depth
  - Value of 0 to 100
  - Lower values → increased anesthetic depth
- **Spectral edge** is the EEG frequency below which 95% of the power exists

NERVOUS SYSTEM MONITORING

- Evoked potentials
  - Used to monitor the integrity of the nervous system during surgery
    - May be sensitive to anesthetic drugs, perfusion pressure, and surgical insult
  - Order of sensitivity to volatiles (most sensitive to least sensitive)
    - **Visual evoked potentials**, motor evoked potentials, somatosensory evoked potentials, **brain stem auditory potentials**
  - **Somatosensory evoked potentials (SSEP)**
    - **Transmission pathway for sensory inputs**
      - Peripheral nerve → dorsal column → brain stem → medial lemniscus → internal capsule → contralateral somatosensory cortex
    - **Monitoring**
      - Peripheral nerve is stimulated → amplitude and latency are measured
        - Amplitude: peak response
        - Latency: time from stimulus to peak response
      - Decrease in amplitude of >50% or latency increase of 10% is significant
        - Represents hypoperfusion, ischemia, temperature, drugs
      - Incidence of sensory deficit without SSEP changes was 0.6% in scoliosis surgery
    - **Effects of drugs**
      - Midazolam: decreases amplitude
      - Etomidate: increases latency and amplitude
      - Opioids: small increases in latency, decreases in amplitude
      - Ketamine: increases amplitude
      - Volatiles, barbiturates: decreases amplitude, increases latency
        - Up to 0.5 to 0.75 MAC can be used for SSEPs
        - If SSEP is difficult to obtain, consider switching to IV anesthetic
      - Neuromuscular blockers: no effects
        - May reduce muscle movement artifact and improve SSEP quality
  - **Motor evoked potentials (MEP)**
    - **Transmission pathway for motor response**
      - Electrical or magnetic stimulation of the motor cortex → evoked potential sent descending motor pathways → recorded at muscle, nerve, or spinal cord
    - **Monitoring**
      - Motor cortex is stimulated → amplitude and latency measured at peripheral muscle
      - Increased mean arterial pressure may improve perfusion
    - **Effects of drugs**
      - Volatiles, IV anesthetics decrease amplitude, increase latency
        - Total IV anesthetic (TIVA) advocated for all MEP testing due to increased sensitivity of MEPs to volatiles
        - 0.25 MAC or less of volatile likely will not influence readings
      - Do not use neuromuscular blockers
- Electroencephalography
  - EEG can be used to monitor depth of anesthesia and cerebral hypoperfusion
  - **EEG wave patterns**
    - Delta waves
      - Slow waves with frequency of up to 4 Hz
      - Seen in adult sleep
    - Theta waves
      - Waves with frequency from 4 to 7 Hz
      - Seen in drowsy state

- Alpha waves
  - Waves with frequency from 7 to 14 Hz
  - Seen in relaxed state
- Beta waves
  - Waves with frequency from 15 to 30 Hz
  - Associated with activity and concentration
- Gamma waves
  - Waves with frequency from 30 to 100 Hz
  - Associated with higher-level cognitive or motor activity
- **Changes with anesthesia**
  - **Subanesthetic doses**
    - Increased frontal β activity
    - Diminished α activity in occipital leads
  - **General anesthesia effects**
    - Frontal β activity converts to α activity
    - Loss of activity in occipital leads
    - Increased anesthetic depth slows EEG and may induce burst suppression
- Specific patterns
  - **Convulsions:** spikes may represent seizure activity
  - **Burst suppression**: alternating high-voltage activity with intervals of electrical silence
    - Volatiles, barbiturates, etomidate, and propofol are capable of causing burst suppression
- **Cerebral oxygenation** and blood flow
  - **Jugular venous bulb oxygen saturation**
    - A fiber-optic catheter is placed retrograde through the internal jugular vein into the jugular bulb under fluoroscopic guidance
      - Fiber-optic catheter emits near infrared light and records light reflected back to the catheter
      - Measures the degree of oxygen extraction
    - Reflects balance between oxygen supply and demand
  - **Cerebral oximetry**
    - Noninvasive technique using two sensors applied to the forehead to determine local venous oxygen saturation
    - Can be used to assess both arterial and venous oxygen saturation
    - Low levels reflective of hypoxia or increased oxygen consumption
      - Can be a marker of cerebral ischemia
  - **Transcranial Doppler**
    - Ultrasound technique that measures blood flow velocity at cerebral arteries
      - Commonly utilizes the temporal window to image the middle cerebral artery
    - Used to diagnose vasospasm, emboli, and vascular stenosis
- **Intracranial pressure (ICP)**
  - Frequency monitored in traumatic brain injury to prevent secondary injury
    - ICP can be monitored through a bolt pressure monitor or external ventricular drain
  - Cerebral perfusion pressure = MAP − ICP or CVP (whichever is higher)
- **Electromyography (EMG)**
  - Intraoperative monitoring of EMG responses can be used to detect surgically induced nerve injury

QUESTIONS

1. High-velocity flow in a patient with aortic stenosis is most accurately measured with which of the following modes of Doppler echo?

   A. Pulsed wave
   B. Continuous wave
   C. Color mode
   D. Aliasing

2. Under normal conditions, the mixed venous oxygen partial pressure is:

   A. 30 mm Hg
   B. 40 mm Hg
   C. 50 mm Hg
   D. 60 mm Hg

3. The pulmonary artery wedge pressure associated with the onset of pulmonary edema is:

   A. 0–5
   B. 6–18
   C. 19–24
   D. 25–30

4. The component of the CVP waveform that corresponds to ventricular systole and atrial relaxation is the:

   A. *a* wave
   B. *v* wave
   C. *x* descent
   D. *y* descent

5. Compared with the waveform obtained from a radial artery catheter, the waveform of a catheter placed in the dorsalis pedis artery would be expected to have:

   A. Lower systolic pressure
   B. More prominent dicrotic notch
   C. Lower diastolic pressure
   D. Elevated mean arterial pressure

PHARMACOKINETICS AND PHARMACODYNAMICS

- **Vessel-rich group**
  - Collection of organs including the heart, lungs, brain, liver, and kidneys that receive a disproportional amount of blood flow relative to their mass
  - Intravenous agents reach and distribute in the vessel-rich group rapidly → rapid onset of induction agents
- **Volume of distribution**
  - Amount of volume that dilutes an administered drug
  - Volume of distribution is dependent on the drug's solubility in blood and tissues
- **Context-sensitive half-time** (CSHT; Fig. 3.1)
  - Time required for a 50% decrease in the central compartment drug concentration after a steady-state infusion
  - More reflective of clinical effects than half-life

HYPNOTICS

- **Propofol**
  - Uses
    - Most widely used hypnotic agent for induction of anesthesia in the operating room and sedation in the intensive care unit
  - Mechanism
    - Binds to the β-subunit of $GABA_A$
    - NMDA receptor antagonist

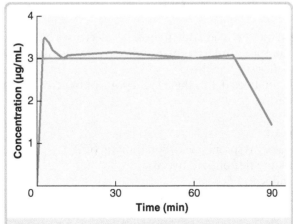

FIGURE 3.1 Context-Sensitive Half-Time. Context-sensitive half-time reflects the drug concentration in the central compartment based on the duration of drug infusion. (Reproduced from Gupta DK, Henthorn TK. Basic principles of clinical pharmacology. In: Barash PG, Cullen BF, Stoelting RK, et al., eds. *Clinical Anesthesia*. 7th ed. Philadelphia, PA: Wolters Kluwer; 2013:178.)

- Direct spinal cord depressant
- Inhibits acetylcholine (ACh) release at the hippocampus and prefrontal cortex
- Increases dopamine concentrations in nucleus accumbens
- Decreases serotonin levels in area postrema
- **Pharmacodynamics and kinetics**
  - Dosing
    - Standard induction dosing is at 2.0 to 2.5 mg/kg, but dosing should be adjusted based on age, desired effect, cardiovascular risk factors, and other drugs being administered
    - Propofol should be used cautiously or avoided entirely in the following situations
      - Severe hypovolemia or hemorrhage
      - Hemodynamically unstable patients
      - Conditions that may not tolerate hypotension (critical aortic stenosis)
  - Formulation
    - 2, 6-diisopropylphenol in a highly lipid soluble solution
      - Contains egg lecithin, glycerol, and soybean oil
    - Disodium edentate or sulfite added to reduce bacterial growth
      - Draw up propofol under sterile conditions and discard after 6 to 12 hours (see individual label)
  - Single bolus injection
    - Propofol levels peak and then rapidly decrease through redistribution and elimination
      - Peak effect from a bolus dose is after ~90 seconds
    - Initial distribution half-time is 2 to 8 minutes, but elimination following redistribution can take hours
  - Prolonged infusion
    - Context-sensitive half-time increases substantially with prolonged infusions due to effects of redistribution
- **Metabolism**
  - Metabolized by conjugation at liver, but extrahepatic metabolism also occurs
  - Eliminated at kidneys
- **Organ system effects**
  - Cerebral
    - Decreases intracranial pressure
    - Decreases intraocular pressure
    - Decreases cerebral perfusion pressure (secondary to hypotension)
    - Increase seizure threshold
    - Less vasodilating than other anesthetics
  - Cardiovascular
    - Vasodilating → decreases preload and afterload → decreases blood pressure
      - Reduces cardiac output, stroke volume, and systemic vascular resistance
    - Mild decrease in cardiac contractility
    - Heart rate generally unaffected, but there are reports of bradycardia or a blunted tachycardic response to hypotension
  - Respiratory
    - Respiratory depressant
      - Decreases ventilatory response to carbon dioxide (CO_2)
      - Decreases ventilatory response to hypoxia
      - Apnea follows induction doses
      - Decreases tidal volume and respiratory rate
    - Bronchodilating
  - Other
    - Decreases postoperative nausea and vomiting
- **Side effects**
  - Hypotension
  - Apnea
  - Pain on injection due to formulation
    - Fospropofol is a prodrug of propofol that is water soluble and does not burn on injection

- Hypertriglyceridemia and pancreatitis with prolonged infusion
  - Avoid in patients with lipid metabolism disorders
- Propofol infusion syndrome
  - Rare condition associated with prolonged propofol infusions (often >48 hours) in pediatric population
    - Theorized to be due to the mitochondrial toxicity of propofol
  - Associated with bradycardia, metabolic acidosis, rhabdomyolysis, and cardiovascular collapse

■ Ketamine
  - **Uses**
    - Can be used for induction and maintenance of anesthesia
    - Used for perioperative and intraoperative pain management
      - Potent analgesic properties
      - Far better for somatic than visceral pain
  - **Mechanism**
    - NMDA receptor antagonist at glutamate receptor
    - Analgesic with dissociative properties
    - Agonist at opioid receptors
      - Decreases opioid tolerance
    - Inhibits nociceptive central hypersensitization
    - Inhibitor of norepinephrine, serotonin, and dopamine uptake
  - **Pharmacodynamics and kinetics**
    - Dosing
      - Induction dosing is 2 mg/kg
    - Formulation
      - Ketamine consists of two stereoisomers, S and R
      - S isomer is more potent with fewer side effects
    - Single bolus injection
      - Levels rapidly peak and ketamine is rapidly redistributed due to high lipid solubility
        - Onset is within 30 to 60 seconds of intravenous administration
        - Onset is within 5 to 15 minutes of intramuscular injection
      - Following induction dose, patients are anesthetized and unresponsive, but may appear awake
        - Eyes open, remains breathing
    - Infusion
      - Ketamine can be infused for general anesthesia, as an adjunct to general anesthesia, or for sedation/pain at subanesthetic doses
  - **Metabolism**
    - Broken down by the liver through demethylation to form norketamine, which is then conjugated to water-soluble products
      - Norketamine has one-third of ketamine's potency
    - Metabolites are excreted in the urine
  - **Organ system effects**
    - Cerebral
      - Creates dissociative anesthesia
        - Depresses cortex and thalamus
        - Stimulates limbic system
      - Corneal, cough, and swallow reflexes are all present
        - Retain pharyngeal and laryngeal reflexes
      - Increases cerebral metabolism, cerebral blood flow, and intracranial pressure
    - Cardiovascular
      - Ketamine stimulates the sympathetic nervous system, but is a direct myocardial depressant
      - Increases cardiac output, heart rate, and blood pressure
        - Increased myocardial oxygen consumption
      - Can increase pulmonary artery pressure

- In stress states where patients are dependent on sympathetic tone (hemorrhage, septic shock) and have depleted endogenous catecholamines, ketamine may decrease blood pressure
  - ◆ Respiratory
    - ➤ Minimal respiratory effects
      - ◆ Transient decrease in minute ventilation and even apnea may occur briefly following a bolus dose
      - ◆ Response to hypercarbia remains intact
    - ➤ Bronchodilator
  - ◆ Other
    - ➤ Increases skeletal muscle tone
- Side effects
  - ◆ Emergence reactions
    - ➤ Hallucinations, illusions, euphoria, and fear
    - ➤ Less common in children
    - ➤ Decreases when administered with a benzodiazepine or other hypnotic
  - ◆ Increased intracranial pressure
  - ◆ Increased intraocular pressure (dose dependent)
  - ◆ Increased pulmonary artery pressure
  - ◆ Nystagmus
  - ◆ Increased salivation
    - ➤ Can cause upper airway obstruction and laryngospasm
  - ◆ Lacrimation
- Etomidate
  - Uses
    - ◆ Primarily used to induce general anesthesia in patients with concern for cardiovascular instability and in whom other hypnotics may not be well tolerated
    - ◆ Used for induction or maintenance of anesthesia
  - Mechanism
    - ◆ Imidazole derivative
    - ◆ Anesthetic mechanism is likely $GABA_A$ related, but understanding remains unclear
  - Pharmacodynamics and kinetics
    - ◆ Dosing
      - ➤ Bolused at 0.2 to 0.6 mg/kg for induction dosing
    - ◆ Formulation
      - ➤ Water insoluble, so formulated in propylene glycol
      - ➤ Hyperosmolar solution
    - ◆ Bolus
      - ➤ Onset and recovery are rapid
      - ➤ Bolus dose quickly redistributes, but even redistributed drug is metabolized quickly by the liver and esterases
    - ◆ Infusion
      - ➤ Can be used, but rare given concerns for increased mortality due to adrenal insufficiency
  - Metabolism/excretion
    - ◆ Metabolized by ester hydrolysis (plasma esterases) or dealkylation at the liver
    - ◆ Excreted by the kidney and in the bile
  - Organ system effects
    - ◆ Cerebral
      - ➤ Decreases cerebral blood flow without altering mean arterial pressure
      - ➤ Decreases intracranial pressure
      - ➤ Increases cerebral oxygen supply due to increased cerebral perfusion pressure
      - ➤ Activates epileptic seizure foci
        - ◆ Use with caution in patients with focal epilepsy
    - ◆ Cardiovascular
      - ➤ Induction doses result in almost no change in mean arterial pressure, heart rate, cardiac output, or pulmonary artery pressure

- ➢ Slight (~15%) reduction in mean arterial pressure
- ➢ Minimal effects on the sympathetic nervous system and on baroreceptor function
- ◆ Respiratory
  - ➢ Decreases respiratory drive, but not as much as propofol or barbiturates
  - ➢ Induction doses cause brief hyperventilation followed by a brief period of apnea
- ◆ Other
  - ➢ Adrenal suppression
    - ◆ Dose-dependent inhibition of 11β-hydroxylase, which is required for cortisol production
    - ◆ Minimal inhibition of 17α-hydroxylase
    - ◆ Effects of adrenal suppression may be minimal in otherwise healthy individuals, but can be contributors to mortality in septic or ICU patients
- ● **Side effects**
  - ◆ Myoclonic activity in up to 70% of patients
  - ◆ Nausea and vomiting in up to 40% of patients
  - ◆ Superficial thrombophlebitis on injection in 20% of patients
  - ◆ Burns on injection due to propylene glycol
- ■ Barbiturates
  - ● **Uses**
    - ◆ Used for induction and maintenance of anesthesia
  - ● **Mechanism**
    - ◆ Acts to activate or prolong GABA$_A$ effects
    - ◆ May also decrease NMDA activity
  - ● **Pharmacodynamics and kinetics**
    - ◆ Dosing
      - ➢ Induction dosing for methohexital is 1 to 1.5 mg/kg
      - ➢ Induction dosing for thiopental is 3 to 4 mg/kg
    - ◆ Formulation
      - ➢ Combined with sodium salts
      - ➢ Highly alkaline solutions → may precipitate in acidic solutions (e.g., succinylcholine)
    - ◆ Bolus
      - ➢ Induction dosing leads to rapid onset (30 to 45 seconds) and redistribution for termination of action
    - ◆ Infusion
      - ➢ Infusions can lead to prolonged effects due to lipid solubility and slow rate of hepatic clearance
  - ● **Metabolism/excretion**
    - ◆ Hepatic metabolism via oxidation, dealkylation, and desulfuration
    - ◆ Renal elimination
  - ● **Organ system effects**
    - ◆ Cerebral
      - ➢ Decreases cerebral metabolic oxygen consumption, cerebral blood flow, and intracranial pressure
      - ➢ Maintains cerebral perfusion pressure
    - ◆ Cardiovascular
      - ➢ Decreased myocardial contractility
      - ➢ Venodilation → decreased blood pressure and cardiac output
      - ➢ Inhibition of sympathetic nervous system
    - ◆ Respiratory
      - ➢ Respiratory depression with transient apnea following bolus administration
      - ➢ Blunts response to carbon dioxide
  - ● **Side effects**
    - ◆ Induces porphyrin synthesis → worsens porphyrias and precipitates attacks
    - ◆ Hypotension
    - ◆ Respiratory depression
    - ◆ Hiccups and myoclonic activity
- ■ Benzodiazepines

- **Uses**
  - Used for anxiolysis, sedation, general anesthesia, and as antiepileptic agent
- **Mechanism**
  - Interacts with $GABA_A$ receptor to mediate amnesia, anxiolysis, and anticonvulsant properties
  - Drugs are often more amnestic than sedative
    - Provides anterograde, not retrograde, amnesia
- **Pharmacodynamics and kinetics**
  - Induction dosing
    - Midazolam: 0.05 to 0.15 mg/kg
    - Lorazepam: 0.1 mg/kg
    - Diazepam: 0.3 to 0.5 mg/kg
  - Properties
    - Midazolam is water soluble → converted to lipid soluble compound in blood → rapidly cross the blood–brain barrier
    - Midazolam levels are reduced from first-pass metabolism due to liver metabolism
- **Metabolism/excretion**
  - Liver oxidation or glucuronidation
  - Metabolites of benzodiazepines
    - Midazolam forms hydroxymidazolams
    - Lorazepam forms lorazepam-glucuronide
    - Diazepam forms oxazepam and desmethyldiazepam
  - Elimination half-life is varied
    - Midazolam: 2 hours
    - Lorazepam: 11 hours
    - Diazepam: 20 hours
  - Context-sensitive half-time
    - Similar between midazolam, lorazepam, and diazepam with single-bolus dosing due to effects of redistribution
- **Organ system effects**
  - Cerebral
    - Reduce cerebral metabolic rate and cerebral blood flow
    - Increase seizure threshold
    - Will not induce burst suppression
  - Cardiovascular
    - Very minor hemodynamic effects
    - Mild decrease in systemic vascular resistance and blood pressure
  - Respiratory
    - Mild respiratory depressant
    - Decreased response to CO_2 is more profound when combined with other anesthetic agents
- **Side effects**
  - Thrombophlebitis
  - Mild respiratory depressant
  - Prolonged sedation when used as maintenance anesthetic
- Reversal: flumazenil
  - Inhibits benzodiazepine activity at the $GABA_A$-receptor
    - Flumazenil is a competitive antagonist that binds benzodiazepine receptor with high affinity
  - Dose at 0.2 mg and uptitrate gradually for suspected overdose
    - Onset is 6 to 10 minutes, with half-life of ~30 minutes
    - Repeated administration may be needed due to short half-life
    - May induce seizures, withdrawal in chronic benzodiazepine users
  - Does not reliably reverse respiratory depressant effects of benzodiazepines
  - Side effects include nausea and vomiting
- **Dexmedetomidine**
  - **Uses**
    - Adjunct to general anesthesia or sedation in the operating room or intensive care unit
    - Provides sedation, hypnosis, and analgesia

- ➤ Decreases MAC by up to 90%
    - ◆ Can also be used for withdrawal of alcohol, opioids, and cocaine
    - ◆ May reduce perioperative cardiovascular risk
- **Mechanism**
    - ◆ α_2-adrenergic agonist that acts at the locus coeruleus,
        - ➤ 1,600× more selective for α_2 than α_1
        - ➤ 8× more selective than clonidine for α_2
    - ◆ Activates sleep pathways
    - ◆ Analgesic effects are likely at the spinal cord
- **Pharmacodynamics and kinetics**
    - ◆ Often bolused at 0.5 to 1 µg/kg over 10 minutes and then infused at a rate of 0.1 to 1.0 µg/kg/hr
        - ➤ Onset is at 5 minutes, peaks at 15 minutes
        - ➤ No bolus necessary if rapid onset is not desired
            - ❖ Can also be started as a continuous infusion without a bolus dose
    - ◆ Highly protein bound (94%)
        - ➤ CSHT ranges from 4 minutes after a 10-minute infusion to 3 hours following an 8-hour infusion
- **Metabolism/excretion**
    - ◆ Metabolized at liver by conjugation, methylation, or hydroxylation
    - ◆ Excreted in kidneys and GI tract
- **Organ system effects**
    - ◆ Cerebral
        - ➤ Sedative effects through the locus coeruleus
        - ➤ Dose-dependent decrease in cerebral blood flow and cerebral metabolic rate
    - ◆ Cardiovascular
        - ➤ A bolus injection causes an initial increase in blood pressure and decrease in heart rate due to vasoconstrictive effects at peripheral α_2 receptors
        - ➤ Prolonged infusion causes bradycardia and hypotension through central α_2 receptors
        - ➤ Decreases systemic vascular resistance and myocardial contractility
        - ➤ Reduces perioperative myocardial ischemia
    - ◆ Respiratory
        - ➤ Reduces minute ventilation, but respiratory changes are similar to normal sleep
        - ➤ Mild increase in $Paco_2$
- Side effects
    - ◆ Bradycardia
    - ◆ Hypotension
    - ◆ Prolonged sedation

OPIATES/OPIOIDS (TABLE 3.1)

- **Opioid receptors and their functions**
    - µ: analgesia, muscle rigidity, constipation, respiratory depression, and prolactin release
    - κ: constipation and shivering
    - σ: hallucinations and dysphoria
- **Mode of delivery**
    - Opioids can be delivered intravenously, intramuscularly, in the epidural space, or in the intrathecal space
    - Potency
        - ◆ **Intrathecal > epidural > intravenous > intramuscular**
- Non-analgesic effects
    - Respiratory depression
        - ◆ Effects increased with age, reduced clearance, and synergy with other anesthetics
    - Bradycardia
        - ◆ Direct inhibition of cardiac pacemaker cells
    - Hypotension
        - ◆ Secondary to bradycardia and/or histamine release

TABLE 3.1 Opioid equivalents		
Drug	IV/IM/SQ	Oral (mg)
Morphine (MS Contin)	10 mg	30
Hydromorphone (Dilaudid)	1.5–2 mg	6–8
Hydrocodone (Vicodin)	NA	30–45
Oxymorphone (Opana IR and ER)	1 mg	10
Oxycodone (Percocet, Oxycontin)	10–15 mg	20
Levorphanol (Levo-Dromoran)	2 mg	4
Fentanyl	100 µg	NA
Meperidine (Demerol)	100 mg	300
Codeine	100 mg	200
Methadone	The conversion ratio for methadone is variable.	

IV, intravenous; IM, intramuscular; SQ, subcutaneous; IR, immediate release; ER, extended release.
(Reproduced from Macres SM, Moore PG, Fishman SM. Acute pain management. In: Barash PG, Cullen BF, Stoelting RK, et al., eds. *Clinical Anesthesia*. 7th ed. Philadelphia, PA: Wolters Kluwer; 2013:1621.)

- Pruritis
  - Histamine release and mast cell activation can be caused by certain opioids
- Muscle rigidity
  - Increase muscle tone, vocal cord closure
- GI effects
  - Constipation through decreased GI motility
    - Constipation persists despite tolerance to analgesic activity
  - Nausea and vomiting through stimulation of the chemoreceptor trigger zone in area postrema of the medulla
  - Increased sphincter of Oddi tone
- **Properties of specific opiates/opioids**
  - Fentanyl
    - Synthetic opioid commonly used for anesthetic induction
      - Highly lipid soluble, rapid onset, and undergoes widespread redistribution following dosing
      - Short-acting, but prolonged effect with higher doses and infusions due to CSHT
    - Metabolized in the liver and excreted in urine
    - Approximately 100× more potent than morphine
    - Fentanyl patches are frequently used for chronic pain
      - Patches require significant amounts of time to become therapeutic, onset is slow
      - Patch removal → serum concentrations require up to 17 hours to be halved
      - Heating patch could increase fentanyl release
  - Hydromorphone
    - Synthetic opioid commonly used for intraoperative and postoperative pain relief
    - Metabolized by glucuronidation at the liver
      - Hydromorphone-3-glucuronide can cause cognitive dysfunction and myoclonus
    - Hydromorphone-to-morphine conversion is ~1 to 8
      - Less histamine release than morphine
  - Morphine
    - Commonly used opioid for intraoperative and postoperative pain relief
    - Metabolized by glucuronidation at the liver
      - Morphine-3-glucuronide with analgesic activity
      - Morphine-6-glucuronide has analgesic activity and requires renal elimination

- ❖ May cause respiratory depression in renal failure
  - ➤ Histamine release can cause hypotension via decreased sympathetic tone
- ❖ PO to IV conversion is 3 to 1
- ● Sufentanil
  - ❖ Synthetic opioid commonly used for intraoperative pain relief
  - ❖ 5× to 10× the potency of fentanyl
  - ❖ Compared to fentanyl, CSHT is shorter and does not accumulate as rapidly with time
- ● Alfentanil
  - ❖ Synthetic opioid commonly used for intraoperative pain control
  - ❖ One-fifth to one-tenth the potency of fentanyl
  - ❖ Rapid onset at 1 to 1.5 minutes
  - ❖ Compared to fentanyl, shorter duration of action and CSHT
  - ❖ Can also be used to induce seizure activity for mapping in neurosurgery
- ● Meperidine
  - ❖ Synthetic opioid used for postoperative pain or to decrease postoperative shivering
  - ❖ Unique features include the ability to cause tachycardia due to atropine-like structure and its depression of myocardial contractility
  - ❖ Metabolite normeperidine can cause seizures and hallucinations → not reversed with naloxone
- ● Remifentanil
  - ❖ Synthetic ultra-short-acting opioid used intraoperatively in cases where high-dose opioids are beneficial, but other opioids may be too long-acting
  - ❖ Ester structure that makes it susceptible to ester hydrolysis
    - ➤ Metabolized by nonspecific plasma cholinesterases
  - ❖ Does not accumulate with prolonged infusion
- ● Tramadol
  - ❖ Mechanism
    - ➤ Centrally acting analgesic that is a weak μ-agonist
      - ❖ One-tenth the potency of morphine
    - ➤ Inhibits serotonin and norepinephrine uptake, enhances serotonin release
  - ❖ Ondansetron may interfere with part of tramadol's analgesic action
  - ❖ Side effects
    - ➤ Decreases seizure threshold
    - ➤ High rate of nausea and vomiting
- ● Codeine
  - ❖ 300× less affinity for μ-opioid receptor
  - ❖ 2% to 3% metabolized to morphine through demethylation via P450 2D6
    - ➤ Must be metabolized for pain control
    - ➤ Some individuals are rapid metabolizers and some are slow metabolizers → unpredictable effects
      - ❖ Rapid metabolism → potent effects
      - ❖ Slow/nonmetabolizers → minimal effects
    - ➤ Possesses cough suppressant properties
- ● Buprenorphine
  - ❖ Partial agonist–antagonist opioid with strong affinity for μ-receptors
    - ➤ 50× greater affinity than morphine with prolonged effects
    - ➤ Due to partial agonist effects, unlikely to cause severe respiratory depression with overdose
  - ❖ Used to treat opioid addiction
  - ❖ Anesthetic implications
    - ➤ Should be discontinued at least 3 days prior to surgery
    - ➤ If not discontinued, opioids administered during the perioperative period will compete with buprenorphine and have fewer therapeutic effects
    - ➤ Buprenorphine is resistant to reversal with naloxone
- ● Methadone
  - ❖ Mechanism
    - ➤ μ-receptor agonist
    - ➤ NMDA receptor antagonist

- ➤ Norepinephrine and serotonin reuptake inhibitor
  - ◆ Risks
    - ➤ QT prolongation
    - ➤ Profound pharmacologic variability based on the individual
  - ◆ Elimination
    - ➤ Cytochrome P4503A4 and 2D6
    - ➤ Half-life varies between 5 and 130 hours based on person
    - ➤ Methadone may induce its own metabolism (half-life decreases with steady state)
- ■ Opioid reversal
  - ● Naloxone
    - ◆ Competitive antagonist at opioid receptors
      - ➤ Used primarily to reverse respiratory depression
    - ◆ Initial doses should be ~40 μg and uptitrated slowly if not an emergent situation
      - ➤ Onset is 1 to 2 minutes and half-life is ~30 minutes
      - ➤ Opioid may outlast naloxone and require repeat dosing
      - ➤ May cause tachycardia, hypertension, and even pulmonary edema if opioid reversal is too rapid
    - ◆ Naloxone can be used to reverse the euphoric effects of alcohol
  - ● Naltrexone
    - ◆ Oral or intramuscular opioid receptor antagonist that has a longer half-life (8 to 12 hours) than naloxone
    - ◆ IM naltrexone dosed monthly
      - ➤ Half-life is 5 to 10 days
      - ➤ Recommend discontinuing 6 to 8 weeks prior to surgery
    - ◆ Uses
      - ➤ Block euphoria for heroin addicts
      - ➤ Block euphoria from alcohol

MUSCLE RELAXANTS

- ■ **Neuromuscular junction** (Fig. 3.2)
  - ● Structure
    - ◆ Nicotinic acetylcholine (ACh) receptor composed of two α-subunits, and one β-, δ-, and ε-subunit
    - ◆ Two α-subunits have ACh binding sites
  - ● **Mechanism of action**
    - ◆ Binding of two ACh molecules to the paired α-subunits → sodium and calcium flow into the cell and potassium flows out of the cell → induces a conformational change in the channel →

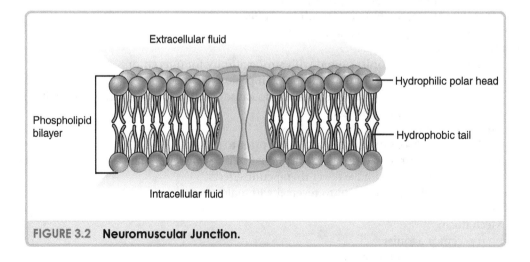

FIGURE 3.2 Neuromuscular Junction.

channel opens and depolarizes → muscle is activated → muscle relaxes when ACh is hydrolyzed by acetylcholinesterase at the neuromuscular junction
- Interference of muscle relaxants
  - Depolarizing muscle relaxants
    - Produces prolonged depolarization of the receptor
    - Action potential fails to generate
  - Nondepolarizing muscle relaxants
    - Competitively binds to the ACh receptor and inhibits channel opening
- Depolarizing muscle relaxant
  - Succinylcholine is the only depolarizing muscle relaxant used clinically
  - Pharmacokinetics and pharmacodynamics
    - Qualities
      - Rapid onset
      - Short duration of action
      - Excellent muscle relaxant conditions
      - Drug of choice for rapid sequence intubation (unless contraindications exist)
    - Dosing
      - Succinylcholine at 1 mg/kg results in good intubating conditions in ~60 seconds
      - An infusion can be used for a brief period of paralysis
        - Prolonged infusions can result in a phase II block of unpredictable duration
          - Normally requires a total dose >4 mg/kg
          - Repeated stimulus of ACh receptor → desensitization at nerve terminal → nerve is less responsive to ACh
        - Phase II blocks take on the properties of a nondepolarizing muscle relaxant
  - Metabolism
    - Rapidly hydrolyzed by butylcholinesterase to succinylmonocholine and choline
    - Butylcholinesterase exists in the circulation and not at the neuromuscular junction
      - Succinylcholine must diffuse from the neuromuscular junction back to the circulation to be metabolized
    - Deficiencies in succinylcholine metabolism
      - **Pseudocholinesterase (butylcholinesterase) deficiency**
        - Butylcholineterase is made by liver, so levels can be low in liver disease, malnutrition, and patients on drugs that affect liver metabolism
        - Must have greater than 75% reduction in butylcholinesterase function to have significant prolongation of neuromuscular blockade
          - Rarely of clinical significance
      - Pseudocholinesterase variation
        - A genetically abnormal butylcholinesterase that cannot metabolize succinylcholine exists in a small population
        - Testing for variation is done with the dibucaine number test
          - Unlike normal butylcholinesterase, the genetic variant is only minimally inhibited by dibucaine
          - Patient's butylcholinesterase is combined with dibucaine
            - If dibucaine inhibits plasma cholinesterase by 80% → dibucaine number 80 (normal)
            - If dibucaine inhibits plasma cholinesterase by 20% → dibucaine number 20 (due to atypical plasma cholinesterase)
          - Dibucaine number represents quality, not quantity, of cholinesterase
        - Duration of succinylcholine bolus in butylcholinesterase variant patients
          - In normal patient, up to 10 minutes
          - In butylcholinesterase heterozygote, paralysis of up to 30 minutes
          - In butylcholinesterase homozygote deficiency, paralysis of up to 3 hours
    - Increased butylcholinesterase
      - Obesity increases concentration of butylcholinesterase
        - Succinylcholine should be dosed by total weight, not ideal weight

- C5 isoenzyme variant
  - Increased plasma cholinesterase activity → rapid breakdown of succinylcholine → shorter duration of action
- Glaucoma patients on ecothiophate
  - Ecothiophate is an organophosphate that irreversibly inhibits acetylcholinesterase
  - Ecothiophate forms complex with acetylcholinesterase → prolongs succinylcholine (up to 25 minutes)
- Side effects
  - Arrhythmias
    - Succinylcholine can cause causes of arrhythmias through the following mechanisms
      - Histamine release from mast cells
      - Stimulation of the autonomic ganglia at the parasympathetic and sympathetic nervous system
      - Stimulation of the cholinergic autonomic receptors at the sinus node
    - Common rhythms are sinus bradycardia, nodal rhythms, and ventricular dysrhythmias
      - Children are more prone to bradycardias
      - Adults are more prone to tachycardias
  - Hyperkalemia
    - Succinylcholine increases K^+ outflow from cells
      - Increases plasma concentration in healthy patients by 0.5 mEq/dL
    - Exaggerated potassium response
      - Increase in potassium can be profound in extrajunctional cholinergic receptor proliferation
        - Cause of hyperkalemic cardiac arrest
      - Spinal cord injury (causing atrophy), burns, strokes, muscle trauma, abdominal infections can result in extrajunctional receptor proliferation
        - Receptor upregulation takes a few days to develop
          - Rare on the first day of injury
        - Peaks at 10 to 50 days after initial injury
      - Succinylcholine should be avoided from 24 hours to 2 years following severe burn injuries
  - Myalgias
    - Succinylcholine causes systemic fasciculations → significant myalgias
    - Approximately 50% of patients are affected
      - NSAIDs and pretreatment with a nondepolarizer prior to succinylcholine decrease myalgias
      - Opioids and propofol do not decrease myalgias
  - Increased intracranial pressure and intraocular pressure
    - Mechanism is not well known, and succinylcholine has been used for emergent neurosurgical and ophthalmologic cases given its brief duration and need to secure the airway rapidly
    - Succinylcholine should be avoided if the anterior chamber of the eye is open
- Nondepolarizing muscle relaxants
  - Nomenclature
    - Classes
      - Aminosteroids: ends with -onium
        - Example: rocuronium, vecuronium
      - Benzylisoquinolinium: ends with -urium
        - Example: cisatracurium, atracurium
    - Pharmacodynamics and kinetics
      - Bolus dosing can be used to create excellent intubating conditions
      - Infusions or intermittent dosing can be used to maintain muscle relaxation during a general anesthetic
    - Dosing (for intubating conditions based on ideal body weight)
      - Rocuronium: 0.6 to 1.0 mg/kg
      - Vecuronium: 0.1 mg/kg
      - Atracurium: 0.5 mg/kg

- ➤ Cisatracurium: 0.2 mg/kg
  - ◆ Specific qualities of muscle relaxants
    - ➤ Rocuronium has the shortest duration for adequate intubating conditions (~60 seconds following 1.0 mg/kg dosing)
    - ➤ Atracurium is associated with histamine release
- **Metabolism**
  - ◆ Nondepolarizing muscle relaxants vary based on their time of onset and clearance
  - ◆ Rocuronium
    - ➤ Metabolized and eliminated by the liver, biliary system, and kidneys
    - ➤ Sugammadex reverses steroidal muscle relaxants at 3 minutes without needing to wait for return of twitches
  - ◆ Vecuronium
    - ➤ Deacetylated at the liver
    - ➤ Metabolite (3-deacetylvecuronium) has 80% of vecuronium's potency and has a longer duration of action
    - ➤ Cleared in bile and kidneys
  - ◆ Atracurium
    - ➤ Metabolized by Hofmann elimination and ester hydrolysis
    - ➤ Laudanosine is a tertiary amine metabolite formed from atracurium that requires liver metabolism and kidney elimination
      - ❖ May cause central nervous system stimulating properties due to ability to cross the blood–brain barrier
      - ❖ Accumulation occurs after prolonged infusion
  - ◆ Cisatracurium
    - ➤ Metabolized by Hofmann elimination, although a small fraction requires renal elimination
    - ➤ Does not create laudanosine due to increased potency compared to atracurium
- ■ **Conditions and drugs that alter muscle relaxant duration**
  - ● Enhancers of muscle relaxants
    - ◆ Drugs
      - ➤ Anesthetics
        - ❖ Volatiles, local anesthetics (quinidine and procainamide)
      - ➤ Antibiotics
        - ❖ Aminoglycosides: gentamicin, tobramycin, streptomycin, neomycin
        - ❖ Lincosamines: clindamycin, lincomycin
      - ➤ Others
        - ❖ Magnesium, furosemide, dantrolene, calcium channel blockers, lithium
    - ◆ Conditions
      - ➤ Acidosis
      - ➤ Hypothermia
  - ● Shorteners of muscle relaxants
    - ◆ Carbamazepine or phenytoin
- ■ Neuromuscular blockade monitoring
  - ● Sequence of neuromuscular blockade
    - ◆ Faster onset, shorter duration
      - ➤ Airway muscles (larynx, jaw, diaphragm), orbicularis oculi
    - ◆ Slower onset, longer duration
      - ➤ Peripheral muscles
  - ● Train of four (TOF) monitoring
    - ◆ Electrical stimulation at peripheral nerves is used to assess neuromuscular recovery
      - ➤ Sequentially provides four stimulations and monitors twitch response at innervated muscle
    - ◆ **Residual blockade**
      - ➤ TOF less than 0.9 is defined as residual neuromuscular blockade
      - ➤ Risks of residual blockade
        - ❖ Pharyngeal dysfunction occurs in 25% of patients with TOF < 0.8 → increased aspiration risk
        - ❖ Upper airway obstruction occurs in 33% of patients with TOF < 0.8

- Increased risk of postoperative pneumonia and atelectasis occurs with TOF < 0.7
  - ➤ Return of function
    - ❖ Swallowing returns at TOF of 0.8
    - ❖ Speaking clearly at TOF of 0.9
    - ❖ Aspiration protection at TOF of 0.9
  - ❖ Extubation timing
    - ➤ TOF of 0.7 considered absolute lowest TOF for safe extubation
      - ❖ At TOF of 0.7, patients can lift their heads for 5 seconds, lift their legs for 5 seconds, have normal tidal volumes with a vital capacity of 15 to 20 cc/kg, and can generate a negative inspiratory pressure of 20 cm H_2O
    - ➤ Provider visual fade assessment is insufficient
      - ❖ 50% of patients are extubated prior to a TOF of 0.7 based on visual fade assessment
- ■ Reversal (Fig. 3.3)
  - ● Specific drugs
    - ❖ Edrophonium works at 1 to 2 minutes
      - ➤ Increases ACh release
      - ➤ Use with atropine because onset is so rapid
    - ❖ Neostigmine at 7 to 11 minutes
      - ➤ Acetylcholinesterase inhibition
      - ➤ Use with glycopyrrolate
      - ➤ Effect inhibited by acidosis, alkalosis, and hypokalemia
    - ❖ Pyridostigmine at 16 minutes
      - ➤ Acetylcholinesterase inhibition
      - ➤ Use with glycopyrrolate
  - ● Timing
    - ❖ Patients should have a TOF of at least 1 twitch prior to reversing neuromuscular blockade
  - ● Specific conditions
    - ❖ Nondepolarizing block and a phase II block can both be reversed with anticholinesterases
    - ❖ If a patient is reversed and then given succinylcholine
      - ➤ Anticholinesterase agents inhibit butylcholinesterase → prolonged succinylcholine effect
  - ● Muscle reversal in parturients
    - ❖ Neostigmine crosses placenta, but glycopyrrolate does not → fetal bradycardia
    - ❖ Neostigmine should be paired with atropine

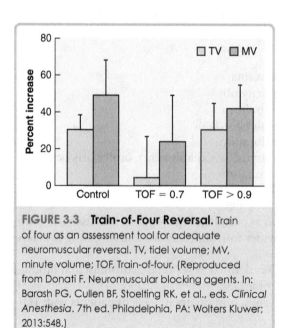

FIGURE 3.3 Train-of-Four Reversal. Train of four as an assessment tool for adequate neuromuscular reversal. TV, tidel volume; MV, minute volume; TOF, Train-of-four. (Reproduced from Donati F. Neuromuscular blocking agents. In: Barash PG, Cullen BF, Stoelting RK, et al., eds. *Clinical Anesthesia.* 7th ed. Philadelphia, PA: Wolters Kluwer; 2013:548.)

- Direct neuromuscular blocker inactivation
  - Sugammadex
    - Modified gamma-cyclodextrin
      - Selective binding agent for aminosteroid neuromuscular blockers
      - Binds and encapsulates aminosteroids within lipophilic core → prevents aminosteroid from binding to neuromuscular acetylcholine receptors
    - Approval
      - Used in other countries, but did not receive FDA approval until 2015
        - Concern for anaphylaxis and arrhythmias delayed approval
    - Use
      - Reverses deep rocuronium or vecuronium neuromuscular blockade rapidly with low incidence of residual blockade
        - Works within 1 to 3 minutes depending on level of blockade
      - Allows rocuronium as an alternative to succinylcholine in cases where succinylcholine may be detrimental due to rapid reversal
- Specific conditions affecting muscle relaxant use
  - Myasthenia
    - Fewer ACh receptors due to autoimmune destruction
    - More resistant to succinylcholine
    - Increased sensitivity to nondepolarizers
  - Myasthenic syndrome (Eaton–Lambert)
    - Decreased ACh release
    - Increased sensitivity to succinylcholine and nondepolarizers
  - Huntington Chorea
    - Degenerative central nervous system disease associated with decreased plasma cholinesterase
    - Prolonged succinylcholine response
  - Duchenne muscular dystrophy
    - Sex-linked recessive trait that affects 1/3,500
      - Presents with proximal muscle weakness, frequent falls, difficulty climbing stairs, abnormal gait
        - Ability to ambulate lost before 12 years of age
      - Other effects
        - Loss of deep tendon reflexes, up to 70% with heart defects, including dilated cardiomyopathy, left ventricular scarring, and mitral regurgitation with papillary muscle dysfunction
        - Decreased respiratory muscle function at third decade of life with increased pneumonias
    - Succinylcholine can cause rhabdomyolysis and hyperkalemic cardiac arrest
    - Nondepolarizers unaffected
  - Myotonic dystrophy
    - Normal muscle contraction followed by inability to achieve muscle relaxation in a normal time frame
      - Episodes of prolonged skeletal muscle contracture
      - Wasting of distal muscles is a common presentation
    - Succinylcholine and reversal agents can precipitate a myotonic crisis
  - Multiple sclerosis (MS)
    - Demyelinating disease of CNS
      - Presents with motor weakness, sensory disturbance, autonomic dysfunction
      - Cranial nerve involvement leads to pharyngeal and laryngeal muscle weakness
      - Stress of surgery and hyperthermia → increases exacerbation of MS
    - Succinylcholine can precipitate hyperkalemic crisis

QUESTIONS

1. Administration of etomidate is most likely to result in which of the following pharmacologic effects?

   A. Decreased aldosterone
   B. Decreased progesterone
   C. Increased histamine
   D. Increased ACTH

2. The "context" in context-sensitive half-time refers to which of the following:

   A. Duration of administration
   B. Method of administration
   C. Clearance of the drug
   D. Elimination half-life

3. A 55-year-old woman with metastatic colon cancer and a bowel obstruction receives succinylcholine for rapid sequence intubation and remains paralyzed for 2 hours. Her blood is sent to the lab for pseudocholinesterase (PChE) testing and the dibucaine number is 80. Which of the following is the most likely abnormality in this patient?

   A. PChE deficiency heterozygote
   B. PChE deficiency homozygote
   C. PChE allergy
   D. Decreased quantity of PChE

4. Sugammadex is most effective at reversal of neuromuscular blockade for which of the following neuromuscular blocking agents?

   A. Cisatracurium
   B. Succinylcholine
   C. Vecuronium
   D. Pancuronium

5. Ondansetron is most likely to antagonize the analgesics effects of which of the following analgesics?

   A. Morphine
   B. Meperidine
   C. Tramadol
   D. Ketorolac

CHAPTER 4   Inhaled Anesthetics

GAS LAWS AND PROPERTIES

- **Gas laws**
  - Boyle law: at constant temperature, pressure and volume are inversely related
  - Charles law: at constant pressure, volume and temperature are directly related
  - Gay-Lussac law: at constant volume, pressure and temperature are directly related
- **Humidity**
  - Absolute humidity is amount of water vapor in a gas
  - Relative humidity is amount of water vapor in a gas expressed a percentage of the amount that would be held if the gas was fully saturated
- **Critical temperature and pressure**
  - Critical temperature is the temperature at which a vapor of a substance can no longer be liquefied
  - Critical pressure is the pressure at which a vapor of a substance can no longer be liquefied

INHALATIONAL AGENT PROPERTIES

- **Mechanism**
  - The mechanism of volatile anesthetics at the molecular level is a well-studied area, but an integrated understanding of how volatiles affect consciousness remains an area under investigation
    - Volatile anesthetics depress excitatory synapses and augment inhibitory synapses
    - Prolong $GABA_A$ inhibitory potentials and act at nicotinic acetylcholine and glutamate receptors
  - Provide amnesia and immobility at therapeutic levels
- **Qualities of an ideal agent**
  - Rapid onset/emergence
  - Muscle relaxation
  - Hemodynamically stable
  - Bronchodilating
  - Not inflammable
  - Lack of biotransformation
  - Ability to estimate concentration at site of action
- **Minimum alveolar concentration (MAC)**
  - Definition
    - Concentration of volatile anesthetic that prevents a motor response to a surgical stimulus in 50% of the population
    - Measure of potency of a volatile anesthetic
      - Low MAC = increased potency
  - Factors that affect MAC
    - Increased MAC
      - Hypernatremia
      - Hyperthermia
      - Chronic opioid, alcohol use
      - Drugs that increase central catecholamines
        - Acute cocaine/amphetamine abuse
        - Monoamine oxidase inhibitors
      - Red hair
      - Infant (highest MAC ~6 months)

- ◆ Decreased MAC
  - ➤ Increased age
  - ➤ Hypotension
  - ➤ Hypothermia
  - ➤ Lithium
  - ➤ Pregnancy
  - ➤ Severe anemia (Hb < 5 g/dL)
  - ➤ Elderly
  - ➤ Hypercarbia
  - ➤ Hyperbaric conditions
  - ➤ Cholinesterase inhibitors
  - ➤ Drugs that lower central catecholamines
    - ❖ Chronic cocaine/amphetamine use
    - ❖ Cholinesterase inhibitors
    - ❖ Clonidine
    - ❖ α-methyl dopa
    - ❖ Reserpine
- ● MAC values for common anesthetics
  - ◆ Halothane: 0.8
  - ◆ Isoflurane: 1.2
  - ◆ Sevoflurane: 1.8
  - ◆ Desflurane: 6.6
  - ◆ Nitrous oxide: 104
- ● Application of MAC
  - ◆ While MAC is derived from population studies, it has been used in research to study the depth of anesthesia
  - ◆ Unconsciousness is generally obtained at a MAC of 0.3 to 0.4
- ● Recall
  - ◆ BIS or Anesthetic Gas to Reduce Explicit Recall (BAG-RECALL) trial showed BIS-guided anesthesia (40 to 60) was not superior to using end-tidal–guided anesthesia (MAC 0.7 to 1.3) for preventing recall in patients at high risk for awareness

VOLATILE UPTAKE

- ■ Alveolar uptake
  - ● F_A/F_I is the alveolar concentration divided by the inspired concentration (Fig. 4.1)
  - ● Increased rate of rise of F_A/F_I → faster inhalational induction and equilibration
- ■ Factors associated with increased volatile uptake
  - ● Increased inspired gas concentration
  - ● High flow rates
  - ● Increased minute ventilation
    - ◆ Neonates have a greater ratio of minute ventilation to functional residual capacity and undergo faster inhalational induction
  - ● Decreased volatile solubility
    - ◆ Blood–gas partition coefficient reflects solubility
      - ➤ Increased value → increased solubility
    - ◆ Blood–gas solubility coefficient for inhalational anesthetics
      - ➤ Halothane: 2.54
      - ➤ Enflurane: 1.9
      - ➤ Isoflurane: 1.46
      - ➤ Sevoflurane: 0.69
      - ➤ Desflurane: 0.42
      - ➤ Nitrous: 0.46
    - ◆ Oil–gas partition coefficient
      - ➤ Oil–gas partition coefficient = 150/MAC
      - ➤ Higher oil–gas partition coefficient → lower MAC

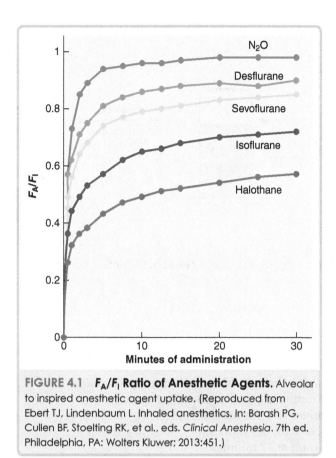

FIGURE 4.1 F_A/F_I **Ratio of Anesthetic Agents.** Alveolar to inspired anesthetic agent uptake. (Reproduced from Ebert TJ, Lindenbaum L. Inhaled anesthetics. In: Barash PG, Cullen BF, Stoelting RK, et al., eds. *Clinical Anesthesia*. 7th ed. Philadelphia, PA: Wolters Kluwer; 2013:451.)

> ➤ Higher partition coefficient indicates greater uptake and lower F_A/F_I
- Reduced cardiac output
  - ✦ Increased blood passing through the lungs lowers the F_A/F_I ratio
- Increased cardiac output
  - ✦ Quicker equilibration of anesthetic, but not speed of induction
- Decreased alveolar to venous partial pressure difference
  - ✦ Gradient of alveolar to venous partial pressure reflects tissue uptake
- Left-to-right cardiac shunt
  - ✦ Associated with more rapid increase in F_A/F_I ratio due to blood from the left side of the heart being shunted back to the right side and pulmonary circulation
- Right-to-left cardiac shunt
  - ✦ Associated with a slower induction
- **Concentration effect** (Fig. 4.2)
  - Increase in rate of alveolar uptake as concentration of a gas is increased
  - Refers to two mechanisms
    - ✦ Increased concentration of inspired gas
    - ✦ Augmentation of inspired ventilation following uptake of the anesthetic gas
  - Primarily applies to nitrous oxide as volatiles are not inspired at a high enough concentration to make the concentration effect clinically significant
- Second gas effect
  - Applies to nitrous oxide administered at a high concentration
  - When nitrous oxide is absorbed into the pulmonary circulation, the concentration of remaining gases in the alveoli is increased
- Time constant
  - Time constant is volume divided by flow
    - ✦ Volume of the lungs at functional residual capacity/minute ventilation

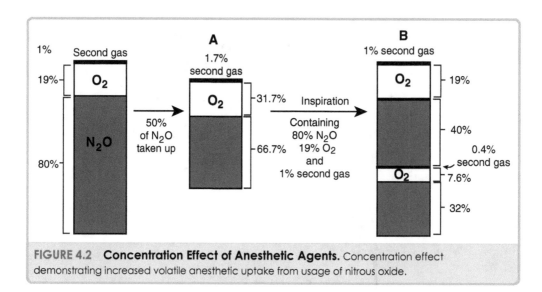

FIGURE 4.2 Concentration Effect of Anesthetic Agents. Concentration effect demonstrating increased volatile anesthetic uptake from usage of nitrous oxide.

- For volatile anesthetics, time constant determined by capacity of a tissue to hold the anesthetic relative to tissue blood flow
    - Brain time constant ~2× brain/blood partition coefficient
    - Sevoflurane and desflurane time constant is 2 minutes
        - Brain equilibrium at 6 minutes
    - Isoflurane time constant is 4 minutes
        - Brain equilibrium at 12 minutes
- Tissue-rich organs
    - Vessel-rich group includes the heart, brain, spleen, liver, kidneys, and endocrine glands
        - Represents 10% of body mass, but 75% of cardiac output
    - Vessel-rich group equilibrates first during induction
        - For sevoflurane, ~12 minutes
    - Fat takes a prolonged period of time to reach equilibrium
        - For sevoflurane, ~30 hours

VOLATILE ELIMINATION

- Elimination
    - Blood/gas partition coefficient correlates with elimination and emergence
        - Higher coefficient = higher dissolved quantity → slower emergence
        - 50% decrement of alveolar partial pressure is similar for most anesthetics
        - 80% to 90% decrement is very different for most volatiles
            - Example: desflurane has a more rapid emergence than isoflurane
    - Increased duration of anesthetic → slower emergence
- Metabolism
    - Halothane: 20% metabolized at liver and lungs
    - Sevoflurane: 5% metabolized
    - Enflurane: 3% metabolized
    - Isoflurane: 0.2% metabolized
    - Desflurane: 0.02% metabolized

ORGAN-SPECIFIC EFFECTS

- **Cardiovascular**
    - Systemic vascular resistance
        - Decreases LV afterload and SVR → decreases MAP

- ➤ 1 MAC isoflurane decreases MAP by ~25%
    - ◆ Decreases stroke volume → decreases cardiac output
  - ● Arrhythmias
    - ◆ Volatiles depress sinoatrial node more than atrioventricular node increased junctional rhythms
    - ◆ Increase QT interval
- ■ **Pulmonary**
  - ● Increase vagal tone
  - ● Bronchodilating
  - ● Activate respiratory centers in central nervous system
    - ◆ Increased respiratory rate
    - ◆ Decreased tidal volume
- ■ **Central nervous system**
  - ● Blood flow
    - ◆ Volatiles possess cerebral vasodilatory activity due to effects on vascular smooth muscle
    - ◆ Volatiles (except for nitrous oxide) produce a dose-dependent decrease in cerebral metabolism; however, they frequently increase cerebral blood flow
      - ➤ Predominate when MAC > 1
      - ➤ "Uncoupling" relationship of cerebral blood flow and metabolic rate
    - ◆ Cerebral autoregulation is dose-dependently altered
    - ◆ Intracranial pressure (ICP) increases at MAC > 1
- ■ **Neuromuscular system**
  - ● Decreased muscle tone through effect on spinal cord
  - ● Reduction in evoked potentials
- ■ **Renal**
  - ● Volatiles tend to decrease glomerular filtration rate
  - ● Volatiles tend to decrease renal blood flow through hypotension
  - ● Sevoflurane is associated with the highest serum fluoride levels, but there is no association with renal failure
- ■ **Hepatic**
  - ● Hepatotoxicity is possible with fluorinated inhaled anesthetics
  - ● Halothane is the most likely agent responsible given its degree of oxidative metabolism

VOLATILES AND UNIQUE PROPERTIES (FIG. 4.3)

- ■ Sevoflurane
  - ● Unique among anesthetics in that sevoflurane's MAC is highest in neonates (0 to 30 days)
    - ◆ Most volatile anesthetics have a higher MAC for infants than neonates
  - ● Minimal airway irritation and lack of unpleasant scent → sevoflurane is the volatile anesthetic of choice for inhalational induction
- ■ Isoflurane
  - ● Coronary vasodilator
    - ◆ Most likely to cause coronary steal syndrome (where atherosclerotic vessels cannot dilate, but normal vasculature can)
  - ● Preserves cardiac output due to preserved carotid baroreceptor reflex that senses a decrease in MAP and increase HR
  - ● Dissolves in rubber and plastic
- ■ Desflurane
  - ● Causes increased airway irritation
    - ◆ Should not be used for inhalational induction
  - ● Increased sympathetic response
    - ◆ May increase HR and BP
      - ➤ Tachycardia rare at <1 MAC
      - ➤ Dose-dependent increase in HR with >1 MAC
    - ◆ Can be blunted by opiates
  - ● Due to vapor pressure of 660 mm Hg (which is near atmospheric pressure), it will boil at room temperature

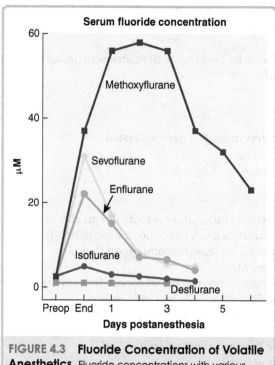

FIGURE 4.3 **Fluoride Concentration of Volatile Anesthetics.** Fluoride concentrations with various volatile anesthetics. Sevoflurane is associated with the highest serum fluoride levels, but enflurane is associated with the highest risk of fluoride-induced nephrotoxicity. (Reproduced from Ebert TJ, Lindenbaum L. Inhaled anesthetics. In: Barash PG, Cullen BF, Stoelting RK, et al., eds. *Clinical Anesthesia.* 7th ed. Philadelphia, PA: Wolters Kluwer; 2013:473.)

- ◆ Heating desflurane to 39°C raises the partial pressure inside vaporizer to 1,500 mm Hg
- Higher elevation → partial pressure of inhaled agent decreases → increase in delivered concentration is required to achieve the same anesthetic effect
  - ◆ Partial pressure of anesthetic gas determines effect on patient, not vapor concentration
- ■ Enflurane
  - Causes fluoride-induced nephrotoxicity
    - ◆ Fluoride inhibits adenylate cyclase activity → inhibits ADH → inability of kidneys to concentrate urine → nephrogenic DI
    - ◆ Presents with polyuria, dehydration, hypernatremia, increased serum osmolality
- ■ Halothane
  - Unique that it is not an ether derivative
  - Halothane hepatitis typically associated with middle-aged obese women exposed to multiple halothane anesthetics over short period of time
  - Cardiovascular effects
    - ◆ Halothane inhibits baroreceptor reflex responses → no reflex tachycardia to decreased BP
    - ◆ Most likely to cause a junctional rhythm
      - ➤ Slows conduction through sinoatrial node → bradycardia
    - ◆ Direct cardiac depressant
    - ◆ Sensitizes the myocardium to epinephrine → avoid excessive doses
  - Metabolism
    - ◆ Oxidative metabolism → trifluoroacetic acid
    - ◆ Reductive metabolism → fluoride ions
  - Stored with preservative (unlike others)—thymol
    - ◆ Therefore, stored in amber-colored bottles

NITROUS OXIDE (N_2O)

- Used for general anesthesia or sedation
  - NMDA receptor antagonists
  - High MAC (104%) requires supplementation with other anesthetics for general anesthesia
- Organ-specific effects
  - Cardiovascular
    - Increases heart rate, increases cardiac output
    - Dose-dependent myocardial depressant, but effects overcome by sympathetic activation
  - Pulmonary
    - Response to CO_2 is mostly unchanged
      - Slight decrease in tidal volume and minute ventilation
    - Dose-dependent decreased response to hypercapnia and hypoxia
    - Potential to expand and rupture blebs in patients with emphysema
    - Can increase pulmonary artery pressures in the presence of severe pulmonary hypertension
  - Cerebral
    - Increases cerebral blood flow
    - Increases cerebral metabolic rate
    - Increases intracranial pressure
- Side effects
  - **Closed air spaces**
    - $34\times$ more soluble than nitrogen in blood
      - Can accumulate in closed air spaces
      - Can accumulate in endotracheal tube cuffs and increase cuff pressure
    - Contraindicated in middle ear surgery, open globe injury, bowel obstruction, and severe emphysema (increased pneumothorax risk)
  - Megaloblastic anemia
    - Nitrous oxide inhibits $B_{12} \rightarrow$ inhibits methionine synthetase and folate metabolism
      - Impaired DNA synthesis and pancytopenia
      - Increased teratogenicity and immunodeficiency
    - Peripheral smear with anisocytosis, macrocytosis, and larger neutrophils
    - Associated with first trimester pregnancy loss, but not teratogenicity
      - Studies have been poor and done before operating room scavenging units
  - Diffusion hypoxia
    - Occurs during emergence from a high concentration of nitrous oxide
      - Shift of NO_2 to lungs $\rightarrow$ reduction of O_2 and reduction in $CO_2 \rightarrow$ reduced drive to breath $\rightarrow$ hypoxia
    - To avoid diffusion hypoxia, 100% O_2 should be administered for at least 10 minutes
      - Saturation more likely drops in patients with some degree of airway compromise
      - Most events occur in operating room en route to PACU (postanesthesia care unit)

QUESTIONS

1. Administration of nitrous oxide is associated with an increased concentration of which of the following metabolites?

   A. Methionine
   B. Homocysteine
   C. Folate
   D. Methemoglobin

2. A 50-year-old man develops transaminitis (elevated AST, ALT) 2 days after undergoing general anesthesia for a shoulder repair. He is least likely to have received which of the following volatile anesthetic agents?

   A. Desflurane
   B. Isoflurane
   C. Halothane
   D. Sevoflurane

3. A patient undergoes general anesthesia with nitrous oxide and desflurane. On emergence from anesthesia her minute ventilation is 5 L/min, and after extubation her oxygen saturation is 99% on 6 L/min oxygen by face mask. The patient is transported to the PACU on room air and her oxygen saturation on arrival is 85%. If her minute ventilation remained constant during transport, what is the most likely explanation for the decreased oxygen saturation?

   A. Second gas effect
   B. Concentrating effect
   C. Diffusion hypoxia
   D. Hypoventilation

4. The MAC of desflurane is 6 vol% at 1 atm. The concentration of desflurane (in vol%) that prevents a motor response to surgical incision in 99% of patients is closest to:

   A. 8
   B. 10
   C. 12
   D. 14

5. The time constant for sevoflurane is ~2 minutes and its MAC is 2. The amount of time required for complete equilibration with the brain is closest to?

   A. 2.5 minutes
   B. 4 minutes
   C. 6 minutes
   D. 10 minutes

CHAPTER 5 Perioperative Management

PREOPERATIVE RISK

- Risk assessment
  - Classifications and scores
    - American Society of Anesthesiologist (ASA) risk classification
      - Higher scores → increased perioperative mortality
      - Stratification
        - ASA 1: healthy without medical comorbidities
        - ASA 2: mild systemic disease that does not impact daily activity
        - ASA 3: significant systemic disease that limits normal activity
        - ASA 4: severe systemic disease that is a constant threat to life
        - ASA 5: moribund patient likely to die within 24 hours with or without surgery
        - ASA 6: brain-dead organ donor
    - Revised cardiac risk index (RCRI)
      - Predicts perioperative risk in patients undergoing noncardiac surgery
        - Created in 1977 with nine risk factors, but revised in 1999 to six factors
      - Predictors
        - High-risk surgery
          - Intraperitoneal, intrathoracic, suprainguinal vascular surgery
        - Ischemic heart disease
        - Congestive heart failure
        - Cerebrovascular disease
        - Diabetes mellitus on insulin
        - Creatinine >2
      - Risk for cardiac event (death, cardiac arrest, or myocardial infarction)
        - One predictor → 0.9%
        - Two predictors → 6.6%
        - Three or more predictors → 11.0%
- Surgical risk
  - High-risk surgery
    - Emergency surgery
    - Vascular surgery (except carotid endarterectomy)
    - Surgeries with large fluid shifts
  - Intermediate risk
    - Carotid endarterectomy
    - Radical neck procedures
    - Short thoracic procedures
    - Abdominal surgery
    - Orthopedic procedures
  - Low-risk surgery
    - Superficial (skin, breast)
    - Endoscopic
    - Cataract
    - Ambulatory procedures
- Functional status
  - Functional status is used as a marker of cardiovascular health and ability to tolerate surgical stress

- Metabolic equivalents of task (MET) is often used to characterize functional status
  - 1 MET = at rest
  - 3 METs = walking
  - 4 METs = climbing one flight of stairs
  - 8 METs = jogging
  - >10 METs = intense aerobic activity
- Patients capable of four or more METs of activity without discomfort are generally able to tolerate the stress of most surgeries

PREOPERATIVE GUIDELINES

- Definitions
  - **Sedation/anesthesia definitions**
    - Light sedation: verbal stimulation → purposeful response
    - Moderate sedation: verbal/tactile stimuli → purposeful response
      - Patent airway without assistance
    - Deep sedation: painful stimulus → purposeful response
      - May need airway assistance
    - General anesthesia: patient cannot be aroused, even with pain
  - Guidelines vs. practice advisories
    - Guidelines
      - Systematically developed recommendations that provide recommendations based on a comprehensive analysis of the literature
        - Often compare two interventions through well-controlled studies
      - Involves statisticians and numerous experts in the field
    - Practice advisory
      - Systematically developed reports that assist decision making based on a comprehensive review of the literature
      - Lack of high-quality studies in the area → practice advisories are not as well supported as guidelines
      - Not intended to define clinical standards
- Preoperative testing
  - **ASA preoperative testing recommendations**
    - History and physical
      - Mandatory for every patient
    - Electrocardiogram (ECG)
      - Age alone is not an indication for ECG testing
      - Indicated for patients with cardiovascular risk factors
    - Chest x-ray (CXR)
      - Recommended for patients >50 undergoing high-risk surgery with cardiovascular or pulmonary risk factors
      - Age, smoking, chronic obstructive pulmonary disease (COPD), cardiac disease, and recent upper respiratory infection may increase the likelihood of an abnormal CXR, but do not mandate a presurgical chest x-ray
    - Preoperative labs indications
      - Type and screen
        - Potential for significant intraoperative blood loss
      - Hemoglobin
        - Preoperative history of anemia
        - Potential for significant intraoperative blood loss
      - Coagulation studies
        - History of bleeding disorders, renal dysfunction, or liver dysfunction
        - Use of anticoagulants (such as Coumadin) that can be monitored by coagulation studies
        - Potential for significant intraoperative blood loss
        - Insufficient data to suggest need for routine coagulation studies prior to regional or neuraxial anesthesia

- ➤ Electrolytes
    - ❖ History of endocrine, kidney, or liver disorders
    - ❖ Use of chronic medications that may cause electrolyte irregularities (e.g., diuretics)
- ➤ Urinalysis
    - ❖ Only indicated for urological procedures or when an infection is suspected
- ➤ Pregnancy testing
    - ❖ May be offered to females of childbearing age, but not mandatory prior to surgery
- ◆ ASA makes no specific recommendations for echocardiography, stress testing, catheterization, or pulmonary function testing
- ● **American College of Cardiology/American Heart Association (ACC/AHA) recommendations for cardiovascular testing for noncardiac surgery** (Fig. 5.1)
    - ◆ Active cardiac conditions
        - ➤ Unstable coronary syndromes such as recent myocardial infarction, angina
        - ➤ Decompensated heart failure
        - ➤ Significant arrhythmias such as Mobitz II, 3rd degree heart block, atrial fibrillation with rapid ventricular rate, and ventricular arrhythmias
        - ➤ Severe valvular disease
    - ◆ Active cardiac conditions → warrant further investigation or postponing surgery
        - ➤ Only order testing or delay surgery if the test will change perioperative management
    - ◆ Surgery risk and decision to proceed
        - ➤ Emergency surgery should proceed without further testing

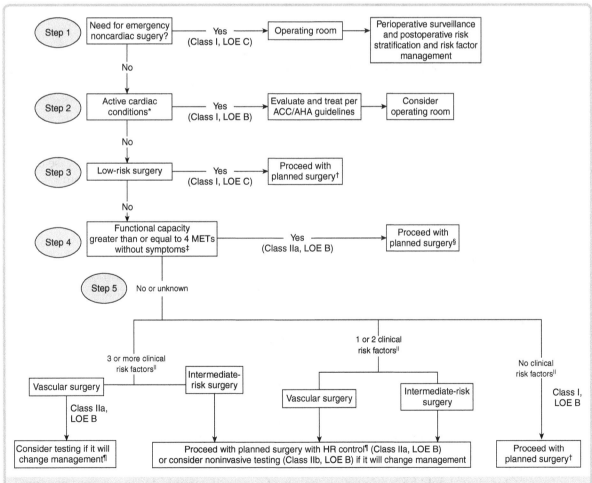

FIGURE 5.1 ACC/AHA Algorithm. (Reproduced from ACC/AHA 2007 Guidelines on perioperative cardiovascular evaluation and care for noncardiac surgery. Circulation 2007;116:e418–e500, with permission.)

- ➢ High-risk and intermediate-risk surgery should be considered on a case-by-case and patient-by-patient basis
  - ✦ Ischemic heart disease, compensated heart failure, cerebrovascular disease, diabetes, and renal insufficiency may warrant additional testing depending on the surgical procedure and whether it will change management
  - ➢ Low-risk surgery in a patient with good functional capacity (>4 METs) can proceed without testing
- ■ **Fasting and NPO recommendations**
  - ● Minimum fasting period
    - ✦ Clear liquids: 2 hours
    - ✦ Breast milk: 4 hours
    - ✦ Infant formula: 6 hours
    - ✦ Nonhuman milk: 6 hours
    - ✦ Light meal: 6 hours
    - ✦ Heavy meal: 8 hours
  - ● **Preoperative antiemetics**
    - ✦ Preoperative antiemetics and anticholinergics should not be routinely administered to patients with no increased risk for aspiration

PREOPERATIVE MEDICATIONS

- ■ **Management of chronic medications**
  - ● Most chronic medications can be continued on the day of surgery, although some medications warrant consideration for whether discontinuation may be beneficial
  - ● Antiplatelets/anticoagulants
    - ✦ Aspirin
      - ➢ A large meta-analysis of periprocedural aspirin withdrawal → increased rate of an acute coronary syndrome perioperatively when aspirin held prior to surgery
      - ➢ Perioperative Ischemic Evaluation 2 (POISE-2) trial → no increase in myocardial infarction or mortality for patients holding aspirin prior to surgery
      - ➢ Aspirin use perioperatively should be considered on a case-by-case basis
    - ✦ Clopidogrel
      - ➢ Commonly prescribed for coronary artery disease or following coronary stent placement
      - ➢ Holding clopidogrel for coronary artery disease should be assessed on a case-by-case basis
      - ➢ Clopidogrel should not be held for recent bare metal stents (at least 6 weeks from placement) and drug-eluting stents (ideally 1 year from placement) due to risk of stent thrombosis
    - ✦ Coumadin
      - ➢ Coumadin for a history of atrial fibrillation or thrombus should be assessed on a case-by-case scenario based on the surgery and patient risk factors
      - ➢ High-risk patients may be transitioned to low-molecular heparin or an intravenous heparin infusion preoperatively to minimize time off anticoagulation prior to surgery
  - ● Antihypertensives
    - ✦ β-blockers
      - ➢ The Dutch Echocardiographic Cardiac Risk Evaluation Applying Stress Echocardiography (DECREASE) trial supported β-blockade in the perioperative period due to decreased mortality and myocardial infarctions → trial recently discredited
      - ➢ Perioperative Ischemia Evaluation (POISE-I) trial showed decreased myocardial events, but increased risk of stroke and mortality with continuation of β-blockade
    - ✦ Angiotensin-converting enzyme (ACE) inhibitors
      - ➢ ACE inhibitors should be held on the day of surgery if possible due to the increased risk of refractory hypotension during general anesthesia
    - ✦ Clonidine
      - ➢ Clonidine should be continued on the day of surgery if possible due to rebound hypertension following withdrawal
  - ● Gastric reflux medication

- Proton pump inhibitors and H2-blockers should be continued on the day of surgery to minimize pulmonary injury in the event of aspiration
- **Management of herbals**
  - Herbals should be stopped ~1 week prior to surgery due to unpredictable antiplatelet effects, alterations in hepatic metabolism, and possible interactions with anesthetics
  - Effects of herbals
    - Ginger: increased bleeding
    - Ginseng: increased bleeding, hypertension, hypoglycemia, interference with Coumadin
    - Garlic: increased bleeding
    - Gingko: increased bleeding
    - Kava: potentiates sedation
    - Valerian: potentiates sedation
    - St. John's wort: inhibits serotonin, norepinephrine, and dopamine reuptake; induces hepatic enzymes
    - Saw Palmetto: increased bleeding due to cyclooxygenase inhibition
    - Echinacea: inhibits hepatic enzymes and alters drug metabolism

PREMEDICATIONS

- **Anxiolysis and analgesia**
  - Adults
    - Preoperative anxiolysis frequently utilizes midazolam and fentanyl for their pharmacokinetic predictability, rapid onset, rapid clearance, and minimal hemodynamic effects
    - **Patient age, comorbidities, and substance use history should guide dosing**
  - Pediatrics
    - Intravenous access may not be available
    - **Oral midazolam, intramuscular ketamine, and intramuscular or rectal methohexital are non-IV options**
- Gastric reflux
  - **H2-blockers**
    - Examples: cimetidine, ranitidine, famotidine, nizatidine
    - Increases gastric pH → decreases pulmonary injury if aspiration occurs
    - Side effects: bradycardia (cardiac H2 receptors), elevated liver function tests, impaired liver metabolism, change in mental status or delayed awakening
  - **Metoclopramide**
    - Increases lower esophageal sphincter tone
    - Stimulates gastric, upper gastrointestinal motility
    - Side effects
      - Extrapyramidal symptoms
      - Mild sedation, dysphoria, agitation, dry mouth
  - **Sodium citrate**
    - Oral antacid
      - 30 cc neutralizes 250 cc of HCl at a pH of 1.0
    - Onset time of 5 minutes
    - Effective 1 hour
- Deep vein thrombosis (DVT) prophylaxis
  - Subcutaneous heparin
    - Administered 2 hours prior to surgery and every 8 or 12 hours postoperatively decreases DVT risk from 30% to 10%
  - Early ambulation is the best prophylaxis for DVT

TYPES OF ANESTHETICS

- **Monitored Anesthesia Care (MAC)**
  - Anesthesia care where the anesthesiologist provides sedation, analgesia, and supports vital functions

- ◆ Utilizes the same medications as general anesthetics, but often at lower doses
- ● Distinguished from sedation
  - ◆ Must have ability to convert to a general or neuraxial anesthetic if needed
  - ◆ Level of sedatives may require airway support
  - ◆ Anesthesiologist also supports vital functions through hemodynamic management
- ■ General anesthesia
  - ● Anesthesia to produce a state of unconsciousness
    - ◆ Uses drug(s) with hypnotic and analgesic qualities
    - ◆ Concentrations and potency of anesthetics often result in blunting of airway reflexes and respiratory depression → airway management often necessary
  - ● **Airway assessment**
    - ◆ Assess for history and signs associated with difficult mask ventilation or intubation
      - ➤ Exam findings
        - ❖ Limited mouth opening
        - ❖ Limited jaw protrusion
        - ❖ Limited neck extension
        - ❖ Limited neck mobility
        - ❖ Short thyromental distance
        - ❖ Increased neck girth
        - ❖ Dentition increases the difficulty of intubation, but facilitates mask ventilation
        - ❖ High Mallampati class
          - ⟩ Technique: visualize the oropharynx with the patient's mouth wide open and tongue protruded while the patient is sitting in an upright position
          - ⟩ Class is determined by structures seen (Fig. 5.2)

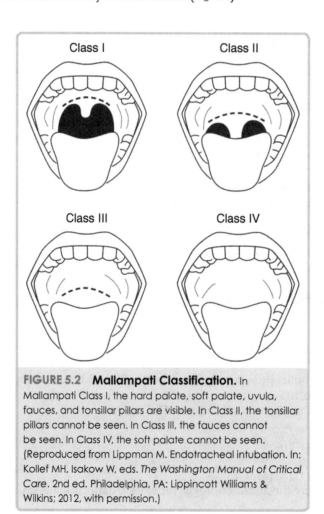

FIGURE 5.2 Mallampati Classification. In Mallampati Class I, the hard palate, soft palate, uvula, fauces, and tonsillar pillars are visible. In Class II, the tonsillar pillars cannot be seen. In Class III, the fauces cannot be seen. In Class IV, the soft palate cannot be seen. (Reproduced from Lippman M. Endotracheal intubation. In: Kollef MH, Isakow W, eds. *The Washington Manual of Critical Care*. 2nd ed. Philadelphia, PA: Lippincott Williams & Wilkins; 2012, with permission.)

- Mallampati I: hard palate, soft palate, faucal pillars, uvula
- Mallampati II: hard palate, soft palate, faucal pillars
- Mallampati III: hard palate, soft palate
- Mallampati IV: only hard palate visible
  - ➤ Medical history suggesting airway difficulty
    - ❖ Documented history of difficult intubation or mask ventilation
    - ❖ Head and neck tumor
    - ❖ History of head and neck radiation
    - ❖ Obstructive sleep apnea
    - ❖ Obesity
    - ❖ Voice changes or hoarseness
  - ◆ ASA difficult airway definitions
    - ➤ Difficult laryngoscopy: unable to visualize any portion of the vocal cords after multiple attempts
    - ➤ Difficult tracheal intubation: unable to intubate after multiple attempts despite no evidence of tracheal pathology
  - ◆ ASA closed claim findings of airway lawsuits
    - ➤ 76% of claims involved substandard care
      - ❖ Death or brain damage in half of cases
    - ➤ 38% of claims were for inadequate ventilation
    - ➤ 185 of claims were for difficult intubation
    - ➤ 17% of claims involved an esophageal intubation
- **Preoxygenation**
  - ◆ Preoxygenation **washes out nitrogen** → reduces likelihood and duration of hypoxia during securing the airway
  - ◆ Deep breathing for 1.5 minutes or tidal volume breathing for 3 minutes is sufficient for preoxygenation
    - ➤ Expired oxygen concentration >80% is often accepted as sufficient
- Induction
  - ◆ Intravenous or inhaled (see Chapters 3 and 4)
  - ◆ **Muscle relaxants can be used to facilitate mask ventilation and intubation**
    - ➤ Selection of muscle relaxant may depend on ability to mask ventilate/intubate
    - ➤ A short-acting muscle relaxant (succinylcholine) may be used for difficult airways to minimize the duration of a "cannot intubate, cannot ventilate" scenario if the airway cannot be secured
- Airway management: supraglottic airways
  - ◆ **Laryngeal mask airway (LMA)**
    - ➤ Laryngeal mask airways can be used for general anesthesia or as a rescue technique
    - ➤ Since the vocal cords are not manipulated, paralysis is not needed for placement
    - ➤ Not a definitive airway
      - ❖ Laryngospasm and vocal cord closure can still occur
      - ❖ Improper seating may limit ability to adequately ventilate
      - ❖ Does not prevent aspiration since the esophagus lies within the opening of the LMA
  - ◆ **Esophageal obturator devices**
    - ➤ A tube with a closed distal end designed for passage into the esophagus
    - ➤ Proximal holes in the tube allow gas delivery to the airway
- Airway management: endotracheal tubes
  - ◆ A secure airway through the trachea
  - ◆ Types of endotracheal tubes
    - ➤ **Cuffed vs. uncuffed**
      - ❖ Cuffed tubes are almost always used
        - › High-volume, low-pressure cuffs
          - ▸ Large size, increased compliance, thinner cuff wall
          - ▸ Exerts lower pressure on the lateral wall of the tracheal
        - › Low-volume, high-pressure cuffs
          - ▸ Smaller size, less compliant

- Associated with increased risk of sore throat and tracheal distortion
    - Uncuffed tubes generally reserved for neonates due to differences in airway anatomy
  - **Orotracheal vs. nasotracheal**
  - **Single lumen vs. double lumen**
  - **Plastic vs. armored**
  - Antibacterial coated vs. non-coated
- Airway management: endotracheal tube placement
  - **Direct laryngoscopy**
    - Miller blade (straight) lifts the epiglottis to reveal the cords
    - Macintosh blade (curved) is placed in the vallecula to reveal the cords
    - A bougie can be bent anteriorly and passed into the cords if a tube is difficult to pass
  - **Video-assisted laryngoscopy**
    - Uses a camera attached to the end of a laryngoscopy blade to visualize the cords
    - Does not require a direct line of site to visualize the cords
  - **Fiberoptic intubation**
    - Can be done **awake or asleep**
    - A bronchoscope with an endotracheal tube loaded on the scope is passed through the cords and the tube advanced off the scope
  - **Retrograde intubation**
    - A percutaneous wire is inserted into the trachea through the cricothyroid membrane and advanced cephalad
    - The wire is passed into the oropharynx and connected to an endotracheal tube
    - The endotracheal tube is passed into the trachea and the guidewire removed
  - **Lighted stylet**
    - An endotracheal tube is loaded on to a lighted stylet
    - The stylet transmits light through the skin of the neck
      - A localized glow at the midline indicates the location of the trachea
    - The tube is passed off the lighted stylet
- Difficult intubation strategies
  - In a scenario where a difficult intubation is anticipated, maintaining spontaneous respirations may be beneficial to prevent a "cannot intubate, cannot ventilate" scenario
  - Strategies to maintain spontaneous respirations
    - Awake intubation
      - Requires adequate topical anesthetic of the airway with/without sedation
    - Inhalational induction with nitrous and/or sevoflurane
  - **Tube exchangers**
    - Can be used when a difficult extubation is anticipated
      - Smaller diameter allows spontaneous respirations around the tube
    - Can be used to switch an endotracheal tube (e.g., double-lumen tube to single-lumen tube) that was difficult to place
  - Translaryngeal or transtracheal **jet ventilation**
    - Methods to deliver oxygen to the lungs
    - Does not guarantee adequate ventilation
- Difficult airway algorithm
  - Decisions to make
    - Awake vs. asleep intubation
    - Noninvasive or invasive airway during initial attempt
    - Preservation of spontaneous breathing vs. muscle relaxation
  - General principles
    - If mask ventilation is adequate → no longer emergency
    - Consider an LMA if intubation is unsuccessful
    - Consider aborting the airway attempt and allowing the patient to awaken if possible
    - Call for help early
- **Surgical airways**
  - **Tracheostomy**
    - Can be performed percutaneously or open

- ➢ Indicated to gain access to the airway during an emergency or for prolonged mechanical ventilation
  - ◆ **Cricothyroidotomy**
    - ➢ Performed during need for emergent airway by making an incision through the cricothyroid membrane
- ● Lung protective ventilation
  - ◆ Low-tidal volume ventilation using 6 to 8 cc/kg may decrease lung injury associated with mechanical ventilation
- ● **Extubation criteria**
  - ◆ Vital capacity > 15 cc/kg
  - ◆ $Pao_2 > 60$
  - ◆ $Paco_2 < 50$
  - ◆ A-a gradient less than 350 at 100%
  - ◆ pH > 7.3
  - ◆ Dead space/tidal volume ratio <0.6
  - ◆ Maximum inspiratory pressure of –20 cm water
  - ◆ Rapid Shallow Breathing Index = RR/TV Less than 105
- ■ Neuraxial
  - ● Use of neuraxial anesthesia
    - ◆ **Indications**
      - ➢ Neuraxial blockade (spinal, epidural, or caudal) can create a sensory block sufficient for the surgical procedure
      - ➢ Choice of neuraxial (spinal vs. epidural) depends on the patient's cardiovascular risk factors, expected surgical duration, urgency of surgery, desired areas of sensory coverage, and strategy for postoperative pain management
      - ➢ Neuraxial blockade can be used as the primary anesthetic or as an adjuvant to general anesthesia
    - ◆ **Contraindications**
      - ➢ Anticoagulation status or use of certain antiplatelet agents
      - ➢ Neurological disease that may be worsened by the placement of the neuraxial or the use of a local anesthetic
      - ➢ Soft tissue infections at the site of placement is a relative contraindication
    - ◆ **Anesthetic considerations and risks all neuraxial procedures**
      - ➢ Cardiovascular instability
        - ❖ A neuraxial block that reaches the sympathetic nervous system may cause a sympathectomy → hypotension
        - ❖ A neuraxial block reaching T1-T4 may block the cardioaccelerator fibers → bradycardia
      - ➢ Infection
        - ❖ Bacterial meningitis presents with fever, altered mental status, neck pain, headache
          - ⟩ Most cases develop 6 to 36 hours after dural puncture
        - ❖ Most common organism is strep viridians from oral bacteria of medical personnel (49%)
      - ➢ Pruritus
        - ❖ Common following the administration of opioids into the intrathecal or epidural space
        - ❖ Treatment options
          - ⟩ Nalbuphine as agonist-antagonist
          - ⟩ Diphenhydramine and hydroxyzine as antihistamines
          - ⟩ Low-dose propofol
  - ● Spinal anesthesia
    - ◆ Procedure
      - ➢ A spinal needle is inserted into the intrathecal space at the lower lumbar level
      - ➢ When cerebrospinal fluid (CSF) returns from the needle, local anesthetic is injected into the intrathecal space
    - ◆ Anatomy
      - ➢ Spinal cord extends to L1-2 in adults (L2-L3 in children), dural sac extends to S3
    - ◆ **Duration and drugs**
      - ➢ Drugs

- Local anesthetic
- Opioids
  - Opioids with $100\times$ potency of IV opioids
- Clonidine
  - Duration is dependent on
    - Local anesthetic selected
    - Local anesthetic concentration
    - Local anesthetic volume
    - Use of a vasoconstrictor
    - Patient characteristics
- Coverage
  - Block height and sensory coverage are determined by the baricity of the solution, volume of injection, and patient positioning
- **Side effects and intraoperative problems**
  - High spinal
    - A spinal level that reaches into the cervical spine can block the phrenic nerve and cause respiratory distress
    - A spinal level that reaches the brain can cause unconsciousness and hemodynamic instability
  - **Transient neurological syndrome (TNS)**
    - Pain or sensory abnormalities at the back, buttocks, or lower extremities following a spinal anesthetic
    - Risk factors
      - Lidocaine use
      - Increased local anesthetic dose
      - Lithotomy position
    - Treatment
      - NSAIDs
      - Nearly all cases of TNS resolve with time
  - **Cauda equina**
    - Symptoms included low back pain, sensory disturbances, leg weakness, and bowel/bladder dysfunction following a spinal anesthetic
    - Attributed to 28 to 32G microcatheters used to deliver a continuous, a concentration (5% lidocaine) spinal anesthetic
      - Suggested mechanism: microcatheter $\rightarrow$ pooling of local anesthetic in intrathecal space $\rightarrow$ neurotoxicity $\rightarrow$ irreversible conduction block
    - Further studies suggested that nearly all cases of reported cauda equina were not attributable to the spinal anesthetic
  - Post-dural-puncture headache (PDPH)
    - Risk factors
      - Increased needle size
      - Cutting needles
      - Young age
      - Females
      - Pregnancy
      - Increased dural punctures and attempts
    - Less common with modern 25G pencil point needles
- Epidural anesthesia
  - Procedure
    - An epidural needle is inserted into the epidural space at the lumbar or thoracic level
    - Local anesthetic is directly injected into the epidural space or a catheter is threaded into the epidural place for prolonged use/infusion
  - Anatomy
    - The epidural space lies between the ligamentum flavum posteriorly, posterior longitudinal ligament anteriorly, and intervertebral foramina and pedicles laterally
  - Drugs/duration

- Drugs
  - Local anesthetics
  - Opioids
    - Opioids with $10\times$ the potency of IV opioids
  - Clonidine
- Continuous catheters allow prolonged drug infusions and use for postoperative analgesia
  - Duration is dependent on
    - Local anesthetic selected
    - Local anesthetic concentration
    - Local anesthetic volume
    - Use of a vasoconstrictor
    - Patient characteristics
  - Onset is slower than spinal anesthesia
    - Allows gradual titration of medications to avoid hemodynamic compromises and minimize side effects
- Coverage
  - Dependent on level of epidural, volume of drug used, and patient age
  - Level of epidural
    - Two-third of segments above the epidural are blocked
    - One-third of segments below the epidural are blocked
  - Increased volume → increased spread
  - Increased age → decreased anesthetic requirement
- Thoracic epidurals
  - Unique benefits following upper abdominal and thoracic surgery
    - Decreased pain → decreased splinting → improved ability to oxygenate, ventilate, and participate in recovery
  - Pulmonary effects
    - Decrease pulmonary infection, atelectasis, hypoxemia, and duration of mechanical ventilation
    - Decreased mortality following rib fractures
  - Gastrointestinal effects
    - Decreased postoperative ileus
- Side effects
  - PDPH
    - Possible if the intrathecal space is entered
    - PDPH is often worse following epidural placement due to the increased gauge of the needle
  - Cardiovascular instability
    - Like a spinal anesthetic, an epidural block that reaches the sympathetic nervous system or cardioaccelerator fibers can cause bradycardia and hypotension
  - Epidural hematoma
    - Highly rare complication typically occurring in patients on anticoagulation
      - 69% with coagulation deficit at time of placement
    - Presentation
      - Back pain
      - Motor weakness is first sign in 46%
      - Sensory deficit is first sign in 14%
    - Warrants rapid MRI and neurosurgical intervention
- Regional anesthesia
  - Used as a primary anesthetic or to supplement a general anesthetic
  - See Chapter 18 for more information
- **Sedation for nonanesthesiologists**
  - Necessary skills
    - Understand the pharmacology of sedative and analgesic agents
    - Understand the pharmacology of agents to reverse sedatives and analgesics
    - Recognize sedation-related complications and respond appropriately

- Be able to provide positive pressure ventilation
- Preparation
    - Clinicians should be aware of a patient's medical history, medications, allergies, time of last oral intake, and substance use history
    - Patients should undergo a basic physical examination and airway assessment
    - Preoperative labs should be ordered if indicated
- Intraprocedural recommendations
    - The clinician administering sedation should monitor the patient
        - During deep sedation, this clinician should have no other tasks
        - During moderate sedation, this clinician may have a minor role in the procedure
    - Oxygen should be readily available and/or administered to the patient
    - Monitors
        - Pulse oximetry should be used for monitoring oxygenation
        - Ventilation should be monitored through observation or auscultation
        - Blood pressure should be checked at least every 5 minutes
    - Patient responsiveness
        - Verbal response should be sought during moderate sedation
        - Purposeful response to an increased stimulus should be sought during deep sedation
- Drugs and dosing
    - Sedatives and analgesics should be titrated in small, incremental doses
    - Drugs should be administered individually to assess for effect
    - Use of propofol or methohexital should warrant monitoring consistent with deep sedation, even if the patient is only moderately sedated

INTRAVENOUS FLUID SELECTION

- Uses
    - Maintenance fluids
    - Resuscitation from active blood and fluid losses
    - Replace third space losses from surgical swelling
- Adult maintenance: 2 cc/kg/hr
- 3rd Space deficit calculation
    - Minor: 6 cc/kg/hr
    - Moderate: 8 cc/kg/hr
    - Major: 10 cc/kg/hr
- Crystalloid solutions
    - **Lactated ringers (LR)**
        - Properties
            - Na 130, Cl 109, K 4, Ca 3, lactate 28
            - pH 6.5, osm 273
        - Use
            - LR is the primary resuscitation fluid used in the operating room
                - Can be administered in large volumes without causing an acidosis
            - Original intent of LR was to act as a buffer for acidosis
                - Bicarbonate is unstable in electrolyte solutions
                - Lactate → metabolized by the liver to CO_2 and water
        - Contraindications
            - Avoid in a diabetic crisis due to conversion of lactate to glucose
            - Some clinicians avoid LR in renal failure due to concerns for hyperkalemia
                - However, the nongap acidosis created by normal saline likely contributes more to hyperkalemia than the minimal potassium content in LR
    - **Normal saline (NS)**
        - Properties
            - Na 154, Cl 154
            - pH 5, osm 308
        - Use

- ➢ Commonly used as a resuscitation fluid
- ➢ Used preferentially in neurosurgery due to hypertonic properties
  - ✦ Contraindications
    - ➢ May cause a nongap acidosis with significant resuscitation due to the high chloride content
- ■ **Colloid**
  - ● Albumin (5%)
    - ✦ Properties
      - ➢ 50 g/L albumin in NS solution
    - ✦ Use
      - ➢ Used as a resuscitation fluid in cases where maintaining volume in the intravascular space is vital
      - ➢ Used to increase oncotic pressure in patients with low baseline albumin levels
    - ✦ Contraindications
      - ➢ May increase mortality in head injury based on the results of the Saline vs. Albumin Fluid Evaluation (SAFE) trial
  - ● Albumin (25%)
    - ✦ Properties
      - ➢ 250 g/L albumin in a salt poor solution
    - ✦ Use
      - ➢ 25% albumin increases oncotic pressure to pull extravascular fluid intravascularly
    - ✦ Contraindications
      - ➢ Avoid albumin in head injury
  - ● Hetastarch
    - ✦ Properties
      - ➢ 6% solution of hydroxyethyl starch in a sodium chloride solution
    - ✦ Use/contraindications
      - ➢ Used as a volume expander, but has fallen out of favor due to renal failure and effects on co-agulation (reduced factor VIII and von-Willebrand factor (vWF) levels)
  - ● Dextran
    - ✦ Properties
      - ➢ Highly branched polysaccharide molecules
    - ✦ Use
      - ➢ Used as a volume expander, but has fallen out of favor due to side effects
    - ✦ Contraindications
      - ➢ Increased rate of anaphylaxis
      - ➢ Increased bleeding and coagulopathy through antiplatelet activity and antifibrinolytic effects
      - ➢ Increased rates of renal failure
- ■ **Glucose requirements**
  - ● In some patient populations, glucose or a caloric source may be needed
    - ✦ Example: diabetics on insulin
  - ● D5 can be added to NS or LR
- ■ **Free water**
  - ● Free water should not be infused intravenously
  - ● If free water is desired (e.g., hypernatremia), D5W may be administered at a slow rate to prevent rapid corrections in electrolyte levels

TEMPERATURE REGULATION

- ■ **Intraoperative heat loss mechanisms**
  - ● Radiation
    - ✦ Most significant form of heat loss perioperatively
    - ✦ Magnitude of heat loss is proportional to temperature differential to the 4th power
  - ● Conduction
    - ✦ Due to contact with cooler surfaces
  - ● Convection
    - ✦ Due to air movement in room

- Evaporation
  - Due to sweating or open procedures
- Consequences of hypothermia
  - Increased wound infections
  - Increased coagulopathy
  - Delayed emergence
  - Increased shivering and metabolic demands
- Mechanisms to counter heat loss
  - Increase temperature of operating room
  - **Forced air heating blankets**
  - **Insulation devices**
  - **Heat lamps**
  - **Blankets** to minimize uncovered skin
- **Malignant hyperthermia**
  - Life-threatening condition of uncontrolled skeletal muscle activation triggered by succinylcholine or volatile anesthetics
    - Patients can have an anesthetic with a nontriggering reaction and then trigger on the second anesthetic
  - Mechanism
    - Hypothesized to be due to decreased control of intracellular calcium stores
    - Inherited as an autosomal dominant disorder attributed to the ryanodine receptor
    - Risk increased with central core disease and King-Denborough syndrome
  - Symptoms and detection
    - Most sensitive finding: hypercarbia
      - Metabolic disorder with increased CO_2 → significant ETCO$_2$ rise
        - Paco$_2$ can be 100 to 200 mm Hg range
    - Most specific finding: muscle rigidity
      - Masseter muscle rigidity
        - Masseter muscle spasm following succinylcholine administration represents malignant hyperthermia in 30% of cases
          - If surgery is not emergent or urgent, it should be delayed
        - Masseter muscle spasm can occur with or without triggering agents
          - Not improved with neuromuscular blockers
      - Despite muscle rigidity, peripheral nerve stimulator shows flaccid paralysis
    - Associated findings
      - Hypertension
      - Tachycardia
      - Dysrhythmias
      - Respiratory acidosis
      - Metabolic acidosis
      - Rhabdomyolysis
      - Fever
      - Disseminated intravascular coagulation (DIC)
        - DIC due to shock and core temperature $>41\,°C$
    - Unlike neuroleptic malignant syndrome (NMS)
      - NMS responds to muscle relaxation from neuromuscular blockers and succinylcholine
  - Testing
    - Rule out malignant hypothermia with muscle biopsy and caffeine-halothane contracture testing
      - Four testing centers in United States
      - Biopsy is only good for 5 hours, so must test near a center
    - Sensitivity ~100%, but specificity is only 80%
      - Lots of false positives
  - Treatment and monitoring
    - Avoid triggering agents
    - If history of malignant hyperthermia, but no symptoms during anesthetic
      - Maintain in PACU for 6 hours prior to discharge

- ◆ Dantrolene
  - ➤ Used to treat malignant hyperthermia
  - ➤ Mechanism
    - ❖ Binds at RYR1 receptor → blocks calcium release at the sarcoplasmic reticulum of smooth muscle → decreases muscle contractility
  - ➤ Formation
    - ❖ 20 mg dantrolene with 3 g mannitol in vials
      - › Mix with sterile water
      - › Dose at least 1 mg/kg to start and continue up to 10 mg/kg total dose
    - ❖ Target adequate urine output
      - › May need to alkalinize urine
  - ➤ May need postop infusion or oral conversion (4 mg/kg) for several days
    - ❖ Malignant hyperthermia symptoms may recur following initial treatment
  - ➤ Side effects
    - ❖ Weakness, nausea, diarrhea, blurred revision
    - ❖ Hepatitis in 0.5% receiving dantrolene for >60 days
    - ❖ Increased aspiration and respiratory weakness
    - ❖ Pleural effusion, fibrosis, pericarditis, and hearing loss

POSITIONING INJURIES

- ■ Visual injuries
  - ● **Corneal abrasions**
    - ◆ Causes
      - ➤ Chemical (antiseptics), trauma, pressure from instruments, self-infliction when emerging from anesthesia
    - ◆ Risk factors
      - ➤ Dry corneas
      - ➤ General anesthesia associated with less tearing
    - ◆ Presentation
      - ➤ Ocular pain with sensation of foreign body in eye
      - ➤ Photophobia, tearing, blurred vision
      - ➤ 16% of cases with permanent injury
    - ◆ Diagnosis requires slit-lamp examination with fluorescein
    - ◆ Treatment
      - ➤ Topical ketorolac
      - ➤ Topical antibiotic may be helpful to decrease further ulceration
      - ➤ Eye patch not helpful
      - ➤ Mydriatic agents not helpful
      - ➤ Topical local anesthetics inhibit healing
  - ● Ischemic optic neuropathy
    - ◆ Mechanism
      - ➤ Lack of perfusion to optic nerve from ischemia → axonal swelling → vision loss
    - ◆ Presentation
      - ➤ Painless loss of visual acuity
      - ➤ Typically presents after surgery, but presentation could be delayed up to 24 hours postoperatively
      - ➤ 43% of patients show visual improvement in symptoms
    - ◆ Types
      - ➤ Anterior ischemic optic neuropathy
        - ❖ Associated with cardiac surgery
        - ❖ Due to watershed infarct at short posterior ciliary arteries
      - ➤ Posterior ischemic optic neuropathy
        - ❖ Associated with back surgery and steep Trendelenburg position
          - › Often bilateral visual loss
        - ❖ Surgical risk factors

> Increased length of surgery
> Increased blood loss
- ❖ Patient risk factors
  > Diabetes
  > Coronary artery disease
  > Smoking history
  > Hypotension
  > Anemia
- ❖ Fundoscopic examination cannot immediately diagnose posterior ischemic optic neuropathy, but it can diagnose anterior ischemic optic neuropathy
- Retinal vessel occlusion
  - ❖ Central retinal artery occlusion often with carotid, spine, and cardiac surgery
  - ❖ Central retinal vein occlusion: follows low long back surgeries with facial edema
- ■ **Upper extremity injuries**
  - Ulnar neuropathy (Fig. 5.3)
    - ❖ Cause
      - ➤ Direct pressure to the ulnar nerve at the medial epicondyle of the humerus
        - ❖ Associated with male gender, extremities of body mass index (both high and low), and prolonged hospital stay
      - ➤ Not associated with case length
    - ❖ Prevention
      - ➤ Limit arm abduction to less than 90° at the shoulder
      - ➤ Hand and forearm should be in neutral position or supinated
      - ➤ Adequately pad the elbow
  - Brachial plexus neuropathies
    - ❖ Cause
      - ➤ Compression of brachial plexus, commonly occurring in the lateral position
    - ❖ Prevention
      - ➤ Avoid high axillary rolls when placing patient in the lateral position
      - ➤ Minimize head rotation
  - Suprascapular nerve and long thoracic nerve injury
    - ❖ Cause
      - ➤ Suprascapular nerve is injured when the patient is shifted ventrally in the lateral position

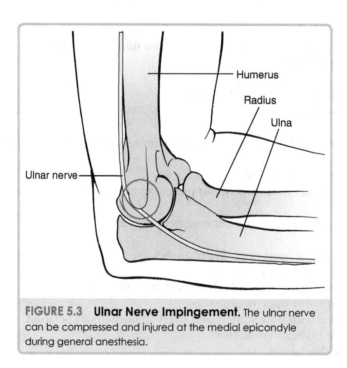

FIGURE 5.3   Ulnar Nerve Impingement. The ulnar nerve can be compressed and injured at the medial epicondyle during general anesthesia.

> ➤ Long thoracic nerve is injured during stretch or direct trauma in the lateral position
  - ◆ Prevention
    - ➤ Move entire body carefully when shifting a patient in the lateral position
- ■ **Lower extremity nerve injuries**
  - ● Common peroneal nerve injury (Fig. 5.4)
    - ◆ Cause
      - ➤ Direct trauma or compression of the nerve at the lateral head of the fibula, commonly during **lithotomy** positioning
    - ◆ Prevention
      - ➤ Avoid lateral compression of the knee or fibula in lithotomy
  - ● Sciatic nerve injury
    - ◆ Cause
      - ➤ Hyperflexion of hips and extension of knees in **lithotomy**
    - ◆ Prevention
      - ➤ Avoid hyperflexion of the hips in lithotomy
  - ● Femoral and obturator nerve injury
    - ◆ Causes
      - ➤ Traction on the nerves from **retractors** used in abdominal surgery
      - ➤ Femoral injury presents with decreased extension at the knee, sensory loss on anterior thigh
      - ➤ Obturator injury presents with inability to adduct the leg and numbness over the medial thigh
    - ◆ Prevention
      - ➤ Surgical care when placing retractors near the lower extremity nerves
  - ● Lateral femoral cutaneous nerve
    - ◆ Cause

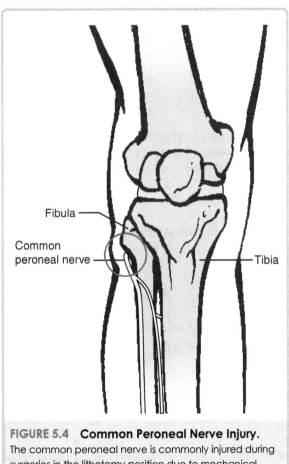

FIGURE 5.4 Common Peroneal Nerve Injury.
The common peroneal nerve is commonly injured during surgeries in the lithotomy position due to mechanical compression of the lateral leg.

- ➤ Excessive hip flexion
- ➤ Presents with numbness of the lateral thigh
  - ◆ Prevention
    - ➤ Avoid excessive hip flexion, especially in **lithotomy**
- ■ Special cases
  - ● **Tourniquets**
    - ◆ Often used in orthopedic, vascular, and general surgery to create a bloodless field
    - ◆ Mechanism of injury to structures
      - ➤ Cuff may cause direct pressure to underlying structures
      - ➤ Cuff restricts blood flow to distal structures → ischemia and anoxia
    - ◆ Prolonged and frequent use can cause skin, nerve, and muscle injury
  - ● Intravenous access
    - ◆ The **median nerve** can be injured at the antecubital fossa through intravenous access
    - ◆ Mechanism
      - ➤ Direct trauma
      - ➤ Drug extravasation
    - ◆ Presents with motor weakness for thumb abduction, flexion, wrist flexion, and forearm protonation due to innervation of the abductor pollicis brevis, flexor pollicis brevis, opponens pollicis, and forearm flexor muscles
    - ◆ Presents with sensory deficit to palmar surface and the lateral three-and-half fingers
  - ● **IV infiltration**
    - ◆ Most cases can be treated supportively by discontinuing use of the IV, raising the extremity, and warm compresses
    - ◆ Hazardous drugs
      - ➤ $CaCl_2$, $NaHCO_3$, or other vesicant → blistering
        - ✦ Treat with injection of hyaluronidase to promote absorption
      - ➤ Phenylephrine → vasoconstriction
        - ✦ Treat phenylephrine infiltration with an injection of phentolamine

ALLERGIC REACTIONS

- ■ **Anaphylaxis**
  - ● Mechanism
    - ◆ Life-threatening allergic reaction mediated by an IgE reaction
    - ◆ Allergen binds to IgE antibodies on surface of mast cells and basophils → histamine and eosinophilic chemotactic factors released (leukotrienes, kinins, tryptase, chymase, and prostaglandins)
    - ◆ Effects of released factors
      - ➤ Urticaria
      - ➤ Bronchospasm and laryngeal/airway edema
      - ➤ Systemic vasodilation
      - ➤ Pulmonary vasoconstriction
      - ➤ Cardiovascular instability
  - ● Predicting severity
    - ◆ Rapid → more severe
    - ◆ Rash is not required for an anaphylactic reaction
    - ◆ Bradycardia is predictive of severe reaction
  - ● Grades
    - ◆ I: cutaneous-mucous signs
    - ◆ II: multivisceral signs (GI upset, dyspnea, rash)
    - ◆ III: life-threatening
    - ◆ IV: CV collapse
  - ● Tryptase
    - ◆ Neutral protease stored in mast cells → released during anaphylactic (but not anaphylactoid) reactions
    - ◆ Measure within 1 to 2 hours of suspected onset

- Treatment
  - Antihistamines
    - Do not stop the release of histamine, but they compete with histamine at the receptor sites
    - Aid in the attenuation of the response and can decrease the severity of the cardiovascular reaction (i.e., hypotension from vasodilatation)
  - Steroids
  - Epinephrine
    - Vasopressor (increases contractility and vasoconstriction)
    - Bronchodilator
    - Decreases the release of vasomotor mediators in the mast cells
- **Anaphylactoid**
  - Presentation similar to anaphyalatic reactions, but not IgE mediated
    - Pretesting is not helpful because tests are for IgE reactions
  - Can be similarly severe and life-threatening due to mast cell release of histamine, proteoglycans, and inflammatory mediators
    - Pretreatment with steroids and histamine blockers may be beneficial in preventing reactions
    - Intravenous contrast most likely agent of anaphylactoid reactions
- **Drugs**
  - Muscle relaxants
    - >60% of allergic reactions in perioperative period
    - 70% cross-reactivity between different muscle relaxants
  - Latex
    - 15% of allergic reactions
      - Cornstarch added to gloves is associated with leaching of allergenic proteins from the gloves and increased aerosolization → increased latex reactions
      - At-risk populations include those with congenital urinary tract infections, spina bifida, spinal cord injury, multiple childhood surgeries, and food allergies (banana, passion fruit, pineapple, mango, kiwi)
      - Health-care workers have twice the risk as the general population
    - Reactions take 30 minutes to develop
    - Types of reactions
      - Irritant contact dermatitis
        - Local rash
      - Allergic contact dermatitis
        - Type IV cell mediated immune response
        - Type I IgE mediated hypersensitivity reactions
  - Antibiotics
    - 14% of allergic reactions
    - 2% to 10% cross-reactivity between cephalosporins and penicillin
      - Older cephalosporins (first generation) more likely to cross-react
    - Skin testing for a penicillin allergy is specific, but not sensitive
  - Local anesthetics
    - Local anesthetic esters more likely to cause allergies than amines
      - Esters cause allergies through p-aminobenzoic acid (PABA) metabolites
    - Methylparaben is preservative in both esters and amides that may cause allergic reactions
  - Sulfites
    - 5% to 10% of patients with asthma may have a sulfite allergy
    - Examples of drugs that may be made with sulfite
      - Proprofol (generic), dexamethasone, epinephrine, hydrocortisone, meperidine, norepinephrine, and tobramycin
  - Propofol
    - Often avoided for egg allergies
      - Propofol is made with egg phosphatide
      - Most egg allergies are due to egg albumin in egg whites, not the component in Propofol
    - Generic Propofol is made with sodium metabisulfite → allergic reaction in those with sulfite allergy
    - Diprivan is made with EDTA and not sulfite

AIRWAY COMPLICATIONS

- Airway injuries
  - **Facial ulcerations**
    - Prolonged pressure from a mask to create a tight seal can cause facial ulceration
    - Most common source is prolonged continuous positive airway pressure (CPAP) or biphasic positive airway pressure (BiPAP) in an intensive care unit, but can also happen with prolonged mask ventilation in the operating room
  - **Tracheal injury**
    - Causes: direct trauma (during intubation), prolonged elevated tracheal **cuff pressures**
    - Trauma to the trachea can cause tracheomalacia or tracheal stenosis
  - Prevention
    - Endotracheal tube cuff pressures should be between 15 and 25 cm H_2O
    - LMA cuff pressures should not exceed 60 cm H_2O
    - Minimize nitrous oxide use or check cuff pressures frequently when using nitrous oxide
- Intraoperative complications
  - **Laryngospasm**
    - Uncontrolled closure of the vocal cords that persists after the stimulus is removed → obstructs ventilation
    - Causes
      - Airway manipulation, secretions, regurgitation, moving the patient, and stimulation of the superior laryngeal nerve
      - Commonly occurs during light planes of anesthesia (induction and emergence)
    - Prevention
      - Minimize airway irritation
      - Intravenous lidocaine
      - Consider deep extubation
    - Treatment
      - Remove stimulus (suction fluid and debris at airway)
      - Provide positive pressure ventilation
      - Consider muscle relaxation
  - **Negative-pressure pulmonary edema**
    - Complication of laryngospasm when a patient generates a high negative inspiratory pressure against closed vocal cords
      - Occurs in 4% to 6% of those that experience laryngospasm
      - Hydrostatic exudation of plasma through capillary membrane and alveolar basement membrane → pulmonary edema, shear forces damage pulmonary basement membranes
    - Mortality between 10% and 40%
    - Treatment
      - Supportive
      - Consider diuretics
      - Most cases resolve in less than 24 hours
  - **Bronchospasm**
    - Spasm and constriction of the bronchiolar wall muscles
      - Causes: reactive airway disease, airway irritation, allergic reactions
    - Presentation
      - Wheezing, decreased expiratory flow, shortness of breath, difficulty ventilating
      - Could become an emergency if ventilation is impossible
    - Treatment
      - β-agonists, anticholinergics, and steroids
      - Deepen anesthetic level
        - Volatiles are bronchodilators
  - **Aspiration**
    - Patients under anesthesia are at greater aspiration risk due to the blunting of airway reflexes
      - Aspiration volumes greater than 0.4 cc/kg with pH < 2.5 → potential for pneumonitis with high morbidity

- ✦ Effects of aspiration: bronchospasm, hypoxemia, atelectasis, hypotension, and lung injury
- ✦ Treatment
  - ➤ Minimize gastric flow to the lungs
    - ❖ Trendelenburg position
    - ❖ Head to the side
    - ❖ Suction gastric contents
  - ➤ Secure the airway (if not already secured)

UNIQUE ANESTHETIC CONSIDERATIONS

- **Controlled hypotension**
  - ● Controlled hypotension must be done carefully and with consideration of the risks
  - ● Risks
    - ✦ Decreased perfusion may increase the risk of stroke, renal injury, and splanchnic hypoperfusion
  - ● Beneficial scenarios
    - ✦ Surgeries where bleeding cannot be controlled with pressure or vascular control (e.g., orthopedic surgery, maxillofacial surgery)
    - ✦ Aneurysm surgery to prevent rupture
    - ✦ Trauma to minimize bleeding while hemostasis is obtained
- **Controlled hypothermia**
  - ● Suggested benefits
    - ✦ Hypothermia decreases metabolic rate → decreases oxygen consumption → protects against ischemia
    - ✦ Reduces inflammation and cytokine release
    - ✦ Therapeutic hypothermia following ventricular fibrillation arrest improves mortality
  - ● Anesthetic implications
    - ✦ Hypothermia may be intentionally induced when circulatory arrest is necessary or be used during cardiac surgery for its protective effects
    - ✦ Paralysis is often needed to prevent shivering and minimize oxygen consumption
- **Hyperbaric oxygen**
  - ● An environment of >1 atmospheric pressure
    - ✦ Provides increased pressure and increased oxygen concentration
  - ● Indications
    - ✦ Air embolism
    - ✦ Decompression sickness
    - ✦ Profound hypoperfusion
    - ✦ Severe carbon monoxide poisoning
    - ✦ Poor wound healing
  - ● Anesthetic affects
    - ✦ Decreases MAC due to increased partial pressure of volatiles at higher barometric pressure
    - ✦ Intravenous anesthetics are unaffected

POSTOPERATIVE ISSUES

- Respiratory
  - ● Airway edema
    - ✦ Anesthetic and surgical factors
      - ➤ Large fluid shifts
      - ➤ Massive resuscitation
      - ➤ Long prone procedures
      - ➤ Surgery on the head, neck, or airway
    - ✦ Intervention
      - ➤ Airway edema should warrant prolonged intubation or repeat visualization of the airway to assess if extubation would be tolerated
      - ➤ Placing patients in an upright position
      - ➤ Consider steroids and/or diuresis on a case-by-case scenario

- Hypoxemia
  - Anesthetic and surgical factors
    - Anesthetic agents are associated with inhibition of hypoxic drive
    - General anesthesia is associated with atelectasis
    - Diffusion hypoxia is possible with the use of high nitrous oxide concentrations
    - Pneumothorax and pulmonary embolisms should be considered in the differential
  - Preexisting comorbidity factors
    - Reactive airway disease → bronchospasm and hypoxemia
    - Heart failure → pulmonary edema
  - Intervention
    - Treat any reversible causes
    - Supplemental oxygen may treat hypoxemia, but may also mask hypoventilation
    - In cases of severe hypoxemia, consider noninvasive ventilation or re-intubation
- **Hypoventilation**
  - Anesthetic and surgical factors
    - Anesthetic agents inhibit hypercapnic ventilatory drive
    - Opioids and benzodiazepines decrease respiratory drive and increase the apneic threshold
    - Residual neuromuscular blockade
    - Splinting due to pain
  - Preexisting comorbidity factors
    - Patients with severe COPD or obstructive lung disease may have a higher resting Pa_{CO_2}
    - Sleep apnea may predispose patients to airway collapse and hypoventilation
  - Interventions
    - Treat any reversible causes
      - Consider naloxone or flumazenil if drugs are the likely culprit
    - Consider noninvasive ventilation such as BiPAP or repeat intubation
- Cardiovascular
  - **Hypertension**
    - Anesthetic and surgical factors
      - Pain
      - Fluid overload
      - Hypothermia and shivering
      - Increased intracranial pressure
    - Preexisting comorbidity factors
      - Patients with preexisting hypertension are likely to have postoperative hypertension, especially if medications were withheld preoperatively
    - Interventions
      - Treat underlying cause
      - Consider antihypertensive agents
  - **Hypotension**
    - Anesthetic and surgical factors
      - Hypovolemia following inadequate resuscitation or continued fluid sequestration
      - Hypovolemia due to active hemorrhage
      - Vasodilation due to inflammatory response
      - Residual anesthetic effects
    - Preexisting comorbidity factors
      - Cardiogenic cause should be considered in patients with a history of coronary artery disease or arrhythmias
      - Vascular tone may be affected by chronic medications
    - Interventions
      - Dependent on likely cause
      - Consider a fluid bolus or inotropic support
- **Renal dysfunction**
  - Anesthetic and surgical factors
    - Hypovolemia (pre-renal) and hypotension are the most likely causes of renal injury in the perioperative period

- Surgical causes of decreased renal perfusion include renal clamping, renal artery stenosis, abdominal compartment syndrome, or ureteral obstruction
  - Interventions
    - Determine if the likely cause is prerenal, intrarenal, or postrenal, and address appropriately
    - Treat any electrolyte disturbances
    - Consider dialysis if medical management is insufficient
- Neurologic
  - Delirium
    - Presents as disorientation and inappropriate behavior on emergence from anesthesia
    - Risk increased in elderly and in those with dementia
    - Nearly all anesthetic drugs can precipitate delirium
    - Interventions
      - Treat underlying cause
        - Infection, hypoglycemia, or electrolyte disturbances
      - Adequate analgesia
      - Antipsychotics
      - Minimizing polypharmacy
      - Supplemental oxygen
  - Postoperative cognitive dysfunction
    - Decline in cognitive function following surgery
      - Cause is not clear
        - May be due to inflammatory response following surgery
        - Not linked with hypotension
      - Risk equal under regional and general anesthesia
    - Risk factors
      - Age
      - Cardiac surgery
      - High-risk or major surgery
      - Significant alcohol use
      - Lower educational levels
      - History of stroke
      - History of cognitive impairment (such as Alzheimer disease)
      - Prolonged hospitalization
  - Central anticholinergic syndrome
    - Patients present postoperatively with symptoms that resemble atropine intoxication
      - Dizziness, blurred vision, nausea, dilated pupils, photophobia, dissociative hallucinations, seizure, and disorientation
      - Diagnosis is difficult and other causes of disorientation must be considered
      - If symptoms resolve with physostigmine, central anticholinergic syndrome is likely the cause
      - Physostigmine
        - Anticholinergic
        - Lipid soluble, tertiary structure allows it to cross the blood–brain barrier (neostigmine is quaternary)
        - Side effects: bradycardia, salivation, vomiting
        - Metabolized by plasma cholinesterases
          - Only works 20 minutes, so repeat dosing may be needed
- Hypothermia
  - Common following anesthetics due to the cold temperature of the operating room, skin and visceral exposure, and room temperature IV fluids
  - Effects
    - **Postoperative shivering**
      - Shivering increases metabolic rate → increases oxygen consumption
      - Benign in healthy, but may be detrimental in those who will not tolerate an increased heart rate
      - Shivering can also occur without hypothermia after anesthetics
    - Impairs platelet function

- ◆ Decreased drug metabolism
- ◆ Immune suppression
- ● Treatment
  - ◆ Increase ambient temperature
  - ◆ Use fluid warmer
  - ◆ Forced air blankets
  - ◆ Medications to reduce shivering include opioids, clonidine, dexmedetomidine, propofol, meperidine, and physostigmine
- ■ **Postoperative nausea and vomiting (PONV)**
  - ● Common following general anesthetics
  - ● Predicting risk
    - ◆ Apfel score predicts PONV
      - ➤ Four factors
        - ❖ Nonsmoker
        - ❖ Female
        - ❖ History of PONV/motion sickness
        - ❖ Intraoperative opioids
      - ➤ Risk of PONV is dependent on number of positive factors
        - ❖ 0 factor = 10%
        - ❖ 1 factor = 20%
        - ❖ 2 factors = 40%
        - ❖ 3 factors = 60%
        - ❖ 4 factors = 80%
  - ● Risk factors
    - ◆ Anesthetic risk factors
      - ➤ Use of volatiles, nitrous oxide, opioids, neostigmine
    - ◆ Surgical risk factors
      - ➤ Strabismus surgery, tonsillectomy, breast surgery, gynecological surgery, orchiopexy, otolaryngology surgery
    - ◆ Patient risk factors
      - ➤ Female, nonsmoking, history of PONV and motion sickness
      - ➤ Risk not gender-related until puberty
  - ● Preventative techniques
    - ◆ Administer prophylactic antiemetics, supply adequate hydration, and modify anesthetic plan to minimize anesthetic risk factors
      - ➤ Gastric evacuation does not help
    - ◆ Drugs
      - ➤ Antiemetics
        - ❖ **Ondansetron**: serotonin antagonist
        - ❖ **Droperidol/haloperidol**: dopamine antagonist
        - ❖ **Metoclopramide**: dopamine and serotonin antagonist
        - ❖ **Dexamethasone**: central inhibition of prostaglandin synthesis
        - ❖ **Scopolamine**: block muscarinic cholinergic emetic receptors at pons and cortex
        - ❖ **Phenothiazines**: dopamine antagonist
      - ➤ **Antacids**
        - ❖ **Proton pump inhibitors**
        - ❖ **H2-blockers**
        - ❖ Sodium citrate
    - ◆ Acupuncture
      - ➤ Works at P6 site to reduce PONV, but only if done prior to anesthesia

PACU DISCHARGE

- ■ Phase
  - ● I: OR to PACU discharge
  - ● II: PACU discharge to home discharge

- III: home discharge to resumption of daily activities
- PACU discharge criteria
  - Discharge criteria continues to evolve and are often institution-dependent based on resources and monitoring capabilities
  - Aldrete scoring system
    - Factors (0, 1, or 2 points each)
      - Activity (not moving, moving two extremities, moving four extremities)
      - Breathing (apnea, shallow breathing, deep breathing, and coughing)
      - Circulation (SBP greater than 50 mm Hg off from pre-anesthetic level, SBP within 50 mm Hg of pre-anesthetic level, SBP < 20 mm Hg from pre-anesthetic level)
      - Consciousness (no response, drowsy, alert)
      - Oxygen saturation (cyanotic, pale, normal)
    - Score of 9/10 considered adequate for discharge

ORGAN DONATION

- Donation after brain death
  - Neurologic death criteria
    - Unresponsive
    - No spontaneous motor activity
    - Absent papillary, corneal, oculocephalic/oculovestibular reflexes
    - Absent cough with suctioning
    - No increase in HR with 2 mg of atropine
    - No respiratory efforts on apnea testing ($Paco_2$ > 60 mm Hg)
    - EEG silence
  - **Pathophysiological changes**
    - Decreased SVR → hypotension
    - Central diabetes insipidus
      - Due to injury to neurohypophysis and reduction of vasopressin
      - Presents with polyuria, hypernatremia, hypokalemia, hypocalcemia
        - Treat with DDAVP or vasopressin
    - Myocardial dysfunction
    - Decreased antidiuretic hormone
    - Hypothyroid
    - Adrenal insufficiency
  - **Intraoperative considerations**
    - Hemodynamic goals
      - Systolic BP > 100 mm Hg
      - Pao_2 > 100 mm Hg
      - Urine output > 100 cc/hr
    - Resuscitation
      - IV fluids and vasopressors may be needed to maintain adequate blood pressure and urine output
      - Excessive fluid resuscitation can cause organ swelling and decrease transplant quality
    - Organ procurement
      - Done in order of susceptibility to ischemia
      - Heart removed first, kidneys removed last
    - Fio_2 < 40% for lung retrieval
    - Goal glucose <200 mg/dL
- Donation after cardiac death
  - Due to removal of organs after cardiac arrest, organs have a longer ischemia time that can affect organ quality
    - Controlled donation: transplant team awaits arrest in operating room
    - Uncontrolled donation: unplanned arrest with either unsuccessful resuscitation or no attempted resuscitation

QUESTIONS

1. A 42-year-old man with morbid obesity is scheduled to undergo a right colectomy. He has a history of a silent MI, hypertension, elevated cholesterol, chronic renal insufficiency (Cr, 1.7), and noninsulin-dependent diabetes mellitus. His medications are metoprolol, amlodipine, metformin, and simvastatin. His revised cardiac risk factor score is:

   A. 1
   B. 2
   C. 3
   D. 4

2. A 72-year-old man is undergoing preoperative evaluation for noncardiac surgery. He is able to walk up one flight of stairs without difficulty. This activity is equivalent to which of the following in terms of oxygen uptake?

   A. 3.5 mL O_2 uptake/kg per min
   B. 7 mL O_2 uptake/kg per min
   C. 14 mL O_2 uptake/kg per min
   D. 21 mL O_2 uptake/kg per min

3. Which of the following therapies is contraindicated for the brain-dead patient undergoing lung donation?

   A. Solu-Medrol
   B. Recruitment maneuvers
   C. 10 cc/kg tidal volumes
   D. Fluid restriction

4. Which of the following factors is associated with the development of postoperative cognitive dysfunction?

   A. Intraoperative hypotension
   B. General anesthesia vs. regional anesthesia
   C. Age > 60 years
   D. Higher educational levels

5. Which of the following statements regarding the use of aprepitant compared with ondansetron for PONV is most correct?

   A. It is more effective for prevention of PONV
   B. Its use is associated with greater QT prolongation
   C. It is more sedating than ondansetron
   D. It is most effective when administered at the end of surgery

STRUCTURE AND MECHANISMS

- **Anatomy**
  - Position of the heart (Fig. 6.1)
    - Positioned in the mediastinum at ~T5-8
    - Anchored in pericardium
    - Slightly rotated
      - ➤ Right ventricle is the most anterior structure and lies in the left parasternal area closest to chest wall → most likely injured in trauma
      - ➤ Left atrium is against esophagus → essential for understanding mid-esophageal transesophageal echocardiogram (TEE) views
  - Chambers
    - Right atrium (RA)
      - ➤ Receives deoxygenated blood from the inferior vena cava (IVC) and superior vena cava (SVC)
      - ➤ Fossa ovalis is fetal remnant of foramen ovale
        - ❖ Patient foramen ovale (PFO) exists in ~25% of population
    - Right ventricle (RV)
      - ➤ Receives deoxygenated blood from RA
      - ➤ Contains anterior, posterior, and septal papillary muscles connected to tricuspid valve
      - ➤ Empties into the right ventricular outflow tract to the pulmonary artery
  - Left atrium (LA)
    - Receives oxygenated blood from four pulmonary veins
    - Left atrial appendage is a muscular pouch

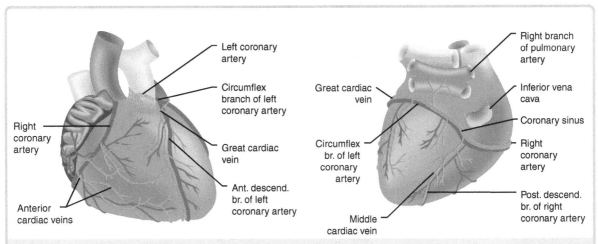

FIGURE 6.1 Position and View of the Heart. Basic cardiac anatomy depicting the chambers and valves of the heart. Ant., anterior; descend., descending; Br., branch; Post, posterior. (Reproduced from Pagel PS, Kampine JP, Stowe DF. Cardiac anatomy and physiology. In: Barash PG, Cullen BF, Stoelting RK, et al., eds. *Clinical Anesthesia.* 7th ed. Philadelphia, PA: Wolters Kluwer; 2013:242.)

> ➤ Location of thrombus formation specifically in low flow states like atrial fibrillation (A-fib) and dilated cardiomyopathy–related heart failure (HF)
- Left ventricle (LV)
  - ◆ Receives oxygenated blood from left atrium
  - ◆ Contains anterior and posterior papillary muscles connected to mitral valve
  - ◆ More muscular and capable of higher pressures than the RV
- ■ **Valves**
  - Tricuspid
    - ◆ Composed of three-valve leaflets → connects RA to RV
    - ◆ Common valve infected in endocarditis
  - Pulmonic
    - ◆ Semilunar valve composed of three-valve leaflets → connects RV to PA (pulmonary artery)
  - Mitral
    - ◆ Composed of two-valve leaflets → connects LA to LV
  - Aortic
    - ◆ Semilunar valve composed of three-valve leaflets → connects LV to aorta
    - ◆ Two percent of the population has a bicuspid aortic valve
- ■ **Coronary vessels** (Fig. 6.2)
  - Aortic sinuses, located just below the aortic valve, give off right coronary artery (RCA) from the right aortic sinus and left coronary artery from the left aortic sinus

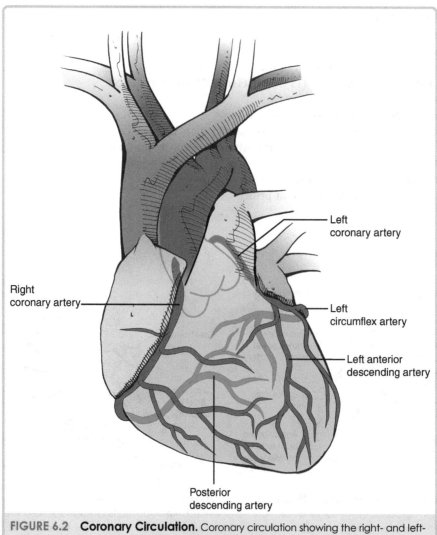

FIGURE 6.2   Coronary Circulation. Coronary circulation showing the right- and left-sided coronary vessels and their associated branches.

- Posterior aortic sinus → no vessel and hence called the noncoronary sinus
- Coronary arteries originate at the root of the aorta
  - RCA → supplies blood to the RA, RV, as well as a minority of the LV
    - Branches into posterior descending artery (PDA) in the right-dominant system and the right marginal artery
    - PDA runs along the posterior interventricular sulcus to the apex
      - Supplies posterior one-third of the interventricular septum
      - Supplies the sinus node and is implicated in dysrhythmias
    - Right marginal artery
      - Supplies blood to the RV
  - Left coronary artery (left main) divides into left anterior descending (LAD) and circumflex (Cx) → supplies blood to majority or left heart and septum
    - LAD supplies blood to anterior, lateral, and apical LV
      - LAD branches into diagonal arteries and septal perforators
        - Diagonal arteries travel from the anterior interventricular groove toward the anterolateral heart
        - Septal perforators travel into the septum
    - Cx supplies blood to the LA and posterior LV
      - Cx branches into obtuse marginal (OM) arteries
      - Obtuse marginal arteries travel from the interventricular sulcus to the apex
  - Coronary veins return deoxygenated blood to the coronary sinus at the right atrium
- Coronary artery dominance
  - Vessel that supplies PDA determines dominance
    - RCA supplies PDA → right dominant
      - Majority of population
    - Cx artery supplies PDA → left dominant
    - RCA and Cx both supply PDA → codominant
- **Cardiac cycle**
  - **Sinoatrial (SA)** node in the right atrium is the pacemaker of the heart
    - SA node transmits signal to both atria → atrial systole (ECG [electrocardiogram] P wave)
    - Right vagus and sympathetic chain supply the SA node
      - Right carotid massage more effective than left carotid massage
  - **Atrioventricular (AV)** node receives signal at junction of atria and ventricles (ECG R wave)
    - AV node transmits signal to Bundle of His and Purkinje fibers
    - Left vagus and sympathetic supplies the atrioventricular node
  - **Purkinje system** sends signal to ventricular myocytes → ventricular systole (ECG QRS complex)
- **Blood flow**
  - Flow into the atria is passive through venous return
    - Venous return equals cardiac output
    - Negative intrathoracic pressure during the spontaneous inspiratory phase aids venous return
  - Flow into ventricle is both passive and active
    - Eighty-five percent of flow into ventricle is passive
    - Fifteen percent of flow into ventricle is active through atrial systole
  - Flow into pulmonary artery and aortic valve is active
    - Ventricles undergo isovolemic contraction → increased pressure opens PV or AV → ventricular ejection
  - Flow into coronary vessels occurs during diastole
    - Ventricles undergo isovolemic relaxation after contraction → pulmonic and aortic valves close
- **Cardiac action potential**
  - Cardiomyocytes are the muscle cells of the heart
    - Depolarization of plasma membrane → calcium enters the plasma membrane across receptors on T-tubules → activate ryanodine receptors on sarcoplasmic reticulum to open → calcium releases into cell → bind to troponin C → actin–myosin contraction → ATP-ase dependent relaxation and uptake of calcium back into the sarcoplasmic reticulum
  - Volatile anesthetics decrease calcium release from the sarcoplasmic reticulum

CARDIAC PHYSIOLOGY

- Definitions of heart function
  - Inotropy: strength of muscular contraction
  - Chronotropy: heart rate
  - Dromotropy: conduction speed of impulses
  - Bathmotropy: threshold for excitation
  - Lusitropy: myocardial relaxation
- Preload, afterload, and contractility
  - **Preload**
    - Ventricular load at end-diastole
      - Determined by **stretching of cardiomyocytes** prior to contraction
      - Linear relationship between sarcomere length and myocardial force
    - Determinants
      - Increased venous return (both venous pressure and volume) → increased preload
      - Increased intrathoracic pressure (mechanical ventilation, mass effect) → decreased preload
  - **Afterload**
    - Systolic load on left ventricle after contraction is initiated
      - Determined by resistance to contraction
    - Determinants
      - Increased hypertension → increased afterload
      - Increased aortic stenosis → increased afterload
      - Increased aortic compliance → decreased afterload
  - **Contractility**
    - Contractile strength of the heart
    - Determinants
      - Increased adrenergic input → increased contractility
      - Aberration in pH → decreased contractility
- **Frank–Starling relationship** (Fig. 6.3)
  - Relationship between myocardial work and preload
  - Increased load on heart → increased myocardial stretch → increased myocardial contraction
    - Force of cardiac muscle fiber proportional to sarcomere length

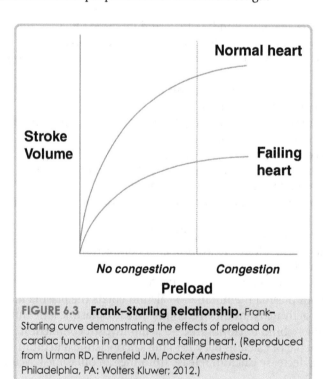

FIGURE 6.3 Frank–Starling Relationship. Frank–Starling curve demonstrating the effects of preload on cardiac function in a normal and failing heart. (Reproduced from Urman RD, Ehrenfeld JM. *Pocket Anesthesia.* Philadelphia, PA: Wolters Kluwer; 2012.)

- Frank–Starling curve
  - Graph
    - X-axis: ventricular end-diastolic volume
    - Y-axis: ventricular performance
  - Normal performance: increased ventricular end-diastolic volume → increased ventricular performance
  - Heart failure: increased ventricular end-diastolic volume → limited increase in ventricular performance
- Cardiac work
  - Cardiac oxygen consumption determined by stroke work and energy required to change shape to fill and relax
  - Cardiac work determined by heart rate, stroke volume, and myocardial wall tension
    - Heart rate has most significant impact on oxygen consumption (then afterload, then preload)
    - Wall tension is determined by end-diastolic ventricular pressure, preload, and systemic vascular resistance
      - Tension = pressure × radius/(2 × wall thickness)
  - Heart failure increases wall stress → increases oxygen consumption
- **Oxygen consumption**
  - Normal heart: 8 to 10 cc/100 g/min
  - Cardioplegic fibrillating heart: 2 cc/100 g/min
  - Cardioplegic quiescent heart: 0.3 cc/100 g/min
- **Metabolic equivalent of task (MET)**
  - Used to assess energy consumption
  - Ratio of metabolic rate during activity to baseline metabolic rate
  - Application
    - 1 MET = amount of energy expended during 1 minute at rest
      - Average value of 1 MET = 3.5 cc O_2/kg/min
    - Example: if patient consumes 250 cc O_2/min at baseline, then a consumption of 2,500 cc O_2/min is 10 METs

BLOOD PRESSURE AND FLOW

- **Blood pressure (BP) modulation**
  - **Sympathetic nervous system**
    - Complex set of nerves that release norepinephrine and epinephrine from the adrenal medulla to produce vasoconstriction and shunt blood to the heart, lungs, and brain
    - Works in response to stress, hypotension, and hypovolemia
  - **Renin–angiotensin–aldosterone system**
    - Signaling pathway that increases aldosterone and sodium retention to increase fluid and blood volume
    - Works in response to hypotension, hyponatremia, and sympathetic nervous system stimulation
  - **Vasopressin**
    - Peptide hormone produced in the hypothalamus that regulates fluid retention at the kidneys and vasoconstriction at the V_1 receptors on vascular smooth muscle
    - Works in response to hypovolemia, hypotension, increased serum osmolality, and increased angiotensin II
    - Does not constrict pulmonary vasculature, hence can be used in pulmonary hypertension
- **Baroreceptors**
  - Sensory neurons that monitor blood vessel stretch and pressure
    - Located at the carotid sinus, aortic arch, and right atrium
    - Carotid baroreceptors send signals via cranial nerve IX
    - Aortic baroreceptors send signals via cranial nerve X
  - Baroreceptor firing slows with decreased BP → initiates baroreceptor reflex to restore BP
  - Baroreceptors adapt with time → patients with essential hypertension may have a higher set point for BP
- **Vascular resistance**

- **Systemic vascular resistance (SVR)** from peripheral circulation
  - SVR = 80 × (MAP – CVP)/cardiac output
  - Reference range: 700 to 1,600 dyn · s/cm^5
- **Pulmonary vascular resistance (PVR)** from pulmonary circulation
  - PVR = 80 × (mean PA pressure – pulmonary artery occlusion pressure)/cardiac output
  - Reference range: 20 to 130 dyn · s/cm^5
- Autoregulation of blood flow
  - Autoregulation is the maintenance of normal blood flow despite variations in BP and volume
  - Brain, heart, and kidneys maintain excellent autoregulation
  - Skeletal and splanchnic organs have moderate autoregulation
  - Uterus and skin has little autoregulation

HEMODYNAMIC DRUGS

- Uppers
  - Primary α-agonists
    - **Phenylephrine**
      - Direct α_1-agonist that increases SVR
      - No direct heart rate effect
        - Can see reflex bradycardia → reduction in cardiac output
    - **Norepinephrine**
      - Direct α_1, α_2, and β_1-agonist that increases SVR, but α-effects predominate
      - Venous return increases
      - Cardiac output is normally unchanged
      - Oxygen consumption increases
      - Increases PVR
      - Decreases blood flow to renal vasculature, mesenteric vascular beds, and peripheral circulation
  - Primary β-agonists
    - **Dobutamine**
      - Primarily β_1 effects, although some α_1 and β_2 agonist effects as well
        - More inotropy than chronotropy (unlike isoproterenol)
        - Increases cardiac output without major alterations in heart rate or blood pressure
      - Effective in low cardiac output states
      - Unlikely to increase size of infarct or cause arrhythmias
      - Useful in cardiogenic shock
    - **Isoproterenol**
      - Nonselective β-adrenergic stimulation
        - $\beta_1 > \beta_2$
      - Primarily used as chronotropic agent after heart transplant
      - Can use to treat hemodynamically unstable bradycardia or 3rd degree heart block when a temporary pacemaker is unavailable
    - **Dopexamine**
      - Synthetic dopamine analog with β_1 and β_2 activity
        - $\beta_2 > \beta_1$
      - β_2 → vasodilation → decrease afterload
      - Vasodilation of renal and splanchnic vessels
      - Increased inotropy
      - Increased diuresis
  - Mixed α and β agonists
    - Ephedrine
      - Indirect α- and β-agonist that increases SVR and inotropy
        - Releases NE at sympathetic nerve endings
      - Depletion of norepinephrine stores may result in tachyphylaxis
      - Do not use in patient's taking monoamine oxidase inhibitors
    - **Epinephrine**

- ➤ Direct α_1, α_2, β_1, and β_2-agonist
- ➤ Increases SVR
- ➤ Increases inotropy
- ➤ Increases chronotropy
- ➤ Compared to norepinephrine, epinephrine vasodilates the pulmonary bed through β_2 receptors and can be used in anaphylactic shock
- ➤ Often diluted
  - ❖ 1:100,000 is interpreted as 1 g per 100,000 mL, or 10 μg/mL
- ➤ Eliminated by reuptake into sympathetic nerve terminals (90%) and diffusion to liver for metabolism (20%)
- ❖ **Dopamine**
  - ➤ α, β, and dopaminergic agonist
    - ❖ At low doses (0.5 to 3 μg/kg/min) → acts at renal receptors to promote renal vasodilation
      - ❭ No evidence of improvement in renal function
      - ❭ May promote diuresis that can worsen hypovolemia in certain shock states
    - ❖ At moderate doses (3 to 10 μg/kg/min), β-agonist and increased chronotropy
    - ❖ At high doses (10 to 20 μg/kg/min), mixed α- and β-stimulation
    - ❖ A very high doses (>20 μg/kg/min), primarily α-stimulation
  - ➤ Increased tendency to cause dysrhythmias
  - ➤ No longer the preferred agent in septic shock
- ● Other
  - ❖ **Vasopressin**
    - ➤ Acts at vasopressin V_1 receptors to increase SVR without increase in PVR
    - ➤ Levels of vasopressin are low in vasodilatory/septic shock
    - ➤ Effective in acidemia
    - ➤ Other receptors include V_2 (water retention) and V_3 (corticotropin secretion)
  - ❖ **Milrinone**
    - ➤ Phosphodiesterase III inhibitor that causes positive inotropy and arterial vasodilation
    - ➤ Used in HF to decrease preload and afterload
    - ➤ Renally excreted; therefore, no need for decreasing dose in renal failure
    - ➤ Adverse effects
      - ❖ Arrhythmias, especially atrial fibrillation
      - ❖ Hypotension if administered too quickly
- ■ Downers
  - ● **β-blockers**
    - ❖ Can be targeted at β_1, β_1 and β_2, or β and α
      - ➤ β-receptors are found on the cells of the heart (β_1) as well as the cells of smooth muscle, airways, and arteries (β_2)
      - ➤ Blocking β-receptors inhibits stimulation from β-agonists, such as epinephrine and other stress hormones
    - ❖ Useful in decreasing myocardial oxygen consumption, arrhythmia management, and hypertension
    - ❖ **Types**
      - ➤ **Selective β_1**: atenolol, bisoprolol, esmolol, metoprolol
      - ➤ **Nonselective (β_1 and β_2)**: nadolol, pindolol, propranolol, timolol
      - ➤ **β and α**: carvedilol, labetolol
    - ❖ Contraindications
      - ➤ Can worsen asthma and bronchospasm through β_2-blockade
      - ➤ Can induce profound unmitigated α-agonism in cocaine use and pheochromocytoma
      - ➤ Can blunt response to hypoglycemia
    - ❖ Glucagon can be used in an overdose
  - ● **Calcium channel blockers**
    - ❖ Target and block the movement of calcium through calcium channels
      - ➤ Effective at reducing heart rate, BP, and cerebral vasospasm
      - ➤ Avoid in patients with congestive heart failure (CHF), cardiogenic shock, low cardiac output states, and AV block

- Classes
  - ➤ **Phenylalkylamine**
    - ❖ Selective for myocardium and reduce myocardial oxygen consumption
      - ⟩ Vasodilatory effects are less than other classes → less reflex tachycardia
    - ❖ Example: verapamil
      - ⟩ Effective for supraventricular tachycardia
        - ▸ AV node depressant, negative inotrope
      - ⟩ Moderate vasodilator on coronary and systemic arteries
  - ➤ **Dihydropyridines**
    - ❖ More selective for vasodilation
      - ⟩ Hypotension may induce reflex tachycardia
    - ❖ Examples: nifedipine, nicardipine, nimodipine, amlodipine
      - ⟩ **Nicardipine**
        - ▸ Arterial vasodilator without negative inotropy, chronotropy
          - ○ Minimal venodilator
          - ○ Increases stroke volume and coronary blood flow
        - ▸ Decreases cerebral and cardiac ischemia
        - ▸ Safer profile than nitroprusside and nitroglycerin
          - ○ Adverse effects: headache (21%), nausea and vomiting (7%), peripheral edema
      - ⟩ Nifedipine
        - ▸ Treats angina as it has powerful effects on coronary artery smooth muscle
        - ▸ Relieves coronary vasospasm
      - ⟩ Nimodipine
        - ▸ Crosses the blood–brain barrier → treats subarachnoid hemorrhage-induced vasospasm
  - ➤ **Benzothiazepine**
    - ❖ Selective for both cardiac depressant and vasodilatory effects
      - ⟩ Vasodilates, but with less reflex tachycardia
    - ❖ Example: diltiazem
      - ⟩ Effective AV nodal drug with mild-to-moderate myocardial depressant effects
- Nitric oxide (NO) releasers
  - **Sodium nitroprusside (SNP)**
    - ❖ Structure
      - ➤ $Na_2[Fe(CN)_5NO]$
        - ❖ Five cyanide moieties for every NO moiety
      - ➤ **Releases NO** as active ingredient
    - ❖ Function
      - ➤ Venodilator and vasodilator
        - ❖ Decreases preload and afterload, but more preload than afterload since it is a venodilator
      - ➤ Rapid onset, effective in hypertensive crisis
      - ➤ Rebound hypertension when discontinued due to increased catecholamine secretion during SNP infusion
    - ❖ Adverse effects
      - ➤ **Metabolism** of SNP requires conversion of Fe^{2+} to Fe^{3+} (oxidation) → methemoglobinemia
      - ➤ Can increase intracranial pressure (ICP)
      - ➤ Can cause coronary steal in patients with CAD (coronary artery disease)
        - ❖ Has been shown to increase mortality when administered to patients following myocardial infarction (MI)
      - ➤ Attenuates pulmonary hypoxic vasoconstriction → decrease in PaO_2
      - ➤ **Cyanide toxicity**
        - ❖ Metabolized to cyanide → metabolized to thiocyanate → excreted by kidneys
          - ⟩ Thiocyanate toxicity can occur with renal failure
          - ⟩ Presents with nausea, vomiting, mental confusion, weakness, and thyroid dysfunction
        - ❖ Cyanide toxicity typically requires doses greater than 2 µg/kg/min
          - ⟩ First sign is resistance to hypotensive effects of drug

- Cyanide binds to iron → inhibits cellular respiration → lactic acidosis and cytotoxic hypoxia
  - Mixed venous PaO_2 elevated in presence of cyanide toxicity
  - Venous blood is well oxygenated and patients are not cyanotic
  - **Treatment options:** sodium nitrate, amyl nitrite, sodium thiosulfate, hydroxycobalamin
    - Sodium thiosulfate (preferred drug) converts cyanide to thiocyanate
  - Light protection
    - Exposure to light → release of cyanide
    - Studies show 8 hours of light exposure does not make much difference in cyanide release
- **Nitroglycerin**
  - Converted to nitric oxide
  - Smooth muscle relaxant and venodilator
  - Decreases angina
    - Decreases myocardial preload → decreased wall tension and oxygen consumption
    - Dilates coronary arteries and improves blood flow
  - Vasodilator at higher doses
- **Other downers**
  - **Fenoldopam**
    - Dopamine-1 receptor agonist with significant vasodilating properties
      - Augments renal blood flow through renal vasodilation
        - Lack of significant systemic vasodilation
        - Increases creatinine clearance and promotes diuresis
      - Metabolized in the liver
    - Used for treatment of severe hypertension (HTN) with to minimize renal insult
      - Reduces acute renal injury, need for hemodialysis, death, and length of stay in ICU after long-term infusion
    - Alternative to SNP and has the advantage of less toxicity, rebound effect, or coronary steal
  - **Hydralazine**
    - Vasodilator via smooth muscle relaxation
      - Works on potassium channels
    - Metabolized at liver
    - Can cause an systemic lupus erythematosus–like syndrome
  - **Nesiritide**
    - Recombinant form of human brain natriuretic peptide that has vasodilatory, natriuretic, and diuretic effects
    - Effective in CHF
  - **Angiotensin-converting enzyme (ACE) inhibitors/Aldosterone receptor blocker (ARB)**
    - Inhibit renin–angiotensin–aldosterone system to prevent hypertension
    - May cause refractory hypotension during general anesthetics

HYPERTENSION

- Types of hypertension
  - Essential hypertension
    - Form of HTN without a clear cause
      - Affects > 95% of hypertensive patients
    - Defined as systolic blood pressure (SBP) > 140 and diastolic blood pressure (DBP) > 90
  - Secondary HTN
    - Clear etiology of HTN
      - Frequently causes more severe forms of HTN that are more refractory to treatment
    - Causes
      - Renal artery stenosis
      - Pheochromocytoma
      - Hyperaldosteronism
      - Cushing syndrome

- ➤ Hyperthyroidism
- ➤ Obstructive sleep apnea
- ➤ Autonomic hyperreactivity
- Hypertension morbidity
  - Systolic and diastolic hypertension are independent predictors of MI, stroke, and renal injury risk
  - Pulse pressure >65 is associated with increased risk of stroke, CHF, and mortality
- Preoperative evaluation
  - Evaluate for causes of HTN, cardiovascular risk factors, signs of end-organ damage, and current medical therapy
    - ◆ Long-standing HTN warrants an ECG and preoperative renal labs
    - ◆ Long-standing HTN with ECG abnormalities may be considered for an echocardiogram
  - Generally recommended to delay surgery for BP >200/115
    - ◆ Goal is to normalize BP as much as possible prior to surgery
    - ◆ No evidence to support cancellation for BP <180/110
  - Urgent/emergent surgery should proceed
- Anesthetic considerations
  - Avoid large fluctuations in blood pressure
    - ◆ Consider arterial line
    - ◆ If not using an arterial line, use appropriate sized BP cuff
  - Relative intraoperative hypotension may cause end-organ damage

CORONARY ARTERY DISEASE AND HEART FAILURE

- **Coronary artery disease**
  - Narrowing of coronary arteries that supply the heart
    - ◆ Plaque buildup along the inner walls of the heart arteries → decreases coronary blood flow
  - Stable angina: chest pain at stable levels of exertion
  - Acute coronary syndrome: chest pain indicative of a MI
    - ◆ Includes unstable angina, non-ST elevation myocardial infarction (NSTEMI), and ST elevation myocardial infarction (STEMI)
- **Coronary perfusion**
  - Difference between aortic diastolic pressure and right and left ventricular end-diastolic pressures
    - ◆ LV is perfused during diastole
      - ➤ During systole, LV pressure increases and occludes intramyocardial portions of coronary arteries
    - ◆ RV is perfused during both systole and diastole
      - ➤ During systole, RV pressure is lower and perfusion pressure is sufficient to supply coronary arteries
- Coronary changes with age
  - Decreased cardiac myocytes, sinus node cells, and conduction fibers
  - Elastic and collagen break down
    - ◆ At large arteries → increase aortic diameter
    - ◆ At venous system → reduce compliance
  - Sympathetic nervous system responsiveness decreases
    - ◆ Lower resting and maximal heart rate
    - ◆ β-receptor responsiveness decreases
- **Myocardial infarction**
  - Occurs when blood stops flowing to part of the heart and causes myocardial ischemia
  - Diagnosis of MI
    - ◆ Symptoms
      - ➤ Chest pain with possible radiation to left arm or neck, shortness of breath, diaphoresis, and exacerbation of symptoms with exertion
      - ➤ Women and diabetics may present with atypical symptoms
    - ◆ **Testing**
      - ➤ **ECG changes**
        - ❖ ST-elevation, ST-depressions may signify acute coronary syndrome

> Transmural MI is due to a major MI that extends through the whole thickness of the heart muscle → ST elevations
> Subendocardial MI is due to ischemia in the subendocardial wall → ST depressions
- ❖ T wave inversions may be a sign of ischemia
- ❖ Q waves may be a sign of a previous ischemic event
- ❖ ECG leads and their heart distribution
  - › Lateral: I, avL, V5, V6
  - › Inferior: II, III, aVF
  - › Septal: V1, V2
  - › Anterior: V3, V4
- ➤ **Enzymes**
  - ❖ Cardiac troponin I is a protein marker for cardiac ischemia
    - › May not increase until 3 hours after coronary event
  - ❖ CK-MB is also a marker for ischemia, but troponin is more commonly used
- ◆ Coronary artery and MI location
  - ➤ LAD: anterior or septal MI
  - ➤ Circumflex: lateral MI
  - ➤ RCA: inferior MI
    - ❖ Often causes heart block due to AV nodal damage
- ● **Antianginal treatment**
  - ◆ Oxygen
  - ◆ Antiplatelet therapy
    - ➤ Aspirin
    - ➤ Clopidogrel
    - ➤ Other antiplatelets agents
  - ◆ Nitroglycerin and/or opioids to decrease sympathetic drive
  - ◆ β-blockers
  - ◆ Statins
  - ◆ Revascularization
    - ➤ Angioplasty
    - ➤ Stent placement
    - ➤ Coronary artery bypass surgery
- ● Complications
  - ◆ Septal rupture
    - ➤ Occurs with the highest frequency within the first week post-MI
    - ➤ More common after a transmural infarction and in an anterior wall MI vs. inferior wall MI
    - ➤ Resulting ventricular septal defect that is created is often irregular in shape
    - ➤ Presents with sudden deterioration and cardiogenic shock
      - ❖ Without corrective surgery, mortality is 100%
      - ❖ With corrective surgery, mortality is still 50% to 75%
    - ➤ Many patients are placed on an intra-aortic balloon pump (IABP) to help decrease afterload
- ■ **Heart failure**
  - ● Defined by inability of the heart to pump a sufficient amount of blood
    - ◆ Can be caused of coronary artery disease, hypertension, cardiomyopathy, valvular disease, or arrhythmias
  - ● Can be caused by systolic or diastolic dysfunction
    - ◆ **Systolic dysfunction:** decreased ejection fraction (EF)
    - ◆ **Diastolic dysfunction:** abnormal heart relaxation
  - ● Symptoms include dyspnea on exertion, orthopnea, peripheral and pulmonary edema (increased peak airway pressures + pink, frothy fluid)
  - ● CXR (chest X-ray) will show cardiomegaly
  - ● Echocardiogram will demonstrate hypokinesis
  - ● Cardiac catheterization
    - ◆ Left ventricular end diastolic pressure (LVEDP) >15
    - ◆ Ejection fraction (EF) <35%
    - ◆ Cardiac Index (CI) <2.5

- Goals
  - Decrease preload and pulmonary blood flow via TNG and morphine
  - Increase LV function via dobutamine
  - Optimization of blood pressure, heart rate, preload, and afterload
- New York Heart Association (NYHA) Classification
  - Class I: no limitation in physical activity
  - Class II: slight limitation in physical activity
  - Class III: marked limitation of physical activity
  - Class IV: inability to perform any physical activity without discomfort
- The most common cause of right heart failure is left heart failure
- Takotsubo cardiomyopathy (broken heart syndrome)
  - Unique case of cardiomyopathy caused by reversible left ventricular dysfunction
  - Common in postmenopausal females under severe and sudden physiological stress
  - Treatment
    - If stable: diuretics, ACE inhibitors, β-blockers, and anticoagulation
    - If unstable: consider balloon pump or mechanical support
      - Epinephrine may increase stunned heart since condition may be mediated by increased catecholamines
    - Full recovery is common after a few months
- Preoperative evaluation
  - Identify heart disease risk, physical symptoms, need for interventions, and medical management
  - Risk factors and stratification
    - **Risk factors for coronary artery disease**
      - Hypertension
      - Hyperlipidemia
        - High LDL, low HDL
      - Diabetes
      - Smoking
      - Obesity
      - Family history
    - Revised cardiac risk index
      - Scoring system to predict perioperative risk in patients undergoing noncardiac surgery
      - Predictors
        - High-risk surgery
        - Ischemic heart disease
        - CHF
        - Cerebrovascular disease
        - Diabetes mellitus on insulin
        - Creatinine >2.0
      - Risk for cardiac event (death, cardiac arrest, or myocardial infarction)
        - 1 predictor → 0.9%
        - 2 predictors → 6.6%
        - 3 or more predictors → 11%
    - Physical symptoms
      - Chest pain and its qualities
      - Dyspnea and its qualities
      - Exercise tolerance
        - 4 METS or ability to walk a flight of stairs is generally a good marker of functional capacity
  - Interventions
    - **12-lead ECG testing**
      - Not needed in patients without risk factors or symptoms regardless of age
      - Worth consideration in patients with one or more risk factors undergoing nonvascular surgery
      - Recommended in patients with one or more risk factors undergoing vascular surgery
      - Pulsus alternans: small and larger waves seen in severe LV dysfunction

- ◆ **Stress testing**
  - ➤ Stress testing can be combined with ECG and/or echocardiography to assess wall motion and coronary vessels
  - ➤ Types
    - ❖ **Exercise testing** on a treadmill or bicycle
      - ⟩ Patients should be able to reach 85% of their maximum heart rate (220 − age) for test to be valuable
    - ❖ Chemical stress test for those who cannot exercise
      - ⟩ **Dobutamine stress test**
        - ▷ Dobutamine increases heart rate
        - ▷ Test uses rapid heart rate to assess for ischemia
        - ▷ Cannot be used in patients on high-dose β-blockers or in those who use pacemakers for bradycardia
      - ⟩ **Adenosine radionucleotide imaging**
        - ▷ Adenosine vasodilates vessels
        - ▷ Uptake of isotope is normal in patent vessels, but vasodilation and uptake of isotope is limited in stenotic vessels
        - ▷ Not dependent on heart rate
  - ➤ Abnormalities
    - ❖ Wall motion abnormalities can indicate active ischemia from increased chronotropy/inotropy or a site of previous infarction
    - ❖ Decreased radionucleotide uptake during adenosine stress testing indicates stenotic lesion
- ◆ **Coronary catheterization**
  - ➤ Invasive procedure to assess coronary vessels with contrast agent
  - ➤ Can be used for intervention → angioplasty or stent placement
    - ❖ Due to need for antiplatelet therapy, stent placement may delay surgical intervention
- ● **Medical management**
  - ◆ Continuation or initiation of antiplatelets agents, statins, β-blockers, diuretics, nitrates, ACE inhibitors, ARBs, and anticoagulants must be made on a case-by-case scenario based on the patient and surgery

VALVULAR DISEASE

- ■ Aortic stenosis
  - ● Presentation
    - ◆ Angina, syncope, HF, or decrease in exercise tolerance
      - ➤ Heart failure symptoms are secondary to a combination of ischemia, left ventricular hypertrophy (LVH), and LV dysfunction
      - ➤ Syncope is secondary to decreased carbon monoxide (CO)
    - ◆ Systolic ejection murmur at right upper sternal border
    - ◆ ECG
      - ➤ Pulsus parvus: diminished pulse wave
      - ➤ Pulsus tardus: delayed upstroke
  - ● Causes
    - ◆ Calcific degeneration, bicuspid or unicuspid aortic valve, rheumatic heart disease, history of chest radiation
  - ● Classification
    - ◆ Normal: valve area >2.5 cm^2, mean pressure gradient <5 mm Hg
    - ◆ Mild: valve area >1.5 cm^2, mean pressure gradient <20 mm Hg
    - ◆ Moderate: valve area 1 to 1.5 cm^2, mean pressure gradient 20 to 40 mm Hg
    - ◆ Severe: valve area 0.7 to 1.0 cm^2, mean pressure gradient >0 mm Hg
    - ◆ Critical: valve area <0.7 cm^2, mean pressure gradient >50 mm Hg
  - ● Pathophysiology
    - ◆ Coronary perfusion is compromised and many patients have coexisting CAD
    - ◆ Aortic stenosis causes compensatory LVH to preserve EF

- LVH will reduce the compliance of the LV and can lead to LA hypertrophy and increased LA pressures
- Increased left atrial and ventricular pressures can transmit and cause elevated pulmonary and right heart pressures
- Anesthetic strategies
  - Adequate preload necessary to maintain forward flow during anesthetic induction
  - Maintain sinus rhythm to preserve atrial kick and ventricular filling
    - Atrial fibrillation prevents adequate preload
  - Minimize tachycardia to allow time for adequate ventricular filling
    - HR <80 to 90 bpm
  - Maintain contractility
    - Use caution with beta blockers and calcium channel blockers
  - Maintain SVR and afterload
- Cardiac intervention
  - Aortic valve replacement (AVR) should be considered in symptomatic severe aortic stenosis, moderate aortic stenosis undergoing bypass surgery, or asymptomatic severe aortic stenosis with a decreased ejection fraction
  - AVR can be done through open surgery or a transcatheter approach
- Outcomes
  - Progressive disease
  - Once symptoms are present, without intervention, mean survival is ~2 to 3 years and is predicted on symptoms
    - Angina: ~5 years
    - CHF: ~3 years
    - Syncope: ~1 year
- Aortic insufficiency
  - Presentation
    - Acute aortic insufficiency (AI): acute weakness, dyspnea, and syncope
      - Elevated SBP and low DBP
      - Bounding pulse
    - Chronic aortic insufficiency: symptoms similar to acute AI, but milder and more prolonged in onset
    - Early diastolic murmur at third left intercostal space
    - Bisferiens pulse: two systolic peaks seen on arterial tracing in aortic insufficiency
      - First wave represents blood ejected with systole
      - Second wave represents reflected peak from the periphery
  - Causes
    - Acute
      - Endocarditis, blunt chest trauma, aortic dissection of a thoracic aneurysm
    - Chronic
      - Biscuspid valve, rheumatoid diseases, degenerative aortic dilatation
  - Classification
    - Severe aortic regurgitation is a regurgitant volume of more than 50%, color jet width of >65% of the left ventricular outflow tract diameter, and Doppler vena contracts width >0.6 cm
  - Pathophysiology
    - Aortic insufficiency causes volume overload and pressure overload from the increased left ventricle volume → LVH
    - Increased left ventricular pressures can cause pulmonary edema and CHF
    - Increased myocardial oxygen requirement secondary to LVH and decreased aortic diastolic perfusion pressure → decreased coronary blood flow → angina (even in the absence of CAD)
  - Anesthetic strategies
    - Increase preload and heart rate to maintain forward flow
    - Reduce afterload and SVR to prevent increased regurgitation
    - Maintain PVR to prevent pulmonary edema
    - Chronic aortic insufficiency is well tolerated, but acute aortic insufficiency can result in significant hemodynamic instability

- Cardiac intervention
  - Surgical AVR is indicated for symptoms of HF or absence of symptoms with a diminished ejection fraction
  - Surgical AVR is indicated over medical management in acute severe AI
- Mitral stenosis
  - Presentation
    - Dyspnea, chest pain, orthopnea, and HF symptoms
    - Mid-diastolic murmur at the apex
  - Causes
    - Almost exclusively rheumatic disease, but other causes are calcifications and endocarditis
  - Classification
    - Normal valve area: 4 to 6 cm^2
    - Mild: 1.5 to 2.5 cm^2
    - Moderate: 1.1 to 1.5 cm^2
    - Severe: normal valve area: 0.6 to 1.0 cm^2
  - Pathophysiology
    - Increased left atrial pressure $\rightarrow$ pulmonary hypertension and CHF
    - Increased left atrial dilation $\rightarrow$ atrial fibrillation
    - Low left atrial flow $\rightarrow$ increased thromboembolism risk
    - Fixed CO and increased pulmonary pressures $\rightarrow$ pulmonary edema and eventual RV failure
    - Left ventricle is protected by the stenotic valve
  - Anesthetic strategies
    - Increased LV preload for forward flow
    - Maintain sinus rhythm
      - Very dependent on their "atrial kick," which accounts for ~35% of their CO vs. ~20% in normal patients
    - Prevent bradycardia to maintain ventricular filling
    - Maintain contractility
    - Maintain systemic vascular resistance
    - Avoid hypoxia and hypercarbia, which can worsen pulmonary HTN
  - Cardiac intervention
    - Percutaneous balloon mitral valvuloplasty can be considered for severe, symptomatic mitral stenosis if no thrombus is present
    - Mitral commissurotomy is indicated for severe, symptomatic mitral stenosis when valvoplasty is not possible
    - Mitral valve replacement (MVR) is indicated for moderate-to-severe mitral stenosis with abnormal valve anatomy
- Mitral insufficiency
  - Presentation
    - CHF, decreased exercise tolerance, palpitations
    - Holosystolic murmur at the apex
  - Causes
    - Cardiac ischemia, rheumatic heart disease, endocarditis, intracardiac tumor, trauma, degenerative tearing of the chordae tendineae
  - Classification
    - Severe when vena contract width >0.7 cm, central mitral regurgitant jet <40% of left atrium, regurgitant volume >50%
  - Pathophysiology
    - Acute mitral insufficiency can cause volume and pressure overload of the left atrium and ventricle $\rightarrow$ pulmonary congestion
    - Portion of stroke volume regurgitated $\rightarrow$ decreased cardiac output
  - Anesthetic strategies
    - Prevent bradycardia and maintain preload for forward flow
    - Decrease afterload and SVR to prevent increased regurgitation
    - IABP may be helpful to prevent hypotension and maintain organ perfusion
  - Cardiac intervention

- Mitral valve repair or replacement indicated for EF <60%, severe pulmonary HTN, or signs of HF
- Tricuspid stenosis
  - Presentation
    - Dyspnea, fatigue, peripheral edema
    - Diastolic murmur over the left sterna border
  - Causes
    - Rheumatic, carcinoid, endocarditis, extracardiac tumors
      - If rheumatic, patients almost always have coexisting mitral disease as well
  - Pathophysiology
    - Increased right atrial pressure → atrial fibrillation
    - Increased venous congestion
  - Anesthetic strategies
    - Increase preload and prevent bradycardia to encourage forward flow
    - Increase systemic vascular resistance
    - Prevent increases in pulmonary vascular resistance
  - Cardiac intervention
    - Tricuspid balloon valvotomy
    - Tricuspid valve replacement
- Tricuspid regurgitation
  - Presentation
    - Right HF, ascites, hepatomegaly, jugular venous congestion
  - Causes
    - Annular dilatation from any process that causes RV dilatation, pulmonary hypertension, rheumatic heart disease, endocarditis, carcinoid heart disease, radiation
  - Pathophysiology
    - Progressive RA and RV pressure and volume overload → right HF
    - Increased RA dilation → atrial fibrillation
  - Anesthetic strategies
    - Prevent volume overload
    - Prevent bradycardia
    - Maintain contractility
    - Maintain systemic vascular resistance
    - Decrease pulmonary vascular resistance
  - Cardiac intervention
    - Tricuspid valve repair or replacement
- Hypertrophic cardiomyopathy
  - Myocardium, especially left ventricle, becomes asymmetrically hypertrophied with a prominent septal knuckle
  - Dynamic outflow obstruction occurs in up to 70% of patients
    - Occurs due to systolic anterior motion of the anterior mitral valve leaflet meeting the anteroseptal segment of the left ventricle → obstructs the left ventricular outflow tract
    - Management
      - Reduce chronotropy to allow diastolic filling
      - Negative inotropy to relieve obstruction
      - Maintain preload
      - Augment afterload
  - Cause of sudden cardiac death
- **Endocarditis prophylaxis**
  - 2007 American Heart Association made recommendations for specific conditions that warranted infectious endocarditis prophylaxis prior to dental procedures
    - Prosthetic heart valves
    - History of endocarditis
    - Heart transplant with abnormal valvular function
    - Congenital heart defects
      - Unrepaired cyanotic defects

- ➢ Repaired congenital heart defects with prosthetic material
- ➢ Repaired congenital heart defects for first 6 months after repair
- ➢ Repaired congenital heart disease with residual defects
- Antibiotic choice
    - ◆ Target gram-positive coverage with amoxicillin, ampicillin, a first generation cephalosporin, a second-generation cephalosporin, or clindamycin

ARRHYTHMIAS AND ELECTRICAL DISORDERS

- ■ Implications of arrhythmias
    - Arrhythmias are associated with increased perioperative risk due to likely association with underlying cardiac disease
    - Consider postponing elective surgery if rhythm is new and underlying cause is not known
- ■ Classification of arrhythmias by location of the electrical disturbance
    - Atrial
        - ◆ Atrial fibrillation, atrial flutter, multifocal atrial tachycardia, premature atrial tachycardia, and sinus bradycardia
    - Atrioventricular node
        - ◆ Heart block
    - Ventricular
        - ◆ Premature ventricular contractions, Long QT syndrome, Wolff–Parkinson–White syndrome, ventricular tachycardia, and ventricular fibrillation (Fig. 6.4)
- ■ **Atrial fibrillation**
    - Defined by irregular rhythm with the absence of P wave on ECG
        - ◆ Disorganized atrial electrical activity → irregular conduction of ventricular impulses
    - Implications
        - ◆ 8× increase in perioperative mortality within 30 days
        - ◆ Loss of atrial kick diminishes cardiac output
            - ➢ Atrial contraction responsible for 15% to 30% of cardiac output
        - ◆ Increased thromboembolic risk due to decreased atrial flow
            - ➢ CHAD2 score
                - ❖ Congestive HF (1 point)
                - ❖ Hypertension (1 point)
                - ❖ Age >75 (1 point)
                - ❖ Diabetes (1 point)
                - ❖ Stroke or transient ischemic attack (2 points)
            - ➢ CHADS2 score and yearly stroke risk
                - ❖ 0 points = 2%
                - ❖ 1 point = 3%
                - ❖ 2 points = 4%
                - ❖ 3 points = 6%
                - ❖ 4 points = 9%

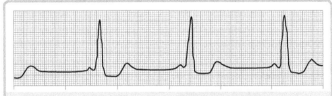

FIGURE 6.4 Wolff–Parkinson–White Syndrome. ECG pattern of Wolff–Parkinson–White with its characteristic delta-wave. (Reproduced from Badescu GC, Sherman B, Zaidan JR, et al. Atlas of echocardiography. In: Barash PG, Cullen BF, Stoelting RK, et al., eds. *Clinical Anesthesia.* 7th ed. Philadelphia, PA: Wolters Kluwer; 2013:1719.)

- ❖ 5 points = 13%
- ❖ 6 points = 18%
- ❖ Rapid ventricular response
  - ➤ Atrial fibrillation can be associated with a rapid ventricular rate that diminishes ventricular filling
  - ➤ Associated with decreased BP, shortness of breath, and lightheadedness
- Causes
  - ❖ An underlying cause of atrial fibrillation is not always found
  - ❖ Associated with heart disease, pulmonary disease, alcohol use, hyperthyroidism, inflammation, and surgical stimulation or stress
- **Treatment**
  - ❖ Rate control and/or rhythm control
  - ❖ Anticoagulation should be considered prior to conversion and immediately after cardioversion if atrial fibrillation has persisted greater than 48 hours
    - ➤ Patients with an elevated CHADS2 score who remain in atrial fibrillation should be considered for long-term anticoagulation
  - ❖ Cardioversion should be considered for hemodynamically unstable patients with acute-onset A-fib
    - ➤ In patients with chronic A-fib, use cardioversion with caution; should ensure there is not a clot in the RA, as cardioversion could cause the clot to embolize
- Atrial flutter
  - Reentrant rhythm caused by a premature atrial rhythm
    - ❖ The ventricular refractory period prevents all impulses from being conducted to the ventricles
  - Complications and treatment are the same as atrial fibrillation
- Multifocal atrial tachycardia
  - Tachycardic rhythm associated with three or more P wave morphologies
    - ❖ Due to clusters of cells initiating electrical impulses
  - Associated with chronic obstructive pulmonary disease and treating the underlying cause can improve rate control
  - Does not respond to direct current (DC) cardioversion because it lacks a reentrant mechanism for termination
- Heart block
  - First-degree AV block
    - ❖ PR interval >0.2 seconds
  - Second-degree AV block
    - ❖ Mobitz type I (Wenckebach): progressive lengthening of the PR interval with missed beats
    - ❖ Mobitz type II: PR interval remains constant with missed beats
  - Third-degree AV block
    - ❖ No association between P waves and QRS complexes
    - ❖ Independent atrial and ventricular rates
- Left bundle branch block (LBBB)
  - RR' in V5 or V6
  - Implies LVH, HTN, and/or CAD
  - Often difficult to diagnose a MI if the patient has a preexisting LBBB
  - Caution should be used in these patients during placement of a pulmonary artery catheter
    - ❖ RBBB can occur during placement (~5%) → complete heart block
- Right bundle branch block (RBBB)
  - RR' in V1 or V2
  - Does not imply cardiac disease
- Unifasicular block
  - Block of one of the fascicles of the left bundle
  - Left anterior hemiblock is more common than a left posterior hemiblock
    - ❖ Left anterior fascicular/hemiblock (LAFB)
      - ➤ ECG: left axis deviation with RBBB
    - ❖ Left posterior fascicular/hemiblock (LPFB)
      - ➤ ECG: right axis deviation with RBBB

- Bifasicular block
  - Presence of an RBBB with involves of one or two of the fascicles from the left bundle
    - RBBB + LAFB is more common vs. RBBB + LPFB
- Junctional escape rhythms
  - Nodal rhythm
  - Impulses can be conducted retrograde (to the atria) and anterograde (normal; to the ventricle)
  - P wave can be close to, precede, or lost in the QRS
  - Commonly asymptomatic, but can be associated with hypotension and reduced cardiac output
  - Common arrhythmia seen under general anesthesia when volatile anesthetics are used
  - Treatment
    - Increase heart rate
      - Ephedrine, atropine, glycopyrrolate
      - Isoproterenol, epinephrine
      - Temporary pacemaker
      - Short-acting β-blockers can be helpful if the arrhythmia is secondary to sympathetic stimulation
- Wolff–Parkinson–White syndrome
  - Preexcitation syndrome with the Bundle of Kent accessory pathway
    - Current is transmitted from the atria to the ventricles, but not through the AV node
  - Induced through sympathetic stimulation and several classes of drugs
    - Sympathetic stimulating drugs: ketamine and ephedrine
    - Rate control drugs: β-blockers, calcium channel blockers, and digoxin
      - May block conduction through the AV node → forces all conduction through the accessory node
  - Procainamide blocks conduction via the accessory pathway
  - EKG findings
    - Short PR interval (<0.12)
    - Wide QRS interval (>0.12)
    - Delta waves
- Brugada syndrome
  - Genetically inherited disease affecting cardiac ion channels (SCN5A sodium channel)
    - Associated with sudden cardiac death
    - Polymorphic ventricular tachycardia can morph into ventricular fibrillation
  - Cardiac testing
    - Baseline ECG may show ST elevations in V1-3, right bundle branch block
    - ECG is negative in 30%
    - Echocardiogram is generally negative
    - Cardiac MRI is useful in diagnosing arrhythmic RV dysplasia
      - Fatty replacement in the RV infundibulum
  - Anesthetic considerations
    - Consider preoperative implantable cardioverter defibrillator (ICD) placement
    - If no internal ICD is present, place pads on patient for possible defibrillation
    - Avoid increased vagal tone and bradycardia
- **QT$_C$ prolongation**
  - Causes
    - **Genetics**
      - Channel alterations that either reduce potassium outflow or increase sodium/calcium inflow
      - **Congenital long QT syndrome**
        - Autosomal recessive syndrome
        - Increased sympathetic activity can precipitate reentrant circuits and cause torsades
        - Only 60% of patients with long QT syndrome show prolongation of QT on screening ECG (QT >420 ms)
        - Strategies to avoid cardiac events
          - β-blockade
          - ICD placement
          - Avoid sympathetic stimulation

- Romano–Ward syndrome
- Jervell and Lange-Nielsen syndrome
- **Drugs that can prolong QT$_C$**
  - Antipsychotics, antidepressants, antibiotics, antifungals, antihistamines
- Electrolytes abnormalities
  - Hypokalemia and hypomagnesaemia can precipitate torsades
- Ventricular tachycardia
  - Classifications
    - Morphology
      - Monomorphic
        - Ventricular tachycardia complexes are identical on ECG
        - Often caused by increased electrical impulses from one ventricular focus
          - Causes include myocardial scarring or irritation during pulmonary artery catheter placement
      - Polymorphic
        - Ventricular tachycardia complexes vary by beat
        - Often caused by problems with repolarization
          - Example: torsades, long QT syndrome
    - Duration
      - Nonsustained: <30 seconds
      - Sustained: >30 seconds
    - Pulse
      - Pulse
        - Cardiac output preserved
      - Pulseless ventricular tachycardia
        - Type of cardiac arrest
        - Shockable rhythm that should warrant immediate Advanced Cardiovascular Life Support (ACLS) treatment
  - Treatment
    - Stable (with pulse)
      - Magnesium
      - Antiarrhythmic agents such as amiodarone
      - Cardiac ablation
      - Cardioversion
      - Overdrive atrial or ventricular pacing
    - Unstable
      - Cardioversion
      - Defibrillation
- Ventricular fibrillation
  - Asynchronous and uncoordinated ventricular activity that is a medical emergency
  - Associated with ischemic heart disease, but cause is not always discernible
  - Treatment
    - Defibrillation
    - Antiarrhythmic agents
- ECG disturbances from electrolyte imbalances
  - Hypokalemia: prolonged PR, T wave flattening, U waves
  - Hyperkalemia: shortened PR, widened QRS, peaked T waves
  - Hypercalcemia: shortened QT

ARRHYTHMIA TREATMENT OPTIONS

- Rate control
  - β-blockers
  - Calcium channel blockers
  - **Digoxin**
    - Cardiac glycoside

- ➤ Commonly used in atrial fibrillation and flutter
- ◆ **Mechanism**
  - ➤ Inhibits myocardial Na-K-ATPase
  - ➤ Increase myocardial inotropy in patients with HF
  - ➤ Slow heart rate through AV node
- ◆ Signs of **toxicity**
  - ➤ Nausea/vomiting
  - ➤ Abdominal pain
  - ➤ Weakness
  - ➤ Confusion
  - ➤ Frequent ventricular ectopic beats
  - ➤ Yellow or green vision changes with halos around lights
- ◆ Predisposing factors → digoxin toxicity
  - ➤ Hypokalemia
  - ➤ Hypomagnesaemia
  - ➤ Hypercalcemia
  - ➤ Hypothyroidism
- ◆ Treatment for ventricular arrhythmias due to digoxin toxicity
  - ➤ Repletion of electrolytes (Mg, K)
  - ➤ Lidocaine, phenytoin, atropine
  - ➤ Digoxin immune fab is extremely effective for severe digoxin toxicity
- ● Adenosine
  - ◆ Nucleoside that produces transient heart block at the atrioventricular node
  - ◆ Used in supraventricular tachycardias to assist in identifying or terminating the rhythm
  - ◆ Undergoes nucleotide metabolism
    - ➤ Inhibited by dipyridamole, so lower adenosine dose should be used to prevent prolonged asystole
- ■ Rhythm control
  - ● Amiodarone
    - ◆ Benzofurane derivative with structure like thyroxine
      - ➤ Prolongs repolarization of cardiac action potential
      - ➤ Prolongs action potential of atrial and ventricular muscle without altering resting membrane potential
        - ❖ Depresses SA and AV node function
      - ➤ Prolongs QT interval
    - ◆ Indications
      - ➤ Used in atrial and ventricular tachycardias
      - ➤ Treatment of choice in cardiac arrest due to ventricular fibrillation
        - ❖ 300-mg intravenous dose
    - ◆ Dosing
      - ➤ Intravenous or oral
        - ❖ Oral dosing has variable bioavailability
      - ➤ Fat soluble with high volume of distribution
        - ❖ Loading dose is ~10 grams
      - ➤ Half-life of up to 1 month
    - ◆ Complications
      - ➤ 2% to 4% with altered thyroid function
        - ❖ Can be hyper- or hypothyroid
      - ➤ 5% to 15% with pulmonary toxicity
        - ❖ Leads to irreversible interstitial pneumonitis
        - ❖ Presents with cough, dyspnea, bilateral diffuse and patchy infiltrates, decreased D_{LCO}
        - ❖ Often in patients who take amiodarone for months or years
        - ❖ Treatment
          - › Discontinue drug, take steroids
      - ➤ Hepatic dysfunction
        - ❖ Can be subclinical or be as severe as cirrhosis

- ➤ Ophthalmologic manifestations
    - ❖ Corneal microdeposits and lenticular opacities
    - ❖ Does not affect visual acuity, but may cause halo vision and photophobia
  - ❖ Side effects
    - ➤ Bradycardia
      - ❖ May cause an atropine-resistant bradycardia due to the anti-adrenergic effects of amiodarone
      - ❖ Treatment involves isoproterenol or a pacemaker
    - ➤ Hypotension through vasodilation and negative inotropy
- ● Procainamide
  - ❖ Sodium channel blocker that prolongs the cardiac action potential
  - ❖ Used for supraventricular tachycardias as well as Wolff–Parkinson–White
- ■ Electrical cardioversion
  - ● A timed electrical current is transmitted during the R wave of the QRS complex
    - ❖ Prevents transmission during the refractory period and ventricular fibrillation
  - ● Used for hemodynamically unstable rhythms including atrial fibrillation, atrial flutter, and ventricular tachycardias
  - ● Energy
    - ❖ 50- to 100-J biphasic energy or 100-J monophasic energy used for atrial flutter
    - ❖ 100- to 200-J biphasic energy or 200-J monophasic energy used for atrial fibrillation and ventricular tachycardia
- ■ Defibrillation
  - ● An electrical current is transmitted and depolarizes cardiac muscle to terminate unstable arrhythmias
    - ❖ Allows normal sinus rhythm to be established
  - ● Used for pulseless ventricular tachycardia or ventricular fibrillation
    - ❖ 200 J biphasic energy or 360 J monophasic energy used
- ■ Invasive interventions
  - ● **Catheter ablation**
    - ❖ Can be done for rate or rhythm control
    - ❖ Targets atria and the pulmonary veins
    - ❖ Complications
      - ➤ Need for pacing mechanism of the ventricle prior to procedure due risk of heart block
    - ❖ Success rate
      - ➤ 50% to 60% in chronic atrial fibrillation
      - ➤ 80% in patients with normal size chambers
  - ● **MAZE procedure**
    - ❖ Surgical procedure to create transmural injury to parts of the myocardium containing electrical pathways
      - ➤ Incise a box around the pulmonary veins and extend the incision toward the left atrium and toward the mitral valve
      - ➤ Scarred tissue is unable to conduct impulses
  - ● **Ligate/excise the left atrial appendage**
    - ❖ Can use heat, laser, cold, or high-intensity ultrasound

OBSTRUCTIVE DISORDERS

- ■ Pericardial effusion and **cardiac tamponade**
  - ● Presentation
    - ❖ Beck triad
      - ➤ Hypotension, jugular venous distention, and decreased heart sounds
    - ❖ Pulsus paradoxus
      - ➤ Inspiratory fall in systolic arterial BP greater than 10 mm Hg
    - ❖ Kussmaul sign
      - ➤ Neck veins become distended during inspiration
      - ➤ More commonly seen with constrictive pericarditis
  - ● Causes

- Trauma, autoimmune disease (SLE, rheumatoid, scleroderma), uremia, cancer, aortic dissection, myocardial infarction, viral, tuberculosis
- Pathophysiology
  - Tamponade is due to accumulation of fluid in the pericardial space
    - If fluid fills faster than pericardial stretch → venous return and chamber filling are compromised during diastole
    - Increased pericardial pressure can shift the interventricular septum toward left → decrease left ventricular filling
  - The magnitude of deterioration and tamponade depends upon how quickly the fluid builds up
    - As little as 100 to 200 cc of fluid or blood can cause acute tamponade
    - In chronic conditions (where there is a slow accumulation of fluid), pericardial effusions up to ~1 L may be asymptomatic
  - Equalization of diastolic pressure due to compression on heart chambers
    - CVP = pulmonary capillary wedge pressure
  - Mechanism of pulsus paradoxus
    - Ventricular filling is limited by blood, thrombus in pericardial space
    - During inspiration, negative intrathoracic pressure enhances filling of RV
      - Due to limited cardiac volume, RV fills, but LV volume drops
    - Late stages of tamponade
      - Hypotension and narrow pulse pressure result in less change in BP for pulsus paradoxus
      - Ratio of paradoxical pulse pressure to arterial pulse pressure more reliable indicator of tamponade severity
- Anesthetic considerations
  - Patients are often reliant on sympathetic tone and have impaired contractility → high risk of cardiovascular collapse on induction
  - Consider volume expansion to augment cardiac filling and vasopressors to maintain contractility
  - Positive pressure ventilation increases PVR and decreases RV outflow → decreases LV filling → decreases BP
    - Ideally the patient should be spontaneously breathing
- Treatment
  - Pericardiocentesis
  - Pericardial window
- **Constrictive pericarditis**
  - Pathophysiology
    - Progressive inflammation of the pericardium that results in a thickened and fibrotic pericardium
      - Normal pericardium is 3-mm thick, but may increase to 6-mm thickness with constrictive pericarditis
    - Diagnosed by a normal medial/septal tissue Doppler with an abnormal or decreased lateral tissue Doppler at the mitral valve annulus on echocardiographic exam. Restricts cardiac filling
      - Physiology is similar to tamponade
  - Causes
    - Idiopathic, inflammatory, autoimmune, uremia, mediastinal radiation
  - Treatment
    - Pericardiectomy is definitive
- **Pulmonary embolism (PE)**
  - **Pathophysiology**
    - A pulmonary embolism is caused by a blood clot that becomes lodged in the pulmonary vasculature and occludes blood flow
    - Increases RV afterload → RV dysfunction → decreased RV output and septal shift toward LV → decreased LV preload → decreased systemic perfusion
  - Presentation
    - Tachycardia, chest pain, dyspnea, cyanosis
  - Predisposing conditions
    - Previous DVT or PE

- ◆ Pregnancy
- ◆ Obesity
- ◆ Cancer
- ◆ Hormone replacement therapy (Tamoxifin)
- ◆ Immobility
- ◆ Surgery
  - ➤ Hip, knee, pelvis
- ◆ Polycythemia vera
- ◆ Antiphospholipid syndrome
- Diagnosis
  - ◆ **ECG**
    - ➤ PE shows **S1Q3T3** pattern on ECG
      - ◆ Finding is not sensitive or specific
    - ➤ ECG is more important to rule out cardiac cause of presentation
  - ◆ CT angiography
    - ➤ Contrast shows impairment of blood flow in the pulmonary vasculature
  - ◆ V/Q scanning
    - ➤ PE presents with areas ventilated, but not perfused
  - ◆ **TEE**
    - ➤ Right ventricular dilation, septal bowing, impaired flow at pulmonary artery
- **Treatment**
  - ◆ Anticoagulation
  - ◆ Thrombolysis
  - ◆ Pulmonary thrombectomy
- **Other types of embolism**
  - ◆ Air embolism
  - ◆ Fat embolism
  - ◆ Amniotic fluid embolism

PULMONARY HYPERTENSION

- Presentation
  - Progressive shortness of breath with exertion, chest pain, fatigue, or syncope
  - Clinical signs include distended neck veins, hepatomegaly, and ascites
  - ECG may show evidence of RV hypertrophy, RV strain, or RA dilation
- Definition
  - Mean pulmonary arterial pressure >25 mm Hg
  - Testing
    - ◆ Echocardiogram where right ventricular systolic pressure is estimated from the tricuspid regurgitant jet
      - ➤ Pressure = $4 \times v_{max}^2$
    - ◆ Right heart catheterization is the gold standard for pulmonary artery pressure
- Pathophysiology
  - Increased pulmonary pressures from vascular remodeling
  - Increased pulmonary artery blood flow (left to right intracardiac shunts)
  - Increased pulmonary vascular resistance
    - ◆ Hypoxic vasoconstriction
    - ◆ Destruction of pulmonary vascular beds
  - Increased left atrial pressure
    - ◆ Mitral stenosis (MS)
    - ◆ Mitral regurgitation (MR)
  - Right ventricle can become volume overloaded and decompensate
  - Pulmonary vascular resistance
    - ◆ Sum of resistance of small and large blood vessels
    - ◆ PVR is least at functional residual capacity (FRC)
    - ◆ If lung volume > FRC → PVR increases due to compression of small intra-alveolar vessels

- ◆ If lung volume < FRC → PVR increases due to kinking of large extra-alveolar vessels
- ■ Treatment
  - ● Prostacyclin analogs (such as epoprostenol)
    - ◆ Epoprostenol is the only drug that has been shown to improve survival
    - ◆ Inhaled prostacyclins have less systemic side effects (such as Iloprost)
  - ● cGMP phosphodiesterase inhibitors (such as sildenafil)
    - ◆ Increase nitric oxide → produce pulmonary and coronary vasodilation
  - ● Endothelin receptor antagonists
    - ◆ Bosentan
      - ➤ Contraindicated in pregnancy
  - ● Milrinone
    - ◆ Decreases pulmonary HTN and adds inotropy
  - ● Inhalational **nitric oxide**
    - ◆ Nitric oxide stimulates cGMP activity → smooth muscle and pulmonary vasodilation → improves V/Q matching
    - ◆ Administered via inspiratory limb of circuit at a concentration denoted in parts per million
    - ◆ Range is 1 to 80 ppm, but typical dose is 20 to 40 ppm
- ■ Anesthetic considerations
  - ● Prevent hypoxia, hypercapnia, and acidosis
  - ● Maintain adequate preload
  - ● Maintain contractility
  - ● Avoid nitrous oxide as it can increase PVR
  - ● Consider drugs listed above
    - ◆ Although norepinephrine increases PA pressures, it may have to be used in severe RV failure

CARDIAC BYPASS

- ■ Purpose
  - ● Cardiac bypass is performed to create a motionless and bloodless field for the cardiac surgeon
  - ● Blood is diverted from the heart and lungs
- ■ Components (Fig. 6.5)
  - ● **Venous line**
    - ◆ Passively removes blood returning to the heart
    - ◆ Drains into a venous reservoir via gravity
      - ➤ An "airlock" can occur if the siphon process is disrupted by a large air bubble
  - ● **Arterial pump**
    - ◆ Roller or centrifugal pump
      - ➤ **Roller pumps** create an occlusive point and then roll the tubing to create forward flow
        - ✧ Capable of generating very positive and negative pressures
        - ✧ Capable of allowing air into the circuit
        - ✧ Thought to cause more trauma to cells
      - ➤ **Centrifugal pumps** generate flow through centrifugal force created through high-speed revolutions
        - ✧ Rotate three disks at 3,000 rotations per minute
        - ✧ Thought to create less trauma to cells
        - ✧ Afterload dependent → prevents line rupture when clamping arterial inflow
        - ✧ Lacks occlusion → risks exsanguinations if disconnected
          - ◦ One-way valve prevents backflow
        - ✧ Will not entrain air into the circuit
    - ◆ Arterial flow pressure should correlate with the peripheral artery tracing
      - ➤ If there are no pulsations, either the cannula was not inserted properly or the attachment of the circuit is backward
    - ◆ Flow rates
      - ➤ Flows >2 L/min/m² associated with
        - ✧ Hematologic trauma
        - ✧ Increased inflammation

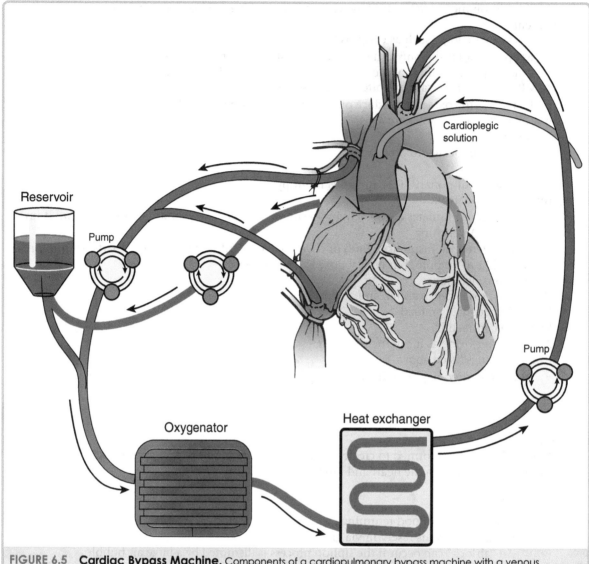

FIGURE 6.5 Cardiac Bypass Machine. Components of a cardiopulmonary bypass machine with a venous reservoir, oxygenator, heat exchanger, and arterial pump.

- ❖ Suture line strain
- ❖ Shunting of blood to lungs
- ❖ Washout of cardioplegia
- ➤ Aim for MAP ~50 mm Hg
  - ❖ Lowest "normal" MAP that still allows for autoregulation
- ● **Heat exchanger**
  - ❖ Regulate body temperature of patient
  - ❖ Cooling is done if hypothermia is protective
    - ➤ Each degree (°C) decrease → 5% to 8% decrease in metabolic rate
  - ❖ Warming is done prior to discontinuation of cardiopulmonary bypass to restore normothermia
- ● **Oxygenator**
  - ❖ A membrane or bubble oxygenator is used to add oxygen and remove carbon dioxide from the circuit
    - ➤ Replaces the function of the native lungs
  - ❖ Membrane oxygenator
    - ➤ Utilizes a blood–membrane–gas interface
    - ➤ The membrane reduces trauma to cells

- ◆ Bubble oxygenator
  - ➤ Utilizes a blood–gas interface
- ● Arterial line filter
  - ◆ Remove potential microemboli from reaching the patient
- ● Arterial line
  - ◆ Transmits blood back to the aorta of the patient
- ■ Anesthetic events
  - ● Induction of anesthesia and securing vascular access
  - ● Preparation for cardiopulmonary bypass
    - ◆ **Prime volume**
      - ➤ Amount of volume to de-air the bypass circuit
      - ➤ Usually done with a crystalloid solution with additives like mannitol, Amicar, albumin, and bicarbonate
        - ◆ **Hemodilutes** the patient's blood
    - ◆ Anticoagulation
      - ➤ Heparin is dosed by body weight assuming no contraindication to heparin
      - ➤ ACT level checked prior to initiation of bypass
    - ◆ **Cannulation**
      - ➤ Arterial cannula placed in the aorta arch above the aortic valve and proximal to the innominate artery
        - ◆ The axillary or femoral artery may be used in procedures involving the aortic arch
      - ➤ Venous cannula placed in right atrium
        - ◆ The IVC and SVC may be cannulated if surgery is done on the right side of the heart
        - ◆ Complications
          - › If the venous return cannula is inserted too far into the SVC → obstructs right innominate vein
          - › If venous return cannula is inserted too far into the IVC → impairs venous return from lower body → causes abdominal distention
      - ➤ Vent cannulas may be placed to decompress the heart
        - ◆ Avoids excessive distention of the LV
        - ◆ Often used for an incompetent aortic valve
        - ◆ Locations for venting
          - › Placement of drain through right superior pulmonary vein and directed at LV
          - › Aspiration of antegrade cardioplegia line placed at proximal ascending aorta
          - › Venting through pulmonary venous drain
  - ● Initiation of cardiopulmonary bypass
    - ◆ Unclamp the venous cannula to allow venous drainage into the venous reservoir
      - ➤ Right-sided heart pressures should be zero
    - ◆ Begin flow through the arterial cannula in the aorta
      - ➤ Flow will be nonpulsatile
      - ➤ Support the mean arterial pressure with vasopressors if needed
    - ◆ Aortic clamping
    - ◆ Cardioplegia is instilled to arrest the heart
      - ➤ Purpose
        - ◆ Immediate and sustained electromechanical quiescence
        - ◆ Myocardial cooling
        - ◆ Washout of metabolic inhibitors
        - ◆ Maintaining therapeutic additives in effective concentrations
      - ➤ Process
        - ◆ Infuse cardioplegic solution into coronary circulation
          - › Cannula inserted between aortic cross-clamp and aortic valve
            - ▹ Requires intact aortic valve
          - › Retrograde delivery in aortic insufficiency
            - ▹ Inserted into coronary sinus via the RA
      - ➤ Solution
        - ◆ High potassium concentration decreases resting potential and prevents repolarization → cells depolarize → intracellular Ca is sequestered → cell relaxes

- **Circulatory arrest**
  - A unique scenario to facilitate aortic root repair since the aortic arch cannot be bypassed
  - Patient is intentionally cooled to 18°C following the initiation of bypass → circulatory arrest
    - The aortic arch is then rapidly repaired
  - Variations exist in the approach, including cannulating the three great vessels to minimize cerebral ischemia and constructing the distal anastomosis under only lower body circulatory arrest
  - Hypothermia causes platelets to be reversibly sequestered at the portal circulation at low temperatures
- Preparation for weaning from cardiopulmonary bypass
  - Warm patient
  - De-air heart
  - Vasopressors should be started, if necessary
  - Epidural pacing wires should be placed, if necessary
    - Placed prior to weaning from CPB (cardiopulmonary bypass) to facilitate heart rhythm intraoperatively and postoperatively
    - Leads placed at epicardium of RA and RV
      - Settings often used are AAI, VVI (for A-fib), DDD
    - If failure to capture
      - Increase output (not sensitivity) to maximum values
      - Reverse the polarity of the leads
      - Convert to unipolar pacing (epidural lead to negative pole of pacemaker) and using a SQ pacing suture for positive lead)
  - Resume ventilation and anesthetic
- Weaning from cardiopulmonary bypass
  - Venous drainage is reduced → heart begins to fill → decreased flow via bypass arterial line
    - Bypass is complete when venous drainage stops and the heart is self-sustaining
  - Removal of cannulas
    - Venous removed first
      - Venous cannula can cause preload drop by physical obstruction
    - Aortic removed last
  - Anticoagulation reversal
    - Protamine administered if heparin used
    - Protamine heparin reaction is an acid–alkali neutralization reaction
  - If there is difficulty in weaning the patient off of CPB, consider MI
  - Ensure the patient is warmed appropriately
    - Esophageal temperature ~37°C
    - Rectal temperature ~33°C
- Complications and considerations of coronary artery bypass graft (CABG)
  - Strokes
  - Renal failure
  - Troponin elevation
    - Often minimal following cardiac surgery
    - Significant troponin rise may indicate an adverse event such as poor cardioplegia, graft occlusion, or poor anastomoses
  - Recall
    - Most likely to occur during the rewarming phase
- Unique surgeries
  - **Off-pump CABG**
    - Coronary artery bypass without the use of cardiopulmonary bypass is possible
    - Recent evidence suggests there is no improvement in mortality, strokes, myocardial infarction, or renal injury at 30 days or 1 year following surgery
  - Robotic-assisted cardiac surgery
    - Surgery is done through a left sided mini-thoracotomy

➤ No need for sternotomy
◆ Requires one-lung ventilation for surgical exposure
➤ Patient must be able to tolerate one-lung ventilation
➤ May increase risk of hypoxia when not on bypass
■ Monitoring during cardiac bypass
● Blood gas analysis
◆ Physiology and temperature
➤ Warming an arterial blood gas (ABG) → gases leave solution → measured gas values higher, measured pH lower
➤ Hypothermia → pH increases, but the transmembrane pH gradient remains constant
◆ Alpha-stat vs. pH stat
➤ **Alpha-stat**
❖ Strategy to maintain intracellular charge neutrality across all temperatures
❖ ABG warmed to 37°C and measured
⟩ Warming takes gases out of solution → measured gas values are higher, pH is lower
❖ Cerebral autoregulation remains largely intact
❖ Alpha-stat often used for adult patients
➤ **pH stat**
❖ Strategy to maintain a constant pH across all temperatures
⟩ Maintains in vivo pH at 7.4 and $Paco_2$ at 40 during hypothermia
❖ Cooling → CO_2 (carbon dioxide) goes into solution → pH increases
⟩ CO_2 is added during bypass to maintain pH of 7.4 → cerebral vasodilation
❖ Produces more homogenous brain cooling
❖ pH stat is often used for pediatric patients
◆ Confounders of ABG analysis
➤ **Delayed measurement**
❖ Metabolism occur by leukocytes and platelets → increases $Paco_2$ (0.1 mm Hg/min)
❖ Place sample on ice to prevent error
➤ Air bubble in syringe
❖ Allows CO_2 to diffuse down concentration gradient → decrease in CO_2
◆ pH, Hb, and other labs should be checked every 30 minutes while on bypass to monitor for acidosis, anemia, and electrolyte disturbances
● Activated clotting time (ACT)
◆ ACT is a point-of-care test to monitor the anticoagulation status of a patient
◆ Set point for an appropriate ACT while on bypass vary by institution
◆ Should be checked prior to initiating CBP and every 30 minutes while on bypass

CARDIAC MECHANICAL SUPPORT

■ IABP (Fig. 6.6)
● Description
◆ A long, thin mechanical balloon that is inserted through the femoral artery
➤ Resides in the aorta and sits 2 cm from the left subclavian artery
➤ Balloon is filled with helium
◆ Inflation and deflation is controlled by a computer
● Function
◆ Inflates during diastole → increases coronary blood flow
◆ Deflates during systole → decreases afterload and improves cardiac output
● Uses
◆ Cardiogenic shock
◆ Valvular lesions
◆ Preoperative or postoperatively for cardiac surgery or angioplasty
● Contraindications
◆ Severe aortic insufficiency
◆ Aortic aneurysm or dissection

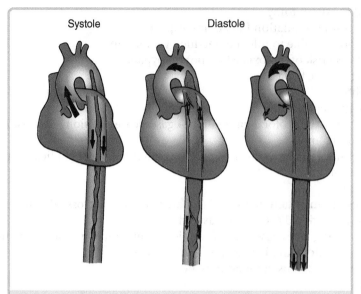

FIGURE 6.6   Intra-Aortic Balloon Pump. IABP that is placed distal to the left subclavian artery. The IABP inflates during diastole to assist coronary perfusion and deflates during systole to assist systemic perfusion. (Reproduced from Cleveland JC Jr, Sun BC, Harter RL, et al. Devices for cardiac support and replacement. In: Hensley FA Jr, Martin DE, Gravlee GP, eds. *A Practical Approach to Cardiac Anesthesia.* Philadelphia, PA: Wolters Kluwer; 2013:643.)

- ◆ Severe aortoiliac or femoral disease
- ■ Left ventricular assist device (LVAD) (Fig. 6.7)
  - ● Description
    - ◆ Mechanical pump that moves blood from the left ventricle into the aorta
  - ● Function
    - ◆ Improves cardiac output in patients who are suffering from severe heart disease
    - ◆ In cases of nonpulsatile flow, arterial line necessary for monitoring pressures
  - ● Uses
    - ◆ Cardiac support following myocardial infarction
    - ◆ Long-term support for cardiogenic shock and bridge to transplantation
  - ● Contraindications
    - ◆ Aortic insufficiency due to worsening stress on left side of heart
    - ◆ LVADs require anticoagulation
    - ◆ LVAD placement may worsen right-sided HF

TRANSPLANTS

- ■ **Heart transplant**
  - ● Performed in end-stage HF or severe coronary artery disease
  - ● Donor heart is denervated and does not respond to vagal inputs
    - ◆ Resting heart rate is ~100 beats per minute
      - ➤ Heart is preload dependent because it cannot stimulate reflex tachycardia in response to hypovolemia
    - ◆ Drugs that inhibit the parasympathetic nerve system are not effective
      - ➤ Example: glycopyrrolate, atropine
    - ◆ Drugs effective at increasing heart rate
      - ➤ Isoproterenol, epinephrine, glucagon, norepinephrine

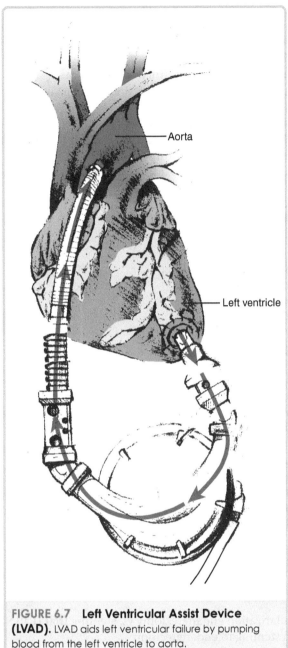

FIGURE 6.7 Left Ventricular Assist Device (LVAD). LVAD aids left ventricular failure by pumping blood from the left ventricle to aorta.

- ❖ Neostigmine can cause bradycardia
- ● Causes of transplant failure
    - ❖ First year
        - ➤ Nonspecific graft failure
        - ➤ Rejection
        - ➤ Infection
    - ❖ After first year
        - ➤ Posttransplant coronary artery disease
            - ❖ Fibroproliferative changes with involvement of all three arterial layers
                - › Narrowing on angiography
            - ❖ Presents with heart fail symptoms due to angina being uncommon in the denervated heart

- ➤ Malignancy
- Right internal jugular is site of choice for surveillance myocardial biopsies to assess for rejection, so its use for central access should be avoided
- Lung transplant
  - Performed in end-stage obstructive and restrictive lung disease
    - ◆ Types of transplantation include single lung, double lung, and heart–lung
  - Postoperative reperfusion injury
    - ◆ Occurs in first 6 hours after transplantation
    - ◆ Transplanted lung receives increased perfusion because of resolution of pulmonary hypertension → pulmonary edema and respiratory failure
    - ◆ Treatment: diuresis, inotropes, nitric oxide, extracorporeal membrane oxygenation
  - Long-term effects
    - ◆ Hypoxic pulmonary vasoconstriction remains intact
    - ◆ Pulmonary pressure immediately normalized
    - ◆ Changes
      - ➤ Mucociliary clearance decreases
      - ➤ No cough reflex at transplanted lung
      - ➤ Lymphatic drainage decreases

VASCULAR SURGERY

- **Carotid endarterectomy (CEA)**
  - **Pathophysiology**
    - ◆ Carotid artery atherosclerosis → decreases cerebral blood flow → associated with strokes, transient ischemic attacks, and amaurosis fugax
    - ◆ Carotid artery emboli can be associated with ischemia or hemorrhage
  - Indications for surgery
    - ◆ TIA
      - ➤ When the deficit is present for >24 hours
      - ➤ >70% stenosis
      - ➤ Ulceration of the plaque
    - ◆ Fluctuating neurological deficits
    - ◆ Acute carotid occlusion
  - Procedure
    - ◆ Removal of atherosclerotic plaque that causes stenosis of the common carotid artery
    - ◆ Indicated for asymptomatic patients with >70% stenosis and symptomatic patients with >50% stenosis
    - ◆ Carotid stenting
      - ➤ Carotid revascularization endarterectomy vs. stenting trial (CREST) demonstrated noninferiority of carotid stenting to endarterectomy
  - Anesthetic
    - ◆ **General or regional anesthesia** are options
    - ◆ Regional anesthesia must cover C2-4
      - ➤ Options
        - ◈ **Deep cervical plexus block** (located at C4-6 at the transverse process)
        - ◈ **Superficial cervical plexus block** (at posterior of the sternocleidomastoid muscle) with infiltration of local anesthesia by surgeon at deeper structures (Fig. 6.8)
      - ➤ Complications
        - ◈ Blocking cervical sympathetic → Horner and blocked recurrent laryngeal nerve
        - ◈ Phrenic nerve palsy
        - ◈ Vertebral artery injection
        - ◈ Deep cervical plexus block more likely to require conversion to general anesthesia than superficial cervical plexus block
        - ◈ Rate of regional to general anesthesia conversion is <6%
    - ◆ **General anesthesia**

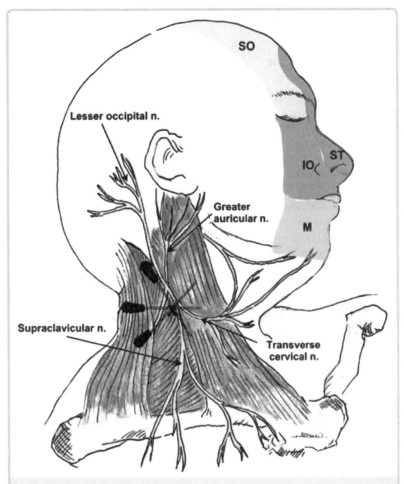

FIGURE 6.8 **Superficial Cervical Plexus Anatomy.** The superficial cervical plexus can be blocked behind the sternocleidomastoid muscle for carotid surgery. N., nerve; SO, supraorbital nerve; ST, supratrochlear nerve; IO, infraorbital nerve; M, mental nerve. (Reproduced from Tsui BCH, Rosenquist RW. Peripheral nerve block. In: Barash PG, Cullen BF, Stoelting RK, et al., eds. *Clinical Anesthesia*. 7th ed. Philadelphia, PA: Wolters Kluwer; 2013:945.)

➤ General anesthesia vs. local anesthesia (GALA) for carotid surgery study showed stroke risk unchanged with general vs. regional anesthesia
➤ Increased cardiopulmonary complications in general anesthesia
➤ EEG (electroencephalogram) monitoring is often used to aid in detection of cerebral ischemia
  ❖ EEG will demonstrate decreased frequency and amplitude over the ischemic hemisphere
    ❯ Intraoperative ischemic EEG changes that last >10 minutes have been shown to be associated with new postoperative neurological deficits
  ❖ Only the cortex is monitored with EEG and deeper brain structures can become ischemic without changes in the EEG tracings
➤ If the patient shows signs of ischemia, the carotid clamp should be released and a shunt should be placed
  ❖ Blood pressure and oxygenation should also be optimized
● Surgical considerations
  ❖ **Denervation of carotid sinus**
    ➤ Patients are prone to significant intraoperative hemodynamic swings

➢ Recommend waiting 1 year prior to correcting stenosis at the other carotid artery to allow for reinnervation of the carotid body
- **Emboli/stroke**
  - ➢ 90% of patients undergoing CEA have embolic events (most not associated with neurologic consequences)
  - ➢ The majority of cerebrovascular accidents (CVA) during CEA are embolic, not ischemic in nature
  - ➢ Transcranial Doppler does not decrease stroke risk, but is the most sensitive emboli monitor
  - ➢ Slow EEG following carotid cross-clamp → need for shunt
    - ❖ Shunts are associated with stroke reduction
    - ❖ 10% of patients with strokes following CEA have normal intraoperative EEGs
  - ➢ Dextran
    - ❖ Possibly decreases thromboembolic events
      - ⟩ Decreases viscosity of the blood
      - ⟩ Decreases platelet aggregation
      - ⟩ Dilutes clotting factors
- **Postoperative hyperperfusion**
  - ➢ Previously maximally vasodilated ischemic area → stenosis relieved → hyperperfusion of previous ischemic area lacking autoregulation → **intracranial hemorrhage**
- Mortality of CEA <2% and the risk of stroke or death <6%
- **Thoracic and abdominal aortic reconstruction**
  - Abdominal aortic aneurysms (AAA)
    - ❖ Causes
      - ➢ Cystic medial necrosis
        - ❖ HTN
        - ❖ Connective tissue disorders
          - ⟩ Marfan, Ehler–Danlos syndromes
        - ❖ Congenital
          - ⟩ Turner syndrome
      - ➢ Inflammatory
        - ❖ Infection
          - ⟩ Mycotic aneurysm
        - ❖ Takayasu arteritis
    - ❖ Most frequent cause of death in patients undergoing major vascular surgery is MI
    - ❖ Dilation of the aorta → increased risk of rupture
      - ➢ Aneurysm defined as diameter >3 cm
      - ➢ Surgical treatment advised when diameter exceeds 5.5 cm
    - ❖ Presentation
      - ➢ More common in men, smokers, and patients with connective tissue diseases
      - ➢ Most are asymptomatic, but chest or back pain may indicate rupture
    - ❖ Classification
      - ➢ **DeBakey classification** (Fig. 6.9)
        - ❖ I: all or most of descending thoracic aorta and upper abdominal aorta
        - ❖ II: all or most of descending thoracic aorta and all or most of abdominal aorta
        - ❖ III: lower thoracic and most of the abdominal aorta
        - ❖ IV: abdominal aorta only
      - ➢ Stanford classification
        - ❖ Type A: affects ascending aorta and arch
          - ⟩ Accounts for ~60% of aortic dissections
          - ⟩ Surgical management
        - ❖ Type B: begins beyond brachiocephalic vessels
          - ⟩ Accounts for ~40% of aortic dissections
          - ⟩ Medical management or endovascular repair (Fig. 6.10)
    - ❖ Surgical options
      - ➢ Open repair or endovascular surgery depends on age, comorbidities, and anatomy
    - ❖ **Cross-clamp physiology**
      - ➢ Effects of aortic cross-clamping

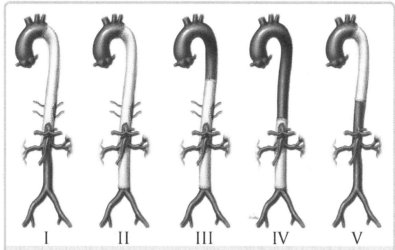

FIGURE 6.9 **Thoracoabdominal Aortic Aneurysm Classification.**
Types of thoracoabdominal aortic aneurysms based on aneurysm location
and the affected visceral organs. (Reproduced from Fox AA, Cooper JR Jr.
Anesthetic management for thoracic aortic aneurysms and dissections. In:
Hensley FA Jr, Martin DE, Gravlee GP, eds. *A Practical Approach to Cardiac
Anesthesia.* Philadelphia, PA: Wolters Kluwer; 2013:718.)

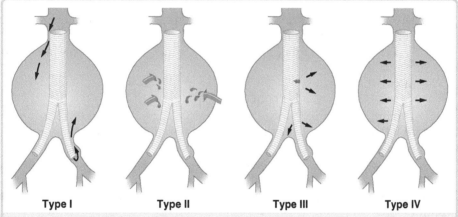

FIGURE 6.10 **Endoleak Classification.** Classifications of endoleaks following
endovascular aortic aneurysm repair. (Reproduced from Smaka TJ, Miller TE, Hutchens MP,
et al. Anesthesia for vascular surgery. In: Barash PG, Cullen BF, Stoelting RK, et al., eds. *Clinical
Anesthesia.* 7th ed. Philadelphia, PA: Wolters Kluwer; 2013:1132.)

- ❖ Acute increase in afterload → increases BP
- ❖ Increased serum catecholamines → increase venous return and preload
- ❖ Depending on location of clamp, decreased splanchnic and renal blood flow
- ❖ Manage with venodilators prior to clamping to minimize effects of afterload increase
  - ➤ Effects of aortic cross-clamp release
    - ❖ Acute decrease in SVR → decrease BP
    - ❖ Manage with IV fluids, calcium, and pressors
- ❖ Paralysis
  - ➤ Paralysis is a feared complication of AAA surgery
  - ➤ Spinal cord is perfused by the anterior spinal artery and two posterior spinal arteries
    - ❖ The **anterior spinal artery** perfuses the motor tracts of the spinal cord
      - ⟩ The thoracic portion of the anterior spinal artery is supplied by the anterior radicular arteries
      - ⟩ Largest radicular artery is the artery of Adamkiewicz
      - ⟩ Located between T9 and T12

- Methods to prevent paraplegia
  - Minimize clamp time
  - Distal aortic perfusion
  - **CSF drainage** through a lumbar drain
    - Increases spinal cord perfusion by decreasing ICP
    - Perfusion pressure = MAP – ICP
- Renal failure
  - Increased risk in this patient population
    - Many have underlying renal insufficiency
      - Further attenuated by IV contrast dye load, intraoperative hemorrhage, and associated hypotension and hypoperfusion
    - Even infrarenal clamping has been shown to decrease renal blood flow
- Aortic dissections
  - Tear or separation of intima and media layers of the aorta
    - Blood enters into the aortic intima and creates a "false lumen"
    - Can lead to decreased perfusion of vital organs, decreased coronary perfusion, aortic rupture, and death
  - Presentation
    - More common in males, those with connective tissue diseases, and those with bicuspid aortic valves
    - Presents with tearing chest pain
  - **Classification** by involvement
    - Stanford A (DeBakey I or II): ascending aorta and possibly the descending aorta
      - Associated features
        - Dissection telescopes down the aorta and results in incompetent aortic valve
        - Pericardial effusion in most patients
          - Do not do pericardiocentesis because it increases blood flow into the pericardial space
        - Myocardial ischemia
          - RCA territory is most frequent
        - End-organ ischemia
    - Stanford B (Debakey III): descending aorta distal to the left subclavian
  - Surgical and medical options
    - Stanford A (DeBakey I or II): surgical emergency requiring cardiopulmonary bypass and often hypothermic circulatory arrest for aortic arch repair
    - Stanford B (Debakey III): medical management through heart rate and blood pressure control

CARDIOPULMONARY RESUSCITATION (CPR)

- In all **ACLS pathways**, **effective CPR** is a critical component
  - Compress 2 in into the chest
  - >100 beats per minute
  - Rotate compressors every 2 minutes
  - Goal end-tidal CO_2 of 10
- Unwitnessed arrest
  - Perform five cycles of CPR before ECG check for defibrillation
    - Shock is more effective after CPR
  - Artificial respirations are no longer recommended for lay responders
    - Respirations increase the time to CPR and increase CPR interruptions → decrease defibrillation success
    - Increases likelihood of lay individuals to perform CPR
    - Hands-free CPR increases survival by 3×
- Witnessed arrest
  - Use automated external defibrillator (AED) if available within moments of cardiac arrest
  - Do not let finding an AED device delay compressions

QUESTIONS

1. A 72-year-old man undergoes cardiac catheterization, which reveals a "left dominant" coronary circulation. Which of the following relationships with the PDA is consistent with this finding?

   A. PDA originates from the left anterior descending artery
   B. PDA originates from the right coronary artery
   C. PDA originates from the left circumflex artery
   D. PDA originates from both the right coronary artery and the left circumflex artery

2. Which of the following terms describing key physiological properties of the heart is correctly paired with its definition?

   A. Lusitropy: myocardial relaxation
   B. Inotropy: heart rate
   C. Chronotropy: conduction speed of impulses
   D. Dromotropy: threshold for excitation

3. A 55-year-old man with septic shock has a blood pressure of 85/55 a CVP of 5 mm Hg and a CO of 10 L/min. His SVR is:

   A. 480 dyn·s/cm^5
   B. 660 dyn·s/cm^5
   C. 810 dyn·s/cm^5
   D. 940 dyn·s/cm^5

4. A 74-year-old woman is receiving sodium nitroprusside for blood pressure control 2 days after undergoing an AAA repair. Which of the following is the earliest sign of sodium nitroprusside toxicity?

   A. Metabolic acidosis
   B. Tachyphylaxis
   C. Cyanosis
   D. Hypotension

5. Which of the following is associated with the "alpha-stat" acid–base management strategy for a patient undergoing deep hypothermic circulatory arrest?

   A. Reduction of CBP gas flow
   B. Addition CO_2 to the CPB circuit
   C. Temperature correction of pH
   D. Respiratory alkalosis

ANATOMY AND INNERVATION

- Airway and respiratory anatomy
  - The **upper airway** can be divided into the nasopharynx, oropharynx, and hypopharynx
    - The pharynx is a muscular tube that connects all three zones to the larynx
  - The **larynx** forms the vocal cords and contains muscles, ligaments, and cartilage
  - The **trachea** (~15 cm long) contains cartilaginous rings on its anterior side and has a posterior membranous wall
    - The trachea separates into the bronchus, bronchioles, and alveoli (see Fig. 7.1)
  - **Right and left mainstem bronchus** (see Table 7.1)
    - The right mainstem bronchus is shorter and more vertical than the left side
      - Three divisions (upper, middle, lower)
      - The middle and lower lobes form the bronchus intermedius
    - The left mainstem bronchus is longer (~5 cm)
      - Two divisions (upper, lower)
- Airway and respiratory muscles
  - **Inspiratory muscles**
    - The diaphragm and external intercostals are the primary inspiratory muscles
    - Accessory muscles for active inhalation: scalene and sternocleidomastoid
  - **Expiratory muscles**

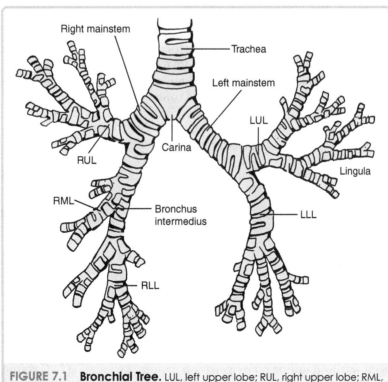

FIGURE 7.1 Bronchial Tree. LUL, left upper lobe; RUL, right upper lobe; RML, right middle lobe; RLL, right lower lobe; LLL, left lower lobe.

TABLE 7.1	Lung lobes and associated segments
Lobe	Segments
Right upper lobe	Apical Posterior Anterior
Right middle lobe	Lateral Medial
Right lower lobe	Superior Medial basal Anterior basal Lateral basal Posterior basal

Left upper lobe	Superior division:
	    Apical-posterior
	    Anterior
	Inferior lingular division:
	    Superior
	    Inferior

Left lower lobe	Superior Anteromedial basal Lateral basal posterior basal

- ◆ Expiration is a passive process
- ◆ Accessory muscles for active expiration: internal and external obliques, transversus abdominus, rectus abdominus, and internal intercostals
- ■ Airway innervation
  - ● The ophthalmic and maxillary divisions of the **trigeminal nerve (CN V)** innervate the nasopharynx while the mandibular division innervates the anterior two-thirds of the tongue
  - ● The **glossopharyngeal nerve** (CN IX) innervates the posterior one-third of the tongue, posterior pharynx, tonsils, vallecula, and anterior epiglottis surface
  - ● The **vagus nerve (CN X)** divides into the superior and recurrent laryngeal nerves
    - ◆ The **superior laryngeal nerve** divides into
      - ➤ Internal laryngeal branch: sensory to posterior epiglottis, arytenoids, and vocal cords
      - ➤ External laryngeal branch: motor to cricothyroid muscle (tenses cords)
    - ◆ The **recurrent laryngeal nerve** innervates all muscles of the larynx (except cricothyroid) and provides sensory input from below the vocal cords
- ■ **Airway nerve injuries**
  - ● Recurrent laryngeal nerve can be injured during neck, thoracic, or cardiac surgery
    - ◆ Innervates the posterior cricoarytenoid muscle. When paralyzed, the vocal cord takes an intermediate position
  - ● The superior laryngeal nerve is rarely injured, but does not lead to displacement of the vocal cords

RESPIRATORY MECHANICS

- ■ Volumes and zones
  - ● **Lung zones** (West Zones)
    - ◆ Zone I: $P_A > P_a > P_v$
    - ◆ Zone II: $P_a > P_A > P_v$
    - ◆ Zone III: $P_a > P_v > P_A$
  - ● **Lung volumes** (see Fig. 7.2)
    - ◆ **Functional residual capacity (FRC)**
      - ➤ **Volume in lungs** at end of normal exhalation
      - ➤ **Nitrogen washout** during preoxygenation requires exchanging FRC volume
      - ➤ Decreased in elderly, women, obese people, supine position, and acute respiratory distress syndrome (ARDS) aptients

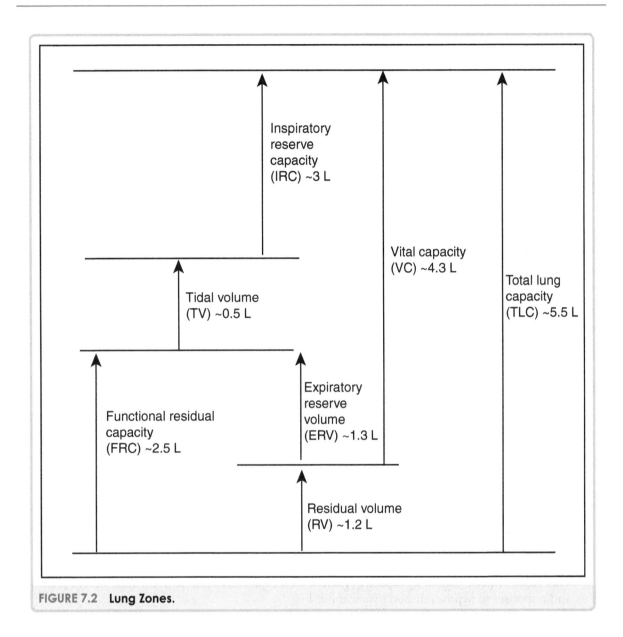

FIGURE 7.2 Lung Zones.

> Increased in obstructive lung disease
- **Closing capacity:** volume of the lungs when the alveoli collapse, causing atelectasis
  - Increases with age, chronic obstructive pulmonary disease (COPD), and bronchitis
  - **LaPlace law:** transpulmonary pressure = $2 \times$ tension/radius
  - **Surfactant** is a lipoprotein that reduces surface tension
- **Dead space**
  - Areas ventilated, but not perfused
  - Begins at oro/nasopharynx and ends at the terminal bronchioles
    - **Dead space fraction = $(PaCO_2 - PetCO_2)/PaCO_2$**
    - Approximately 2 cc/kg in healthy
  - Positive pressure, PEEP (positive end-expiratory pressure), and hypovolemia increase Zone I and dead space
- **Shunt**
  - Areas perfused, but not ventilated
  - **Shunt fraction $Q_s/Q_t = (CcO_2 - CaO_2)/(CcO_2 - CvO_2)$**

- **Pulmonary function testing**
  - Spirometry tests lung mechanics, including forced expiratory volume in 1 second (FEV$_1$) and forced vital capacity (FVC)
    - Obstructive disease: FEV$_1$/FVC ratio <70%
    - Restrictive disease: FEV$_1$/FVC normal, but volumes decreased
  - **Diffusing capacity** of carbon monoxide (D$_{LCO}$) measures tissue function
    - Decreased with emphysema, anemia, hypovolemia, and pulmonary hypertension
    - Increased with higher cardiac output, left-to-right shunt, and supine position

RESPIRATORY PHYSIOLOGY

- **Work of breathing**
  - Elastic work
    - Work against elastic recoil of chest wall and lung parenchyma
    - Work against surface tension of alveoli
  - Nonelastic work
    - **Flow resistance** from obstructive disease or dead space
    - Airway resistance is greatest at medium-sized bronchioles
- **Pleural pressure gradient**
  - Pleural pressure is negative to balance positive pressure from chest wall
    - Sum is 0 at end-expiration
    - Resting intrapleural pressure is -5 cm of H$_2$O
  - Inhalation → negative pressure of pleura increases
  - Exhalation → negative pressure of pleura decreases
- **Compliance**
  - Ability of lungs to expand (↑ compliance = ↑ ease of expansion)
  - Equations
    - **Static:** $V_t/(P_{plat} - PEEP)$
    - **Dynamic:** $V_t/(P_{peak} - PEEP)$
  - **Hysteresis** is the difference in compliance required to recruit additional alveoli
- Effects of aging
  - Cartilage and elastic tissue stiffen → ↓lung volumes
  - Kyphosis ↓lung volumes
  - Functional residual capacity (FRC), residual volume (RV), and closing capacity ↑
  - Vital capacity (VC), total lung capacity (TLC), forced expiratory volume in the first second (FEV$_1$), and responses to hypoxemia and hypercapnia ↓
- **Nonrespiratory functions of lungs**
  - Filtration and removal of foreign and infectious particles
  - Immune defense
  - Drug metabolism

OXYGEN EXCHANGE

- **Oxyhemoglobin dissociation curve** (see Fig. 7.3)
  - Relationship between oxygen partial pressure and oxygen saturation
    - Shifts represent environmental adaptations to increase oxygen uptake (left shift) or delivery (right shift)
      - Left shift causes
        - **Alkalosis, hypothermia, increased 2,3-DPG, fetal hemoglobin**
      - Right shift causes
        - **Acidosis, hyperthermia, decreased 2,3-DPG, volatile anesthetics, pregnancy**
    - **Haldane effect:** when Hb is deoxygenated, it can bind more CO$_2$
    - **Bohr effect:** increased Hb–CO$_2$ binding → right shift → increases oxygen delivery
  - P$_{50}$: partial pressure of oxygen required to saturate 50% of Hb receptors
    - Normal: 27 mm Hg
    - Low conditions (left shift)

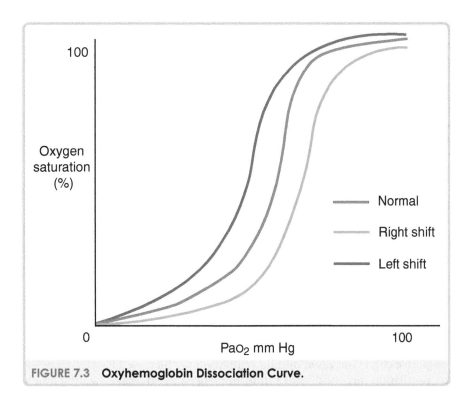

FIGURE 7.3 Oxyhemoglobin Dissociation Curve.

- ➤ Fetal Hb: 20 mm Hg
- ➤ CarboxyHb: 6 mm Hg
- ◆ High conditions (right shift)
  - ➤ Sickle cell: 31 mm Hg
  - ➤ Pregnancy: 30 mm Hg
- ■ Oxygen delivery
  - ● Alveolar gas equation
    - ◆ $PaO_2 = FIO_2 \times (P_b - P_{H_2O}) - PaCO_2/RQ$
    - ◆ RQ = ratio of carbon dioxide elimination to oxygen consumption
      - ➤ 0.7 to 1.0 based on metabolism
        - ❖ Carbohydrate diet → ~1 (6 O_2 → 6 CO_2)
        - ❖ Fat diet → ~0.7 (23 O_2 → 17 CO_2)
  - ● **A-a gradient** and age
    - ◆ A-a gradient is difference between alveolar oxygen and arterial oxygen
    - ◆ $PaO_2 = 102 - age/3$
  - ● **Oxygen delivery**
    - ◆ Oxygen delivery = cardiac output × oxygen content
    - ◆ Oxygen content (O_2 mL/dL) = 1.34 mL × Hb × saturation + 0.003 × PaO_2
- ■ **Oxygen consumption**
  - ● Approximately 3 to 4 cc/kg/min in adults at rest
  - ● Approximately 7 to 9 cc/kg/min in newborns
  - ● Mixed venous saturation
    - ◆ $SvO_2 = SaO_2 - (VO_2/1.39 \times Q \times Hb \times 0.1)$
    - ◆ Improved cardiac output will increase mixed venous saturation
    - ◆ Low mixed venous, high cardiac output → likely to benefit from transfusion
- ■ **Systemic effects**
  - ● **Hypoxia**
    - ◆ Increased lactic acidosis
    - ◆ Increased ventilation via carotid body
    - ◆ Vasodilation to increase perfusion
    - ◆ Hypoxic pulmonary vasoconstriction

- **Hyperoxia**
  - ◆ Atelectasis
  - ◆ Lung injury
  - ◆ CNS toxicity
  - ◆ Oxidative cell damage
- **Hypoxic pulmonary vasoconstriction**
  - Pulmonary arteries constrict in presence of hypoxia → flow redirected to alveoli with higher oxygen content → improves V/Q matching and oxygenation
  - Inhibited by
    - ◆ Drugs: inhalational agents, nitrous, nitroglycerin, nitroprusside
    - ◆ Physiologic factors: hypocapnia, hypothermia, acidosis/alkalosis, increased pulmonary vascular resistance (PVR), PEEP

VENTILATION CONTROL

- Control
  - **Central chemoreceptors** sense and respond to CSF acidosis
  - **Peripheral chemoreceptors** at carotid and aortic bodies sense Pa_{CO_2}
    - ◆ Augmented response when coupled with hypoxia
- Effects of hypercapnia
  - Breathing stimulation
    - ◆ **CO_2 response curve**: increased minute ventilation per increased Pa_{CO_2}
    - ◆ Minute ventilation increases 2 to 3 L/min/mm Hg Pa_{CO_2} in awake, healthy humans
    - ◆ Pa_{CO_2} increases ~6 mm Hg during first minute of apnea, 3 to 4 mm Hg during successive minutes
  - Drug effects
    - ◆ Volatiles, opioids, benzodiazepines, and barbiturates depress response to Pa_{CO_2} in dose-dependent manner
  - **Systemic effects**
    - ◆ Cerebral vasodilation
    - ◆ Myocardial depression and decreased contractility
    - ◆ Pulmonary vasoconstriction
    - ◆ Sympathetic increase and increase in cardiac output

FLOW-VOLUME LOOPS

- **Flow–volume loops** are used to determine lung pathology in obstructive disorders (see Fig. 7.4)
  - Intrathoracic obstruction
    - ◆ Normal inspiration, but expiratory airway obstruction
    - ◆ Examples: mediastinal mass, obstructive sleep apnea
  - Variable extrathoracic obstruction
    - ◆ Normal expiration, but inspiratory airway obstruction
    - ◆ Examples: airway tumors, laryngomalacia, tracheomalacia
  - Fixed obstructions
    - ◆ Both inspiration and expiration are impaired
    - ◆ Example: tracheal stenosis
- **Flow resistance**
  - Reynold number: $Re = Q \times D/\eta \times A$
    - ◆ Q = flow, D = diameter, η = viscosity, A = cross-sectional area
  - **Hagen–Poiseuille: Flow (Q)** $= \pi P r^4 / 8 \eta L$
    - ◆ r = radius, η = viscosity, L = length, P = pressure
  - Types of flow
    - ◆ **Laminar**: resistance depends on gas viscosity (Reynold number <2,100)
    - ◆ **Turbulent**: resistance depends on gas density (Reynold number >2,100)
  - Helium less dense than air and oxygen. Useful for flow through small cross-section

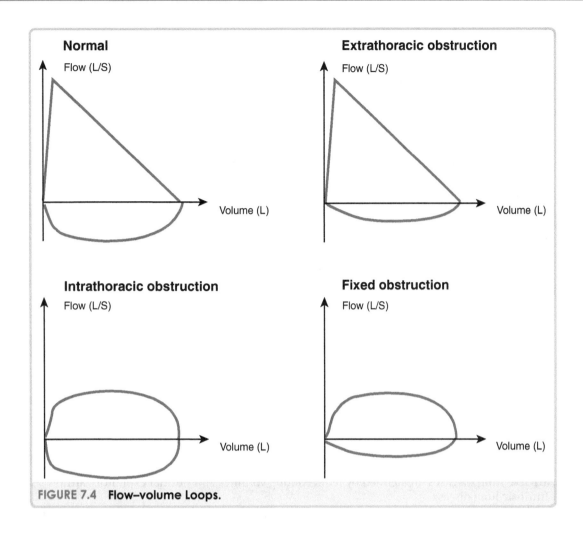

FIGURE 7.4 Flow–volume Loops.

- ◆ → Decreases resistance during turbulent flow
- ◆ → Increases likelihood of being in laminar flow

OBSTRUCTIVE DISORDERS

- ▪ **Anesthetic management**
  - ● **Preoperative airway and respiratory assessment** to assess for potential complications
  - ● **Ventilator settings** should minimize air trapping and avoid barotrauma
    - ◆ Low tidal volumes
    - ◆ Increased expiratory time
    - ◆ Prevention of auto-PEEP
  - ● Preparation for increased airway reactivity and bronchospasm
  - ● Consider **alternatives to general anesthesia**
- ▪ **Obstructive sleep apnea**
  - ● Often due to upper airway obstruction when sleeping or supine
  - ● Increased apneic or hypopneic episodes
    - ◆ Apnea–hypopnea index (AHI) diagnoses severity
  - ● **Anesthetic management**
    - ◆ Proper airway management
    - ◆ Avoidance of oversedation
    - ◆ Extended PACU (postanesthesia care unit) monitoring
    - ◆ Extremely sensitive to opioids

- **Asthma**
  - Inflammatory airway disease with reversible airflow obstruction and bronchospasm
    - Increased smooth muscle contractility
  - Presents with wheezing, coughing, and shortness of breath
  - **Treatment** includes oxygen, bronchodilators, steroids, magnesium, and volatile anesthetics
- **COPD**
  - Chronic incomplete expiration (air trapping)
  - Previously classified into chronic bronchitis and emphysema
    - Chronic bronchitis: inflammation of bronchial airways with frequent cough and mucus production. Presentation includes CO_2 retention, erythrocytosis, and right heart failure
    - Emphysema: lung tissue destruction, small airway narrowing, low D_{LCO}
  - Treatment includes oxygen, bronchodilators, steroids, and potential lung transplantation
- **Bronchiectasis**
  - Inflammatory disease characterized by enlarged bronchi and airflow obstruction
  - Prone to respiratory infections, hemoptysis
  - **Treatment** includes chest physiotherapy, bronchodilators, and potential surgery
- **Cystic fibrosis**
  - Autosomal recessive disorder of a sodium and chloride transmembrane conductance regulator
  - Predisposed to lung infections and pancreatic insufficiency due to impaired ciliary transport
  - Treatment includes prevention and treatment of infections, pulmonary rehabilitation, and organ transplantation
- **Mediastinal masses**
  - Can include neurogenic tumors, thymoma, lymphoma, teratomas, and others
  - Airway management challenging as muscle relaxation or breathing inhibition can make ventilation impossible from airway collapse

RESTRICTIVE DISORDERS

- **Restrictive lung diseases** are defined by reduced lung volumes and normal expiratory airflow
  - Intrinsic lung disease
    - Includes **interstitial lung disease, pulmonary fibrosis, connective tissue diseases, ARDS, and lung parenchymal disease**
  - Extrinsic lung disease
    - Includes **neuromuscular, pleural, mediastinal, and abdominal diseases** that compress or diminish normal lung volumes
- Treatment is difficult and often dependent on underlying cause

PULMONARY HYPERTENSION

- Definition: mean pulmonary artery pressure >25 mm Hg at rest
  - Causes: left-sided cardiac disease, pulmonary disease, collagen vascular disease
- Presentation includes shortness of breath, chest pain, fatigue, and syncope
- Treatment: correct volume status, pulmonary vasodilators, and address cause
- Anesthetic goals
  - Hemodynamic stability: prevent hypotension, dysrhythmias, and hypovolemia
  - Ventilator management: prevent hypoxia, hypercapnia, and acidosis
  - If severe or refractory, consider nitric oxide, inhaled prostacyclin, or phosphodiesterase inhibitors

SMOKING

- Smoking → ↑ airway reactivity, ↑ secretions, and immunosuppression
- **Cessation benefits**
  - 12 to 48 hours: sympathetic response decreases, carboxyhemoglobin level decreases
  - 1 to 2 weeks: sputum decreases
  - 4 to 6 weeks: improved PFTs (pulmonary function tests)
  - >4 to 8 weeks: reduced postoperative infectious and pulmonary complications

CARBON MONOXIDE

- Reduces oxygen-carrying capacity of blood
  - CO with 200× greater affinity for Hb than O_2
  - Breathing not affected because Pao_2 and $Paco_2$ are normal
    - Respiratory rate only increases when lactic acidosis occurs
- Measure carboxyhemoglobin with co-oximeter
- CO Levels
  - 1% to 3% in nonsmoker
  - 10% in smoker
  - >25%, suspect poisoning
- Treatment
  - Depends on severity. At 25%, oxygen is indicated. At 40%, hyperbaric oxygen should be considered
  - Half-time of carboxyhemoglobin on room air is 4 to 6 hours, at 100% O_2 is 1 hour, and in hyperbaric conditions is 15 to 30 minutes

ONE-LUNG VENTILATION

- Endobronchial intubation: lung separation and/or one-sided ventilation are frequently required in thoracic surgery
- **Absolute indications**
  - Exposure: VAT (Video-assisted thoracostomy)
  - Management of underlying condition: bronchopleural fistula, bullae at risk of rupturing, unilateral infection
  - Hemorrhage: massive pulmonary or thoracic bleeding
- **Devices**
  - Double-lumen tube (DLT)
    - Distinct tracheal and bronchial lumen
      - Clamping one lumen and opening it to air will cause passive lung deflation
      - Available in right- or left-sided tubes to conform to the mainstem bronchus
    - DLT placement should be confirmed with a bronchoscope
  - Bronchial blockers
    - An occlusion catheter with a balloon is mainstemmed to operative side
    - Lung deflation occurs slowly through gas absorption
    - Placement should be visualized with a bronchoscope
- **One-lung ventilation management**
  - Prevent barotraumas by maintaining airway pressures <25 cm H_2O if possible
  - After lung isolation, oxygenation ↓ due to shunting
    - Hypoxic pulmonary vasoconstriction ↓ shunting
  - Troubleshooting hypoxemia
    - 100% oxygen
    - Confirm DLT/bronchial blocker position
    - Recruitment maneuver/PEEP to ventilated lung
    - CPAP (continuous positive airway pressure) to nonventilated lung
    - Resume two-lung ventilation
    - Clamp pulmonary artery
    - Cardiopulmonary bypass

THORACIC SURGERY

- Lobectomy/pneumonectomy
  - Factors increasing operative risk
    - FEV_1 <2 L preoperative, <0.85 L postoperatively
    - D_{LCO} <50%
    - RV:TLC >50%
    - $Paco_2$ >45 mm Hg

- Pao_2 <50 mm Hg
- Preoperative testing
  - PFTs and room air arterial blood gases (ABG) (Phase I)
  - If Phase I concerning → split lung V/Q function testing (Phase II)
  - If Phase II concerning → balloon occlusion catheter to measure PA pressures (Phase III)
- Complications
  - Postpneumonectomy pulmonary edema is a feared complication with high mortality
  - Risk factors: right pneumonectomy/lobectomy, excessive IV fluids, airway pressures >25 cm H_2O, preoperative EtOH

- Mediastinoscopy
  - Often performed before lung resection to stage tumor
  - Anesthetic considerations
    - Compression of the right innominate artery causes diminished right-sided blood pressure
    - Use blood pressure monitor or pulse oximetry on right side
  - Complications
    - Hemorrhage from laceration of the innominate vein, pulmonary vein, pulmonary artery, or azygous vein
    - Pneumothorax
    - Venous air embolism
    - Vagal compression and bradycardia

- Bronchopleural fistula
  - Anesthetic considerations
    - Positive pressure to affected side (without chest tube decompression) → tension pneumothorax
    - Secure airway and isolate while spontaneously breathing

- Intrapulmonary hemorrhage
  - Causes: trauma, pulmonary artery rupture, tumors, and arterial fistulas
  - Anesthetic considerations
    - Isolate lung to protect unaffected side
    - In emergency, consider endotracheal tube (ETT) mainstem to unaffected side

- **Lung transplant**
  - Anesthetic considerations
    - Anesthetic best controlled with total IV anesthetic
    - Lung isolation best with contralateral endobronchial tube
    - Cardiopulmonary bypass may be necessary
  - Postoperative considerations
    - Lung reperfusion injury occurs in the first hours after transplantation
      - Transplanted lung receives increased perfusion due to patient history of pulmonary hypertension
      - Treat with diuresis, hemodynamic support
    - Transplanted lungs are denervated and without cough reflex at transplanted portion
      - Mucociliary clearance, lymphatic drainage reduced
    - Hypoxic pulmonary vasoconstriction (HPV) remains intact

QUESTIONS

1. A 57-year-old man with a history of hypertension, coronary artery disease, and an anterior mediastinal tumor is scheduled to undergo a mediastinal mass resection. You decide to pursue an awake fiberoptic intubation. You nebulize and spray lidocaine in the patient's nasopharynx, oropharynx, and vocal cords. As you pass your scope, you contact the patient's arytenoids and he begins to cough uncontrollably. Which nerve needs to be better anesthetized to complete this intubation?

   A. Trigeminal nerve (V)
   B. Facial nerve (VII)
   C. Glossopharyngeal nerve (IX)
   D. Superior laryngeal nerve (X)
   E. Recurrent laryngeal nerve (X)

2. You are providing anesthesia for a 60-year-old woman undergoing a total thyroidectomy for tumor. Following extubation, she becomes stridorous and begins to desaturate. The surgeon tells you he may have transected the recurrent laryngeal during his dissection. You decide to re-intubate for respiratory distress. After an intubating dose of succinylcholine, what position do you expect the vocal cords to be in?

   A. Open
   B. Intermediate
   C. Closed

3. A 52-year-old man is undergoing a pneumonectomy. Following lung isolation with a DLT, the patient's saturation decreases to 86%. You place the patient on 100% oxygen and check your DLT, which is appropriately positioned. Which of the following drug infusions could be worsening your patient's hypoxemia?

   A. Propofol
   B. Remifentanil
   C. Norepinephrine
   D. Nitroglycerin
   E. Vasopressin

4. You are assessing a 38-year-old woman for a laparoscopic hepatectomy in the preoperative area. Her vitals are as follows: HR: 70, BP: 137/80, Sat: 95% on room air. A baseline set of labs off her arterial line shows 7.40/40/70. Her hemoglobin is 10. What is the oxygen content of her blood?

   A. 1.34 L/dL
   B. 13.4 mL/dL
   C. 13.2 mL/dL
   D. 1.39 mL/dL
   E. 1.32 mL/dL

5. You are evaluating a patient with tracheomalacia. Which flow–volume loop do you expect for your patient?

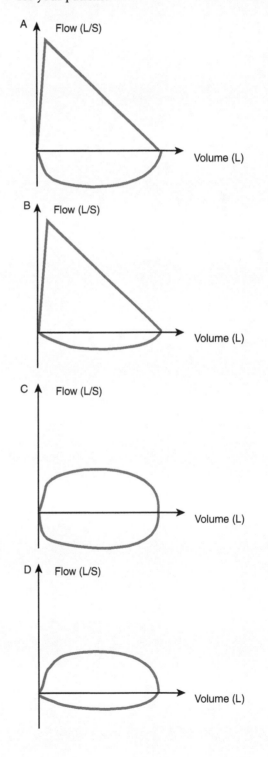

CEREBRAL ANATOMY AND PHYSIOLOGY

- ■ **Cerebral organization**
  - ● **White vs. gray matter**
    - ◆ **White matter** (composed of axons)
      - ➤ Transmits information between gray matter areas
      - ➤ Forms deeper structures of the brain such as the thalamus and hypothalamus
      - ➤ Forms superficial parts of the spinal cord
    - ◆ **Gray matter** (composed of cell bodies, dendrites, and axon terminals)
      - ➤ Forms the cortex of the brain and the deeper parts of the spinal cord
      - ➤ Center for higher processing
        - ❖ Consumes more than 90% of the oxygen in the brain
  - ● Structures
    - ◆ **Cerebral cortex**
      - ➤ Folded outer layer of brain that is 2- to 4-mm thick
      - ➤ Composed of gray matter
        - ❖ Involved in memory, attention, language, and higher level thought processes
      - ➤ Divided into four lobes
        - ❖ Frontal: emotions, planning, problem solving
        - ❖ Parietal: movement, orientation, perception
        - ❖ Occipital: visual processing
        - ❖ Temporal: auditory processing and speech
      - ➤ Right vs. left
        - ❖ Each side has unique functions
        - ❖ Wernicke (sensory speech) and Broca (motor speech) areas → linked to language and speech
          - › Left hemisphere in most individuals
          - › Right hemisphere in 40% of left-handed individuals
        - ❖ Corpus callosum connects two hemispheres
    - ◆ **Cerebellum**
      - ➤ Located posterior to the brainstem and inferior to the cerebral cortex
      - ➤ Composed of white matter
      - ➤ Primarily involved in motor coordination and balance
    - ◆ **Limbic system**
      - ➤ Collection of structures located deep to the cerebral cortex
      - ➤ Structures include the hippocampus, amygdale, hypothalamus, and others
        - ❖ **Hippocampus** is involved in memory formation
        - ❖ Amygdala is involved in emotional memory and processing
        - ❖ Hypothalamus is involved in maintaining homeostasis through hormonal and endocrine regulation
    - ◆ **Thalamus**
      - ➤ Located deep to the cerebral cortex and adjacent to the midbrain
      - ➤ Involved in coordinating sensory and motor signals to the cerebral cortex as well as regulation of sleep
    - ◆ **Basal ganglia**
      - ➤ Collection of gray matter deep to the cerebral cortex in the forebrain

- ➤ Involved in voluntary motor control and procedural learning
  - ◆ **Internal capsule**
    - ➤ Collection of white matter deep in the brain
    - ➤ Contains tracts that carry motor and sensory information between the brain and the spinal cord
  - ◆ **Reticular activating system**
    - ➤ Collection of structures connecting the brainstem and cortex
    - ➤ Critical in regulating sleep–wake cycles and attention
  - ◆ **Medulla oblongata**
    - ➤ Located at the lower part of the brainstem
    - ➤ Controls inspiration and expiration
      - ◆ Inspiratory control center is at the dorsal portion of the medulla
      - ◆ Expiratory control center is at the ventral portion of the medulla
    - ➤ Pneumotaxic center of the pons controls respiratory rate and breathing patterns
- ■ **Cerebral blood flow**
  - ● Brain receives ~15% to 20% of cardiac output despite being only 2% of total body mass
    - ◆ Normal values (average brain ~1,350 g)
      - ➤ Cerebral blood flow (CBF): 50 cc/100 g/min
      - ➤ Cerebral metabolic rate of oxygen ($CMRO_2$): 3 cc/100 g/min
      - ➤ Intracranial pressure (ICP): 8 to 12 mm Hg
    - ◆ CBF and $CMRO_2$ are 4× greater in gray matter than white matter
    - ◆ Brain is dependent on **glucose** for energy
  - ● **Regulation**
    - ◆ Increased cerebral activity or processing → increased cerebral metabolism → increased CBF
    - ◆ Complex mechanism involves interaction between glutamate, nitric oxide, and neurotransmitters
  - ● **Cerebral autoregulation**
    - ◆ CBF remains constant across a wide range of blood pressures
      - ➤ Mean arterial pressure (MAP) of 50 to 150 mm Hg typically associated with unchanged CBF
        - ◆ Some studies report a MAP >70 is necessary
        - ◆ Higher requirements may be necessary in chronic hypertensives
    - ◆ Loss of autoregulation can occur with
      - ➤ Hypoxemia
      - ➤ Hypercarbia
      - ➤ Volatile anesthetics
      - ➤ Cerebral vascular disease
    - ◆ **Cerebral perfusion pressure (CPP)**
      - ➤ CPP = MAP – ICP
        - ◆ ICP should be substituted for central venous pressure (CVP) if CVP > ICP
  - ● Factors that alter or uncouple CBF and cerebral metabolic rate (CMR)
    - ◆ **Anesthetics**
      - ➤ Anesthetics (except ketamine) → decrease neuronal activity → decrease CMR
        - ◆ Burst suppression → profound decrease in CMR
      - ➤ Oxygen still needed for basal and metabolic functions of the brain
    - ◆ Hypothermia
      - ➤ Each degree (°C) lower → reduces CMR by 6%
      - ➤ Total EEG (electroencephalogram) suppression at ~18°C
      - ➤ Decreases oxygen requirements for neuronal activity and basal functions of the brain
    - ◆ Ventilation
      - ➤ Decreased $Paco_2$ → decreases CBF
      - ➤ Increased $Paco_2$ → increases CBF
      - ➤ CBF dependent on degree of ventilator changes
        - ◆ 1 mm Hg change in $Paco_2$ → CBF changes 1 to 2 cc/100 g/min in the same direction
        - ◆ Approximately 2% change in CBF per 1 mm Hg of $Paco_2$
      - ➤ Magnitude of $Paco_2$ effect on CBF greater at gray matter than white matter
        - ◆ $Paco_2$ effect: cerebrum > cerebellum > spinal cord

- ◆ **Oxygenation**
  - ➤ Decreased PaO$_2$ (less than 60 mm Hg) → increases CBF
    - ◆ CBF increases exponentially with further drops in PaO$_2$
  - ➤ Oxygenation has a minimal effect on CBF at PaO$_2$ >60 mm Hg
- ● **Critical levels of CBF**
  - ◆ 50 cc/100 g/min: normal
  - ◆ 22 cc/100 g/min: ischemia begins to occur
  - ◆ 15 cc/100 g/min: isoelectric EEG
  - ◆ 10 cc/100 g/min: critical CBF when under volatile anesthetics
  - ◆ 6 cc/100 g/min: irreversible membrane damage and cell death
- ● **Luxury perfusion**
  - ◆ Ischemia → abolishes CBF autoregulation → CBF becomes passively dependent on the CPP
  - ◆ Acute focal cerebral ischemia → regional vasoparalysis → impaired coupling between CBF and CMR
  - ◆ Blood pressure control important during focal ischemia
    - ➤ Perfusion is dependent on blood pressure
    - ➤ Mild hypertension may be beneficial after ischemic strokes
- ■ **Cerebrospinal fluid (CSF)** (Fig. 8.1)
  - ● Colorless fluid that surrounds the brain and spine
    - ◆ Produced in the choroid plexus

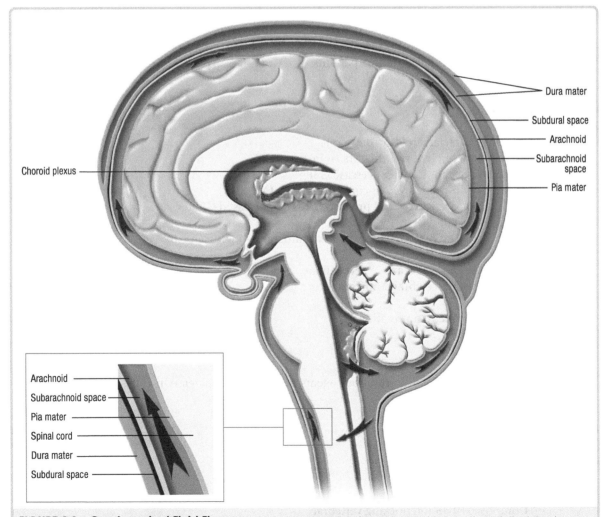

FIGURE 8.1   Cerebrospinal Fluid Flow. Flow of cerebrospinal fluid from the choroid plexus through the lateral ventricles to the subarachnoid space. (Reproduced from Anatomical Chart Company, 2001.)

- ◆ Provides mechanical protection, immunological support, and homeostatic functions
- ◆ Involved in autoregulation of CBF
- **CSF production and volume**
  - ◆ CSF volume ~150 cc in average adult
  - ◆ CSF production is 0.3 to 0.4 cc/min
    - ➤ Approximately 500 cc of CSF produced daily
- **CSF production and pathway**
  - ◆ Produced in choroid plexus → fills lateral ventricles → flows through foramina of Monro → enters third ventricle → flows through aqueduct of Sylvius → enters fourth ventricle → flows through foramen of Magendie and two foramen of Luschka → enters subarachnoid space → absorbed at arachnoid granulations
- **Regulation of CSF volume**
  - ◆ Effects of increased CSF volume
    - ➤ Displacement of CSF below foramen magnum
    - ➤ Increased CSF absorption
    - ➤ Decreased CSF production
    - ➤ Decreased intracranial blood volume

ANESTHETICS AND CBF

- **Intravenous agents**
  - Propofol: decrease CBF and CMR
  - Barbiturates: decrease CBF and CMR
  - Etomidate: decrease CBF and CMR (better at maintaining CPP)
  - Ketamine: increases CBF, CMR, ICP
    - ◆ Contraindication in head trauma patients
  - Benzodiazepines: decrease CBF and CMR
  - Opioids: minimal effects on CBF and CMR
- **Inhaled anesthetics**
  - Volatiles
    - ◆ Competing characteristics (uncouplers)
      - ➤ Volatiles are cerebral vasodilators → increase CBF
      - ➤ Volatiles decrease CMR → decrease CBF
    - ◆ Influence of minimum alveolar concentration (MAC)
      - ➤ MAC <1 → decreased CMR predominates → decreased CBF
      - ➤ MAC = 1 → mild decrease in CBF
      - ➤ MAC >1 → cerebral vasodilation predominates → increased CBF
    - ◆ Potency of vasodilation
      - ➤ Desflurane and isoflurane > sevoflurane
    - ◆ MAC >2 abolishes cerebral autoregulation
  - Nitrous oxide
    - ◆ Increases sympathetic stimulation
      - ➤ Increases CBF
      - ➤ Increases CMR
      - ➤ Increases ICP
    - ◆ When administered with intravenous agents or volatiles → increase in CBF significantly attenuated

SPINAL CORD ANATOMY

- Spine
  - Anatomy
    - **Vertebrae**
      - ➤ Composed of 33 interlocking vertebrae
      - ➤ Cervical: 7 vertebrae
        - ◆ C1-Occiput (connects directly to skull): flexion and extension of head

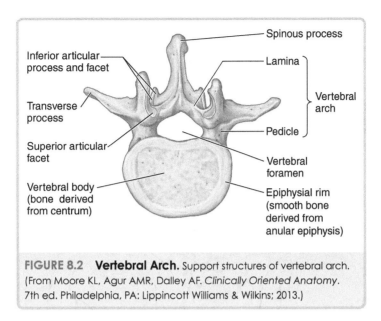

FIGURE 8.2 Vertebral Arch. Support structures of vertebral arch. (From Moore KL, Agur AMR, Dalley AF. *Clinically Oriented Anatomy.* 7th ed. Philadelphia, PA: Lippincott Williams & Wilkins; 2013.)

- ❖ C1-C2 (atlantoaxial joint): lateral rotation of the head
- ➤ Thoracic: 12 vertebrae
- ➤ Lumbar: 5 vertebrae
- ➤ Sacrum: 5 fused vertebrae
- ➤ Coccyx: 4 fused bones
- ❖ Vertebral support
  - ➤ Each vertebral arch contains two pedicles and laminae → structurally support each vertebrae (Fig. 8.2)
  - ➤ Ligamentum flavum, anterior longitudinal ligament, and posterior longitudinal ligament → support the spine
- ❖ Spinal curves
  - ➤ Cervical and lumbar spine: concave curve (lordosis)
  - ➤ Thoracic and sacral spine: convex curve (kyphosis)
- ● **Spinal cord**
  - ❖ Spinal cord structure (Fig. 8.3)
    - ➤ Originates from medulla oblongata and reaches to approximately the L1 level in adults → terminates as conus medullaris
      - ❖ Cauda equina is collection of nerves that travel below the conus medullaris
    - ➤ Filum terminale anchors the spinal cord to coccyx
    - ➤ Dural sac ends at the second sacral vertebrae
  - ❖ Spinal nerves nomenclature
    - ➤ C1-C7 cervical nerve roots exit about their corresponding vertebral body
    - ➤ C8 and other distal spinal nerves exits below their corresponding vertebral body
  - ❖ Spinal nerve structure and function
    - ➤ White vs. gray matter
      - ❖ Outer white mater with sensory and motor neurons
      - ❖ Inner gray matter with cell bodies
    - ➤ Tracts
      - ❖ Sensory relays
        - ⟩ Dorsal column–medial lemniscus tract (touch, proprioception)
          - ▸ Neurons enter dorsal column → travel in fasciculus gracilis or fasciculus cuneatus → ascend to medulla → secondary fibers decussate → ascend up contralateral medial lemniscus → thalamus
        - ⟩ Anterolateral tract (pain and temperature)
          - ▸ Neurons enter spinal cord → ascend one to two levels → secondary fibers decussate → synapse at substantia gelantinosa → ascend through spinothalamic tract

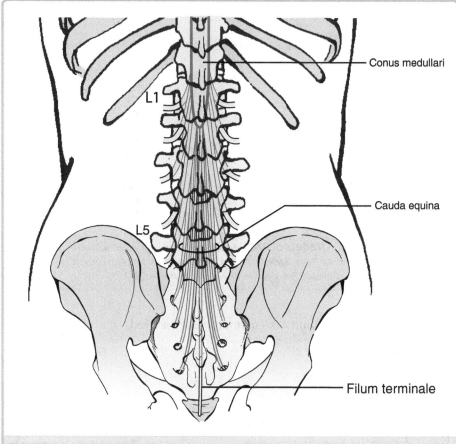

FIGURE 8.3 **Spinal Cord Structure.** Structure and location of the conus medullaris and cauda equine at the distal spinal cord.

- ❖ Motor relays
  - ⟩ Corticospinal tract
    - ▸ Cortical signals descend through internal capsule→ decussate at medullary pyramids → descend at the lateral corticospinal tract → synapse with lower motor neurons in ventral horns of spinal cord
- ❖ **Blood supply**
  - ➤ Arteries
    - ❖ Two posterior spinal arteries
    - ❖ One anterior spinal artery
  - ➤ Branches
    - ❖ Intercostal and lumbar radicular arteries provide anastomoses and supplement blood flow to the spinal cord
    - ❖ Largest anterior radicular artery is the artery of Adamkiewicz
      - ⟩ Originates between T9 and T12 in 75% of cases
      - ⟩ Most likely to be damaged during thoracic aortic repair
- ● Meninges and spinal spaces
  - ❖ **Meninges** protect the spinal cord
  - ❖ Layers
    - ➤ Dura mater
      - ❖ **Epidural space** exists between dura and vertebrae
    - ➤ Arachnoid mater
      - ❖ **Subdural space** exists between dura and arachnoid

➤ Pia mater
  ❖ **Subarachnoid space** exists between arachnoid and pia
  ❖ Tightly covers the spinal cord
❖ CSF is contained in the subarachnoid space

NERVOUS SYSTEMS

■ **Autonomic nervous system** (Fig. 8.4)
  ● Composed of the sympathetic nervous system (SNS) and parasympathetic nervous system (PNS)
    ❖ Regulate hormonal and homeostatic functions
  ● SNS
    ❖ Described as "fight and flight" response
    ❖ Neurons
      ➤ **Preganglionic**
        ❖ Originate at thoracolumbar spinal cord (T1-L2) and travel to paravertebral ganglia
          › Referred to as the **sympathetic trunk** or chain
        ❖ Release acetylcholine at nicotinic receptors on postganglionic neurons
      ➤ **Postganglionic**
        ❖ Originate at paravertebral ganglia and travel to rest of body
        ❖ Release norepinephrine at target receptors
        ❖ Sweat glands and the chromaffin cells also release epinephrine
    ❖ Functions
      ➤ Increase heart rate and contractility
      ➤ Bronchodilating

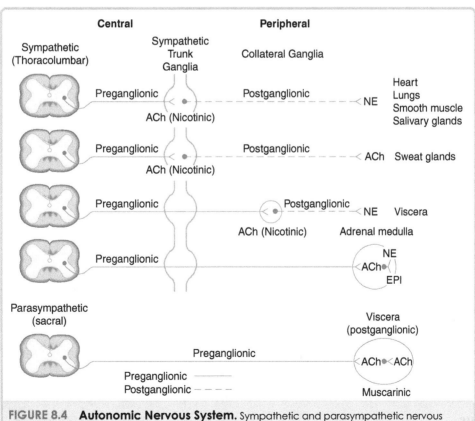

FIGURE 8.4 Autonomic Nervous System. Sympathetic and parasympathetic nervous system and their associated neurotransmitters. Ach, acetylcholine; NE, norepinephrine; EPI, epinephrine. (From Grecu L. Autonomic nervous system: physiology and pharmacology. In: Barash PG, Cullen BF, Stoelting RK, et al., eds. *Clinical Anesthesia.* 7th ed. Philadelphia, PA: Lippincott Williams & Wilkins; 2013:365.)

- ➢ Increases blood flow to skeletal muscle
- ➢ Constricts splanchnic blood flow
- ➢ Activates sweat glands
- ➢ Increases renin secretion
- **PNS**
  - ◆ Described as "rest and digest" system
  - ◆ Neurons
    - ➢ **Preganglionic**
      - ◆ Arise from cranial nerves (CN) and pelvic splanchnic nerves
      - ◆ Release acetylcholine at nicotinic receptors on postganglionic neurons
    - ➢ **Postganglionic**
      - ◆ Release acetylcholine to stimulate muscarinic receptors on target organs
  - ◆ Functions
    - ➢ Decreases heart rate
    - ➢ Bronchoconstriction
    - ➢ Decreases blood flow to skeletal muscle
    - ➢ Increases splanchnic perfusion
    - ➢ Increases renal perfusion
- **Cranial nerves (CN)**
  - Nuclei location of CN
    - ◆ Olfactory bulb: CN I
    - ◆ Lateral geniculate nuclei: CN II
    - ◆ Midbrain: CN III, IV
    - ◆ Pons: CN V, VI, VII, VIII
    - ◆ Medulla: IX, X, XI, and XII
  - CN names
    - ◆ I: olfactory
    - ◆ II: optic
    - ◆ III: oculomotor
    - ◆ IV: trochlear
    - ◆ V: trigeminal
    - ◆ VI: abducens
    - ◆ VII: facial
    - ◆ VIII: vestibulocochlear
    - ◆ IX: glossopharyngeal
    - ◆ X: vagus
    - ◆ XI: accessory
    - ◆ XII: hypoglossal
- **Chemoreceptors and baroreceptors**
  - **Carotid bodies**
    - ◆ Located at the bifurcation of the common carotid artery
    - ◆ Senses PaO_2 and $PaCO_2$
      - ➢ Primarily an oxygen sensor
      - ➢ Decreased PaO_2 or increased $PaCO_2$ → neurons depolarize → relay information to medulla oblongata → stimulate respiration
  - **Aortic bodies**
    - ◆ Located along aortic arch
    - ◆ Sense changes in pressure, oxygenation, and carbon dioxide levels

NEUROMUSCULAR SYNAPSES AND COMMUNICATION

- **Structure**
  - Motor neurons originate from the spinal cord or medulla → diverges into multiple branches → nerve terminals contact muscle fibers
  - Synaptic cleft is space between the nerve and muscle cell
- **Action potential**
  - Acetylcholine is synthesized in the motor neuron → stored in vesicles at the nerve terminal

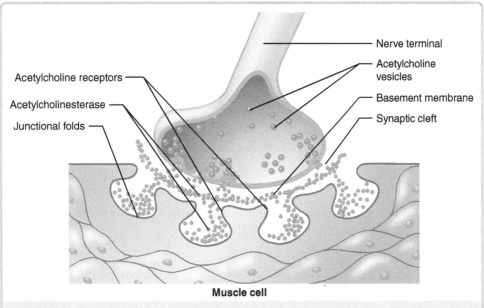

FIGURE 8.5 Neuromuscular Junction. Structure of the neuromuscular junction. (From Donati F. Neuromuscular blocking agents. In: Barash PG, Cullen BF, Stoelting RK, et al., eds. *Clinical Anesthesia*. 7th ed. Philadelphia, PA: Lippincott Williams & Wilkins; 2013:527.)

- Nerve action potential → depolarization across motor neuron → **calcium** enters neuron → acetylcholine released from neuromuscular junction → **acetylcholine** diffuses across junctional cleft → reaches postjunctional acetylcholine receptors → binds to both α-subunits of muscle cell → opens G-protein channel → inflow of **sodium and calcium**, outflow of **potassium** → depolarization of muscle fiber → muscle twitch (Fig. 8.5)

TRAUMATIC BRAIN INJURY (TBI)

- Occurs following traumatic stress to the brain
  - Primary injury: inciting event
    - Direct trauma by mechanical force, torsion, or shear injury
    - Sudden acceleration/deceleration injury
  - Secondary injury: pathophysiological changes following injury that decrease cerebral perfusion
    - Increased ICP
    - Altered CBF
    - Increased CMR
    - Seizures
    - Hypoxia
- Severity classification
  - Glasgow Coma Score
    - Scoring mechanism
      - Verbal
        - 1: none
        - 2: sounds
        - 3: inappropriate words
        - 4: confused speech
        - 5: appropriate
      - Eye
        - 1: none
        - 2: opens to pain
        - 3: opens to voice
        - 4: spontaneous

- ➤ Motor
  - ❖ 1: none
  - ❖ 2: extends
  - ❖ 3: flexes
  - ❖ 4: withdrawals
  - ❖ 5: localizes
  - ❖ 6: obeys command
- ❖ Interpretation
  - ➤ Score of 13 to 15 is mild
  - ➤ Score of 9 to 12 is moderate
  - ➤ Score of 3 to 8 is severe
    - ❖ Warrants intubation
- Intracerebral steal
  - Increased CBF leads to vasodilatation in normal blood vessels but "steals" blood from the ischemic areas, as these areas are already maximally dilated
- Inverse steal ("Robin Hood syndrome")
  - Occurs with relative hypocarbia
  - Normal blood vessel vasoconstriction; however, ischemic vessels remain dilated and therefore receive more blood
- Brain bleeds
  - Intra-axial hemorrhage
    - ❖ Intraparenchymal hemorrhage: occurs within brain tissue
    - ❖ Intraventricular hemorrhage: occurs within ventricles
  - Extra-axial hemorrhage
    - ❖ Subarachnoid hematoma
      - ➤ CT shows bleeding around arachnoid membrane
    - ❖ Subdural hematoma
      - ➤ Common in elderly from tearing of bridging veins
      - ➤ CT shows concave shape that follows the curve of the brain
    - ❖ Epidural hematoma
      - ➤ Commonly occurs from injury to the middle meningeal artery
        - ❖ Does not cross suture lines
      - ➤ CT scan shows convex appearance
      - ➤ Associated with lucid interval before becoming obtunded
- Management
  - Consider neurosurgical intervention
  - Consider airway management if GCS ≤8 or other signs of distress
  - Serial neurological exams
  - Support hemodynamics → prevent hypotension
  - Prevent elevated ICP
    - ❖ Consider hypernatremia
  - Maintain normothermia
  - Maintain normoglycemia
    - ❖ Hyperglycemia worsens outcomes in TBI and spinal cord injury (SCI)
- Steroids
  - Corticosteroid randomization after significant health injury (CRASH) trial showed increased mortality after steroid administration for closed head injuries

DISORDERS ASSOCIATED WITH INTRACRANIAL PATHOLOGY

- Intracranial hypertension
  - ICP can increase following trauma, hemorrhage, or mass effect
    - ❖ Monro–Kellie hypothesis: cranial compartment is a fixed in space
      - ➤ Any increase in space by one component must be compensated by a decrease in space from another component
      - ➤ Components

- ❖ Brain (80% to 85%)
- ❖ CSF (5% to 15%)
- ❖ Blood (3% to 6%)
- ◆ Increased brain swelling → compensated by decreasing CBF and/or CSF
- ◆ If the brain expands beyond the limits of the cranial vault, herniation can occur
  - ➤ Supratentorial or infratentorial
  - ➤ Example: uncal herniation
    - ❖ The brain exerts pressure on the brainstem
    - ❖ Causes significant alteration of function of midbrain structures → can be fatal
  - ➤ Treatment involves maximal medical therapy and possible decompressive craniectomy
- Clinical signs of increased ICP
  - ◆ Altered mental status, headache, nausea, vomiting, or localizing signs
  - ◆ Cushing triad
    - ➤ Increased blood pressure
    - ➤ Decreased heart rate
    - ➤ Irregular breathing
- ICP monitoring
  - ◆ Indications
    - ➤ Severe head injury patient who cannot be followed with serial neurological exams
    - ➤ Consider strongly in elderly and in those who are hypoxemic or hypotensive
  - ◆ Types of ICP monitoring
    - ➤ Intraventricular catheters with external transducer
      - ❖ Most invasive and difficult to place
      - ❖ Most accurate ICP measurement
      - ❖ Offers ability to drain CSF in cases of intracranial hypertension
    - ➤ Intraparenchymal microtransducers
      - ❖ Easier to place and smaller burr hole
      - ❖ Less reliable and cannot be recalibrated once placed
      - ❖ Small risk of intracranial hemorrhage (<1%)
    - ➤ Subarachnoid catheters/subdural bolts
      - ❖ Least invasive with least hemorrhage
      - ❖ Less accurate with greater risk of malfunction or obstruction
- Treatment
  - ◆ Head elevation
  - ◆ Fluids and diuretics
    - ➤ Mannitol
      - ❖ Mechanism
        - ⟩ Osmotic diuretic
        - ⟩ Decreases CSF production
      - ❖ Bolused at 0.25 to 1.0 g/kg
        - ⟩ Effects noted within 15 minutes of administration, peak effects at 1 hour
        - ⟩ Effects last 2 to 6 hours
        - ⟩ Mannitol extravasation is highly dangerous due to high osmolar content (1,098 mOsm/L) → increased risk of compartment syndrome
      - ❖ A rapid bolus may cause hypotension and dilation of intracranial vessels
      - ❖ Requires an intact BBB (blood–brain barrier) to be effective
    - ➤ Furosemide can be used to decrease intravascular volume
      - ❖ Side effect is worsening of hypotension
    - ➤ Hypertonic saline
      - ❖ Hypertonic conditions decreases ICP
        - ⟩ Saline at 3% as infusion or 23% as bolus
      - ❖ Lactated ringers and other hypo-osmolar solutions should be avoided
  - ◆ Hyperventilation
    - ➤ Each 1 mm Hg decrease in $Paco_2$ → CBF decreases 2%
    - ➤ Therapeutic hyperventilation
      - ❖ Target a $Paco_2$ or 30 to 35 mm Hg

- ❖ Pa_{CO_2} values less than 25 mm Hg → risks cerebral ischemia
- ❖ Effects of hyperventilation diminished when Pa_{CO_2} <25 mm Hg
- ❖ Steroids
  - ➤ Do NOT improve outcome
  - ➤ Can help decrease ICP if cellular edema is present
- ❖ Surgical decompression (craniectomy)
  - ➤ Decompressive craniectomy (DECRA) trial showed decompressive craniectomy had worsened long-term outcomes compared to medical management when ICP was resistant to first-tier therapies
- Disorders of fluid regulation
  - Diabetes insipidus (DI)
    - ❖ Types
      - ➤ Central: diminished water reabsorption due to insufficient antidiuretic hormone (ADH)
      - ➤ Nephrogenic: diminished water reabsorption due to defect at ADH receptors
    - ❖ Causes
      - ➤ Central DI can be caused by brain tumors, trauma, hypoxic injury, and infections
    - ❖ Clinical findings
      - ➤ Dehydrated, hypernatremic, high serum osmolality, low urine sodium, low urine osmolality
    - ❖ Treatment
      - ➤ Treat underlying cause
      - ➤ Replace water losses
      - ➤ If central DI, vasopressin or ADH administration
  - Syndrome of inappropriate ADH secretion (SIADH)
    - ❖ Elevated ADH levels despite low osmolality → increases water reabsorption
    - ❖ Causes
      - ➤ Brain tumors, hemorrhage, hypoxic injury, infections, trauma, and drugs
    - ❖ Clinical findings
      - ➤ Low urine output, hyponatremia, low serum osmolality, low serum sodium, high urine sodium, high urine osmolality
    - ❖ Treatment
      - ➤ Treat underlying disorder
      - ➤ Fluid restrict
      - ➤ Hypertonic saline
      - ➤ Diuresis
      - ➤ Demeclocycline
      - ➤ Vaptans
  - Cerebral salt wasting
    - ❖ Increased urinary losses of sodium despite hypovolemia
    - ❖ Causes
      - ➤ Brain tumor, trauma, or infections
    - ❖ Clinical findings
      - ➤ Polyuria, dehydration, hyponatremia, high urine sodium
    - ❖ Treatment
      - ➤ Replace sodium losses
- Sympathetic surge
  - Inappropriate sympathetic outflow often follows subarachnoid hemorrhage (SAH) or brain injury
  - Organ specific effects
    - ❖ Cerebral
      - ➤ Increased ICP
      - ➤ Vasoconstriction and vasospasm
    - ❖ Cardiovascular
      - ➤ ECG (electrocardiogram) with ST and ischemic changes
      - ➤ Troponin elevation
      - ➤ Echo may show left heart strain
        - ❖ Decreased left ventricle contractility
        - ❖ Decreased cardiac output

- ◆ Respiratory
  - ➤ Increased pulmonary vasoconstriction → neurogenic pulmonary edema

SUBARACHNOID HEMORRHAGE

- Presentation
  - Etiologies include brain injury or spontaneous bleed
  - Symptoms
    - ◆ Severe "thunderclap" headache, change in mental status, seizures, stroke
    - ◆ Often fatal
    - ◆ Brain bleed may increase protons and acidosis at brain → acidosis sensed in CSF → stimulate chemoreceptors on anterolateral surface of medulla exposed to fourth ventricle → increased minute ventilation
  - Risk factors
    - ◆ Hypertension, atrial fibrillation, heart failure, coronary artery disease, renal disease, and family history
  - Risk of rebleed
    - ◆ 4% on day one, 1% to 2% daily for next 4 weeks
  - Classification
    - ◆ Fisher grade based on amount of blood seen on CT
      - ➤ 1: no hemorrhage
      - ➤ 2: SAH <1 mm thick
      - ➤ 3: SAH >1 mm thick
      - ➤ 4: SAH with intraventricular hemorrhage or parenchymal extension
    - ◆ Hunt–Hess grade based on clinical symptoms
      - ➤ 1: asymptomatic or minimal headache
      - ➤ 2: moderate headache, no neurologic deficit
      - ➤ 3: drowsy, minimal neurological deficit
      - ➤ 4: minimally responsive
      - ➤ 5: comatose
- Treatment
  - Control bleed
    - ◆ Reverse coagulopathy
      - ➤ Consider fresh frozen plasma (FFP), vitamin K, recombinant factor VIIa
    - ◆ Interventional radiology embolization
    - ◆ Neurosurgical intervention
  - Prevent vasospasm
    - ◆ Timing
      - ➤ Vasospasm commonly occurs 4 to 12 days after initial bleed
    - ◆ Detection methods
      - ➤ Transcranial Doppler
      - ➤ Computed tomography (CT)/Computed tomography angiography (CTA)
      - ➤ Serial neurological exams
    - ◆ Mechanism
      - ➤ Breakdown products of blood → increase endothelin release → vasoconstriction through nitric oxide inhibition → ischemic brain injury
      - ➤ Increased SAH bleed → increased vasospasm risk
    - ◆ Treatment
      - ➤ Triple H therapy: hypervolemia, hypertension, and hemodilution
        - ✤ Now more controversial due to potential side effects including pulmonary edema, myocardial ischemia, electrolyte alterations, and cerebral edema
      - ➤ Nimodipine
      - ➤ Balloon angioplasty or intra-arterial dilation
      - ➤ Avoid sodium nitroprusside as an antihypertensive agent in these patients
        - ✤ Rebound hypertension, platelet dysfunction, and increased pulmonary shunting can occur

- Anesthetic implications
  - Strategies to decrease ICP
    - Limit volatile anesthetic concentration to prevent increased CBF and ICP
      - Total IV anesthetic of propofol and an opioid may be beneficial
    - Consider modest hyperventilation
    - Consider mannitol and hypertonic saline
    - Consider steroids depending on etiology of SAH and swelling
    - Minimize catecholamine release through adequate analgesia
  - Maintain CPP
    - Increase MAP and minimize ICP
    - After aneurysm ablation or clipping, consider moderate HTN (hypertension) to aid perfusion
  - Normothermia
    - Hypothermia does not improve outcomes

SPINAL PATHOLOGY

- Spinal stenosis
  - Mechanism: narrowing of spinal cord that causes neurological deficits
  - Presentation: extremity numbness, weakness, pain (neurogenic claudication)
    - Symptoms may improve when bending forward
      - Examples: symptoms improve with bike riding, walking uphill
    - Symptoms may worsen when standing straight
      - Example: walking downhill
  - Treatment: medical management, physical therapy, or decompressive laminectomy
- Spinal tumors
  - Types
    - Primary tumors: astrocytomas, ependymomas, schwannomas, meningiomas, neurofibromas
    - Metastasis: common from lung, breast, prostate
  - Presentation: neurological deficits, pain
- SCI Injuries
    - Cervical: result in full or partial **tetraplegia**
      - Lesions above C3 require mechanical ventilation due to phrenic paralysis
      - Could result in **neurogenic shock**
        - Loss of sympathetic stimulation → decreased SVR → hypotension
        - Unopposed vagal activity → bradycardia
    - Thoracic: result in **paraplegia**
      - Lesions above T4 can also result in neurogenic shock
      - Lesions above T6 may result in autonomic hyperreflexia
    - Lumbar and sacral: results in bowel and bladder incontinence, weakness of lower extremities
  - Treatment
    - Steroids with mild benefit in neurological function
    - Side effects include increased infection risk and avascular necrosis
  - Cord syndromes
    - Anterior cord syndrome: loss of motor function and loss of pain and temperature sensation due to interruption of anterior spinal artery
    - Posterior cord syndrome: loss of proprioception, but motor function, pain, and temperature are preserved due to interruption of the posterior spinal arteries
    - Central cord syndrome: incomplete injury resulting in upper extremity, but not lower extremity, impairment
    - Brown-Sequard syndrome: hemisection of the spinal cord with ipsilateral loss of motor and proprioception and contralateral loss of pain, temperature, and touch
- Autonomic **hyperreflexia**
  - Involuntary exaggerated hemodynamic response to stimulation following the resolution of SCI and return of spinal cord reflexes
    - 85% of patients with T6 lesion or higher with this response

- ◆ Rare in lesions below T10
- Mechanism of hyperreflexia
  - ◆ Cutaneous or visceral stimulation → afferent impulses to spinal cord → reflex sympathetic activity
  - ◆ Modulation of this reflex is lost from higher structures
- Symptoms
  - ◆ Sweating, headache, severe hypertension, vasodilation above lesion, vasoconstriction below lesion, bradycardia
  - ◆ Hemodynamic changes such as hypertension and bradycardia
- Anesthetic implications
  - ◆ Block sensation of stimulation to prevent hyperreflexia
    - ➤ Deep general anesthetic
    - ➤ Regional anesthesia
    - ➤ Neuraxial anesthesia
      - ❖ Spinal often sufficient
      - ❖ Epidural may be insufficient depending on the procedure due to sacral root sparing
  - ◆ Ganglionic blocking drugs
    - ➤ Trimethaphan, phentolamine, vasodilators

NEUROLOGIC DISORDERS AND ANESTHETIC IMPLICATIONS

- ■ Hereditary conditions
  - Hereditary angioneurotic edema
    - ◆ Mechanism and presentation
      - ➤ C1 esterase inhibitor deficiency → increased vascular permeability
      - ➤ Presents with mucocutaneous swelling that is not pitting and occurs in the skin or mucous membranes
    - ◆ Perioperative implications
      - ➤ Steroids or antifibrinolytic agents decrease attack frequency
        - ❖ Examples: danazol, ε-aminocaproic acid, tranexamic acid
      - ➤ Airway manipulation may precipitate attack
        - ❖ Consider transfusion of FFP to replace C1 esterase
        - ❖ Consider administration of C1 esterase inhibitors
        - ❖ Consider androgens prior to surgery
      - ➤ If airway manipulation
        - ❖ Steroids, FFP, and C1 esterase inhibitor can be administered on the day of surgery
  - Spina bifida occulta
    - ◆ Mechanism and presentation
      - ➤ Incomplete closure of neural tube during development
        - ❖ 60% of deformities between L4 and S2
      - ➤ Meningomyelocele is the most severe form of spina bifida where both meninges and spinal cord protrude through a vertebral defect
        - ❖ Diagnosed at birth and requires urgent intervention
        - ❖ Prone to infection with meningitis
    - ◆ Perioperative implications
      - ➤ Corrective surgery should be performed within 48 hours
      - ➤ Anesthetics for patients with corrected spina bifida occulta
        - ❖ May have bladder incontinence
        - ❖ Increased risk for latex allergy
        - ❖ Neuraxial anesthesia may be unreliable
          - › Epidural space may be discontinuous → incomplete/patchy blocks
          - › Increased risk of dural puncture
- ■ Stroke
  - Mechanism and presentation
    - ◆ Strokes can be hemorrhagic or ischemic

- Strokes should be worked up for an etiology as certain causes can increase perioperative risk factors and affect perioperative management
  - Examples: carotid stenosis, patent foramen ovale (PFO), hypercoagulable condition
- Anesthetic implications
  - Ischemic territory may have loss of autoregulation and normal vasomotor responses
  - Recommended to postpone surgery for at least 4 weeks and preferably 6 weeks after stroke for elective surgery

- Seizures
  - Mechanism and presentation
    - Abnormally excitable neurons → present with symptoms reflecting focal or grand mal seizure
    - Recent undiagnosed seizure → warrants evaluation for etiology
  - Anesthetic implications
    - Many anesthetic drugs increase seizure threshold, so intraoperative seizures are unlikely
      - Examples: benzodiazepines, propofol
    - Antiepileptics should be continued perioperatively
    - Antiepileptics may alter drug metabolism of anesthetics and perioperative drugs
      - Examples: **phenytoin, carbamazepine**, phenobarbital induce cytochrome P450 activity

- Parkinson disease
  - Mechanism and presentation
    - Degenerative disorder of the basal ganglia
      - Dopamine fails to adequately inhibit the extrapyramidal motor system
    - Presents with tremor, rigidity, masked facies, difficulty speaking, and autonomic dysfunction
    - Treatment is with **levodopa with Catechol-O-methyltransferase (COMT) inhibitor** (entacapone, tolcapone)
  - Perioperative implications
    - Continue drug therapy perioperatively
      - Levodopa is an oral medication with a half-life of 1 to 3 hours, so it should be taken prior to induction
    - Avoid dopaminergic drugs (inhibitors like metoclopramide)
    - Increased aspiration risk due to swallowing dysfunction
    - Increased autonomic hyperreflexia

- Pseudotumor cerebri (idiopathic intracranial hypertension)
  - Mechanism and presentation
    - Increased ICP of unclear etiology
    - Presents with headache, nausea, and vision changes (papilledema)
    - Treatment
      - Acetazolamide decreases CSF production
      - Lumbar puncture for diagnosis and therapy
  - Perioperative implications
    - Neuraxial is safe

- Polio
  - Mechanism and presentation
    - Infectious disease caused by poliovirus
      - Largely obliterated due to polio vaccine
      - Polio survivors still seen
    - Presents with muscle weakness
      - Lesions at anterior horn neurons, motor nuclei of CN, and reticular formation
      - 1% to 2% with paralytic polio → asymmetric flaccid paralysis
    - Postpolio syndrome marked by continued weakness years after initial infection
      - 50% patients with pain
  - Perioperative implications
    - Increased sensitivity to anesthetic medications
    - Increased sensitivity to nondepolarizing muscle relaxants
    - Increased postoperative pain
    - Increased autonomic instability
    - Increased aspiration risk due to muscle weakness

ANESTHESIA FOR CRANIOTOMIES

- Anesthetic selection
  - While no anesthetic agent is contraindicated for neurosurgery, the selection of anesthetic drugs should take into account goals for ICP, CPP, and CBF
  - Brain parenchyma is devoid of sensation → minimal anesthetic requirements following dural opening
- **Brain relaxation**
  - Often necessary prior to dural opening
  - Methods
    - Increase osmolality
      - **Mannitol** at 0.5 to 1.0 mg/kg
        - Osmotic diuretic → increase serum osmolality
        - Water passes from brain to intravascular fluid via the blood–brain barrier
      - **Normal saline** or **hypertonic saline**
        - Normal saline is 308 mEq/L, making it hypertonic to serum
    - Furosemide
      - Decreases overall water content
    - Mild hyperventilation
      - Decreases CBF
    - Steroids
      - Dexamethasone and other steroids → decrease vasogenic edema and swelling
- **Fluid regulation**
  - Goal is to choose a fluid that decreases brain water content perioperatively → increases surgical exposure and decrease ICP
    - Mild fluid restriction beneficial to decrease cerebral edema
    - Severe fluid restriction may cause hypotension and cerebral ischemia
  - Normal saline is used for maintenance for its hypertonic qualities
    - Avoid lactated ringers, hypotonic solutions, and glucose solutions
    - If normal saline causes a significant metabolic acidosis, consider another fluid
- **Positioning**
  - Depending on the location of the lesion, craniotomies can be done supine, prone, or sitting
  - **Sitting craniotomy** increases the risk for a **venous air embolism**
    - Venous air embolism can occur when the operative level is above the heart
      - Air can be entrained in a non collapsible vein (venous sinus) → passage to the heart and lungs can cause cardiovascular collapse
      - Patients with a PFO are at risk of a right-to-left shunt → stroke
        - Relative contraindication to the sitting position
    - Methods for air detection
      - Transesophageal echocardiography most sensitive
        - PFO best diagnosed by a transesophageal echocardiogram (TEE) study with agitated saline
        - Bubbles crossing from the right atrium to left atrium within three cardiac cycles suggests a PFO
      - Doppler ultrasound is very close in sensitivity to TEE
        - Can detect as little as 0.25 cc of air
      - Capnography
        - Abrupt decrease in ETCO$_2$ concerning for air embolism
      - End-tidal nitrogen monitoring
    - Treatment
      - The patient should be taken out of the sitting craniotomy position and placed in supine position
      - Surgeons flood field with saline to close sinus
      - Aspirate air if a central venous catheter is present in right atrium
      - Hemodynamic support
      - Discontinue nitrous if used
      - 100% oxygen

- **Mayfield pins**
  - Used to secure the head in place and prevent movement
  - Placement is highly stimulating → consider opioids, lidocaine, or deepening the anesthetic prior to pinning
  - Consider muscle relaxation for pinning and while the head is pinned to prevent coughing and head/neck injury

ANESTHESIA FOR SPECIFIC NEUROSURGICAL PROCEDURES

- **Intracranial aneurysms**
  - Preoperative workup should include assessment for cardiac injury (following SAH), vasospasm, and neurological status
  - Most common site = circle of Willis
  - Vasospasm is a severe complication of ruptured aneurysms and is seen in up to 30% of patients
  - Hemodynamic management
    - Prior to clipping
      - Avoid significant intraoperative HTN to prevent rupture
      - Avoid significant hypotension since injured brain may have altered autoregulation
    - During temporary clipping
      - Induce mild hypertension to improve collateral flow around clipped vessel
      - Adenosine may be used to open cerebral aneurysm instead of temporary clip ligation
        - Dose of 6 to 12 mg causes brief period of asystole
        - Hypotension follows the asystole
        - Allow hemodynamics to return to normal prior to next dose
        - Pacing pads should be available prior to adenosine use
    - Following permanent clipping
      - Mild hypertension may be beneficial to improve perfusion around the aneurysm
- **Transsphenoidal resection**
  - Performed for pituitary tumors
  - In patients with acromegaly, airway may be challenging due to difficult mask ventilation and intubation
    - Increased difficulty with mask ventilation
      - Increased head size may make finding an adequately sized mask difficult
      - Increased head size may make it difficult to position hands around the mouth and jaw
      - Larger tongue increases airway obstruction
    - Increased difficulty with intubation
      - Anatomical changes include narrower airways, larger tongue, larger epiglottis
      - Longer laryngoscope blade may be needed
- **Stereotactic surgery**
  - Access to airway may be compromised by stereotactic apparatus
  - Gamma knife is a type of procedure that utilizes a stereotactic device to direct high-intensity radiation to a target lesion
- **Deep brain stimulator**
  - Microelectrodes are inserted through burr holes to the subthalamic nuclei, globus pallidum, or thalamus
  - Patients are not sedated to prevent interference with electrode readings
- **Ventriculostomy**
  - Acute hydrocephalus warrants careful attention to minimize ICP while increasing CPP during surgery

ANESTHESIA FOR ELECTROCONVULSIVE THERAPY (ECT)

- Physiologic disturbances of ECT
  - Goal of ECT is to generate a brief tonic clonic seizure
  - Initial vagal stimulation → bradycardia, hypotension
  - Subsequent sympathetic discharge → tachycardia, hypertension

- Contraindications
  - Inability to tolerate intracranial hypertension
    - ICP increases during the sympathetic discharge
  - Major cardiovascular comorbidities
    - Rapid hemodynamic fluctuations in heart rate and blood pressure during ECT
- Drug selection
  - Hypnotics
    - Methohexital, propofol, and/or benzodiazepines commonly used
    - Selection between propofol and methohexital depends on desired seizure intensity and duration
      - Propofol increases the seizure threshold more than methohexital
    - Benzodiazepines used to terminate a seizure that is extending beyond therapeutic duration
    - Etomidate and IV caffeine can lengthen seizure duration
  - Muscle relaxants
    - Succinylcholine preferred for short duration and ability to monitor fasciculations
    - Used to prevent injury during induced seizure
  - Hemodynamic agents
    - Vasopressors, antihypertensives, anticholinergics, and other hemodynamic drugs should be available for hemodynamic fluctuations

QUESTIONS

1. A 50-year-old man is undergoing mechanical ventilation for acute respiratory distress syndrome (ARDS). A lung-protective strategy of ventilation is employed, which results in the Pa_{CO_2} increasing from 42 to 47 mm Hg. The patient's estimated CBF with this ventilation strategy is:

   A. 67–71 cc/100 g/min
   B. 61–66 cc/100 g/min
   C. 55–60 cc/100 g/min
   D. 45–54 cc/100 g/min

2. A 74-year-old woman is undergoing CSF drainage to optimize spinal cord perfusion during a thoracic aortic aneurysm repair. If the management plan is to close the CSF drain when CSF drainage exceeds normal production, then it should be closed when the hourly drainage exceeds:

   A. 20–25 cc
   B. 30–35 cc
   C. 40–45 cc
   D. 50–55 cc

3. A 24-year-old woman was a pedestrian struck by a car while crossing the street. On arrival in the emergency department she opens her eyes to verbal stimuli. Her speech is incoherent and she withdraws from painful stimuli. Which of the following is the patient's Glasgow Coma Scale (GCS) score?

   A. 7
   B. 10
   C. 12
   D. 14

4. A previously healthy 55-year-old patient underwent craniotomy and resection of a brain tumor 2 days ago. His examination is notable for somnolence, dry mucus membranes, and postural hypotension. His laboratory values reveal that serum sodium is 129 mEq/L and the urinary sodium is 105 mEq/L. The most likely diagnosis is:

   A. SIADH
   B. Cerebral salt wasting
   C. Nephrogenic DI
   D. Central DI

5. A 25-year-old man is admitted to the ICU after sustaining TBI and a pelvic fracture in a motor vehicle accident. He receives lactated ringers and blood transfusion over the next 1 day with evidence of adequate resuscitation. On post-trauma day 2 his urine output decreases. His vital signs are T, 99; HR, 80; R, 22; BP, 145/84, with O_2 saturation of 99% on mechanical ventilation. His laboratory values reveal a serum sodium of 130 mEq/L, serum osmolality of 270 mOsm/kg, and the urinary sodium is 20 mEq/L and dark urine with a specific gravity of 1.020. The most appropriate therapeutic intervention for this patient is:

   A. Fluid restriction
   B. Fluid replacement with 0.45% saline
   C. Fluid replacement with 3% saline
   D. Desmopressin administration

OPHTHALMIC ANATOMY AND PHYSIOLOGY

- ■ Anatomy (Fig. 9.1)
  - ● Three layers of the eye are the sclera, the uveal tract, and the retina
    - ◆ Sclera is the outermost layer and contains the cornea
    - ◆ Uveal tract contains the choroid iris and ciliary body
    - ◆ Retina is the innermost layer
  - ● Fluid
    - ◆ Types
      - ➢ Vitreous humor fills the center of the eye
      - ➢ Aqueous humor fills the anterior portion of the eye between the cornea and the iris
    - ◆ Pathway of flow
      - ➢ Aqueous fluid produced by ciliary body and created by filtration of vessels on the iris →
        flows over lens and through pupil → enters angle of anterior chamber → flows through
        trabecular meshwork → canal of Schlemm
  - ● Ophthalmic artery supplies most structures of the eye
  - ● Cranial nerve (CN) II carries signals from the retina while CN III, IV, and VI control eye movement

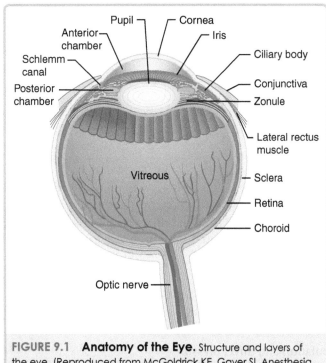

FIGURE 9.1 Anatomy of the Eye. Structure and layers of
the eye. (Reproduced from McGoldrick KE, Gayer SI. Anesthesia
for ophthalmologic surgery. In: Barash PG, Cullen BF, Stoelting RK,
et al., eds. *Clinical Anesthesia*. 7th ed. Philadelphia, PA: Wolters
Kluwer; 2013:1374.)

- Intraocular pressure (IOP)
  - Globe is a fairly noncompliant compartment (similar to brain)
    - IOP is determined by globe contents
    - Production and drainage of aqueous humor, extraocular muscle tone, and fluid content in the eye (choroidal blood volume) are the major factors influencing IOP
  - Carbonic anhydrase converts CO_2 and $H_2O \rightarrow$ carbonic acid $\rightarrow HCO_3^-$
  - Aqueous fluid volume and choroidal blood volume are variable $\rightarrow$ primary intrinsic factors determining IOP
    - Changes that increase aqueous fluid
      - Impaired aqueous drainage
      - Sclerosis of the trabecular meshwork (open-angle glaucoma)
      - Closure of anterior chamber angle and obstruction of aqueous drainage (closed-angle glaucoma)
    - Changes that increase choroidal blood volume
      - Cough, straining, vomiting
      - Hypoxia
      - Hypercapnia
      - Hypertension
  - Extrinsic factors that increase IOP
    - Blinking
    - Forceful eyelid closure
    - Compression from mask ventilation
    - Laryngoscopy
      - Administration of lidocaine or narcotics can minimize this effect
    - Venous congestion
    - N_2O
      - Can diffuse into an intraocular bubble $\rightarrow$ increase IOP $\rightarrow$ compromise retinal blood flow $\rightarrow$ retinal detachment
  - Drugs
    - Succinylcholine causes a brief and mild increase in IOP
    - Ketamine can increase IOP and intracranial pressure (ICP)
  - Equation
    - Intraocular perfusion pressure (IPP) = mean arterial pressure − intraocular pressure
    - Normal IOP is 10 to 22 mm Hg
  - Strategies to decrease IOP
    - Head up
    - Hyperventilation
    - Muscle relaxants
    - Anesthetics
    - Acetazolamide
    - Diuretics
- Oculocardiac reflex (OCR)
  - Pathway
    - Pressure on eye $\rightarrow$ afferent input from the ciliary ganglion $\rightarrow$ transmitted via ophthalmic division of trigeminal nerve $\rightarrow$ efferent output from vagus nerve $\rightarrow$ bradycardia, atrioventricular block, or asystole
    - Trigeminal vagal reflex is precipitated by
      - Preoperative anxiety
      - Hypoxia/hypercarbia
      - Light general anesthetic (GA)
  - Triggers
    - Surgical manipulation and direct pressure
    - Traction on extraocular muscles
      - Medial rectus > lateral rectus
    - Increased IOP
    - Ocular pain
    - Placement of regional blocks

- Prevention and treatment
  - Consider pretreatment with intravenous anticholinergics
  - Stop surgical stimulation
  - Although regional blocks or local anesthetic may precipitate the OCR, it can also prevent it during the surgery

PREOPERATIVE OPHTHALMIC ASSESSMENT

- Ophthalmic surgery is low risk, but the patient population is often older with more cardiovascular risks
  - Very few reasons should result in case cancellation or warrant additional testing, but a careful history and physical examination should be done to prevent any perioperative problems
- Chronic medications and anesthetic interactions
  - Glaucoma drugs
    - Topical β-blockers: systemic absorption → bradycardia, hypotension, bronchospasm
    - Acetazolamide: systemic absorption → diuresis, hyponatremia, hypokalemia
  - Mydriasis-inducing drugs
    - Atropine: systemic absorption → tachycardia, anticholinergics symptoms
    - Phenylephrine: systemic absorption → hypertension, bradycardia
  - Miosis-inducing drugs
    - Echothiophate (topical anticholinesterase inhibitor): Systemic absorption → inhibits plasma cholinesterase → prolonged muscle paralysis following succinylcholine and may inhibit metabolism of ester local anesthetics
    - Pilocarpine: systemic absorption → bronchospasm, bradycardia
    - Acetylcholine: systemic absorption → bronchospasm, bradycardia

OPHTHALMIC ANESTHESIA

- Decision
  - General, regional, local, and topical anesthesia are options depending on the surgery
  - Regional anesthesia offers the benefits of less postoperative nausea and vomiting, shorter time to discharge, and improved postoperative pain relief
  - Surgeries are often ambulatory, so anesthetic plan should take into account short discharge duration
- General anesthesia
  - Unique goals of ophthalmic anesthesia include smooth induction and emergence
    - Coughing can increase IOP
    - Stimulation can trigger the OCR
  - Scopolamine should be avoided in patients with glaucoma due to papillary dilation
  - Nitrous oxide contraindicated in vitreoretinal procedures
    - Surgeon injects intravitreal air bubble to tamponade the retina against the wall
      - SF_6, C_3F_8, or room air used for bubble
    - Nitrous oxide causes bubble expansion → increase IOP → blindness
    - Avoid nitrous postoperatively for at least a month to allow bubble reabsorption
- Regional blocks
  - **Retrobulbar block** (Fig. 9.2)
    - Technique
      - Local anesthetic injected through the inferotemporal quadrant of eye in neutral position to the muscular cone behind the eye
        - Anesthetizes the three cranial nerves for eye movement (CN III, IV, VI)
        - Anesthetizes sensation to the eye (CN V)
        - Blocks ciliary nerves for anesthesia to the conjunctiva, cornea, and uvea
      - Must also block accessory facial nerve to block blinking
    - Complications
      - Injury to globe or muscular cone
      - Retrobulbar hemorrhage → IOP increase warrants lateral canthotomy

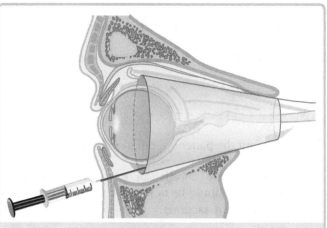

FIGURE 9.2   **Retrobulbar Block.** Location and anatomy for performing a retrobulbar block. (Reproduced from McGoldrick KE, Gayer SI. Anesthesia for ophthalmologic surgery. In: Barash PG, Cullen BF, Stoelting RK, et al., eds. *Clinical Anesthesia*. 7th ed. Philadelphia, PA: Wolters Kluwer; 2013:1384.)

- ➤ Injection into optic nerve sheath →
    - ❖ Local anesthetic tracks to subdural to midbrain to respiratory centers → respiratory arrest
    - ❖ Optic nerve sheath continuous with subarachnoid space → altered mental status
- ➤ Injection at ophthalmic artery → seizures due to retrograde flow to carotid artery
- • **Peribulbar blocks** (Fig. 9.3)
    - ❖ Technique
        - ➤ Two injections needed
            - ❖ One inferotemporally and one superonasally
                - › Requires injection of a larger volume of local anesthetic behind the eye; the injection is outside of the muscular medullary cone
                - › Equally effective, similar degree of akinesia
            - ❖ Blocks the orbicularis oculi muscles of eyelid
            - ❖ Longer onset time (10 minutes) and decreased rate of complete akinesia compared to retrobulbar block

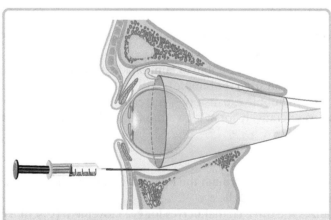

FIGURE 9.3   **Peribulbar Block.** Location and anatomy for performing a peribulbar block. (Reproduced from McGoldrick KE, Gayer SI. Anesthesia for ophthalmologic surgery. In: Barash PG, Cullen BF, Stoelting RK, et al., eds. *Clinical Anesthesia*. 7th ed. Philadelphia, PA: Wolters Kluwer; 2013:1384.)

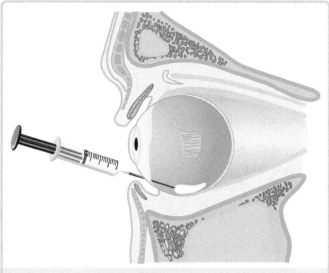

FIGURE 9.4 Sub-Tenon Block. Location and anatomy for performing a sub-Tenon block. (Reproduced from McGoldrick KE, Gayer SI. Anesthesia for ophthalmologic surgery. In: Barash PG, Cullen BF, Stoelting RK, et al., eds. *Clinical Anesthesia*. 7th ed. Philadelphia, PA: Wolters Kluwer; 2013:1386.)

- ◆ Complications
  - ➤ Easier, safer, and less painful than retrobulbar block
  - ➤ Intravascular injection or direct injury to underlying structures still possible
- ● **Sub-Tenon block** (Fig. 9.4)
  - ◆ Technique
    - ➤ Under topical sedation, an incision is made in the conjunctiva through Tenon fascia
    - ➤ Injection of local anesthetic into the sub-Tenon space using a blunt needle→ blocks sensory nerves around the globe
- ■ Topical anesthesia
  - ● Many ophthalmic surgeries can be performed solely under topical anesthesia
  - ● Does not prevent eye movement

SPECIFIC OPHTHALMIC SITUATIONS

- ■ Open-eye injury
  - ● Follows penetrating trauma
  - ● Anesthetic considerations
    - ◆ May require general anesthesia due to surgical duration, surgical complexity, full stomach, and inability to lie still
    - ◆ Increased IOP → risks extrusion of eye contents → permanent vision loss
      - ➤ Succinylcholine may increase IOP, but often used given full stomach and aspiration risk
      - ➤ Minimize IOP associated with laryngoscopy with adequate depth of anesthesia
- ■ Strabismus
  - ● Surgery to alter length of extraocular muscles
  - ● Anesthetic considerations
    - ◆ Avoid succinylcholine due to short-term effects on extraocular muscles
    - ◆ Significant risk for PONV (postoperative nausea and vomiting)
      - ➤ Consider pretreatment, stomach decompression, adequate hydration, and total IV anesthetic

OTOLARYNGOLOGY SURGERY

- Anesthetic considerations for airway and oral surgery
  - Laryngeal surgery
    - Complex airway
      - Depending on the surgical indication, the patient may have a difficult airway
      - Risk factors
        - History of head and neck radiation
        - Congenital malformation
        - Previous surgical manipulation
        - Cancer or obstruction
      - Extubation may be challenging based on airway edema and the surgical procedure
    - Unsecured airway
      - Depending on the location of the lesion or surgery, an endotracheal tube may interfere with the surgery
      - Options include spontaneous respirations, jet ventilation, or intermittent positive pressure ventilation
      - Jet ventilation
        - Jet needle is placed on end of rigid laryngoscope
        - Utilizes high pressure, but smaller tidal volumes
        - Relies upon the Venturi effect to entrain room air and dilute the gas mixture
        - Must observe for chest rise and excursion for ventilation quality
    - **Airway fire**
      - Triad for fire: ignition, fuel, oxidizer
        - Most airway fires start on the outside of an endotracheal tube
        - If fire burns to inside of tube → blowtorch effect
      - **Strategies to minimize risk**
        - Minimize oxidizer
          - Avoid high oxygen concentration (keep F_{IO_2} <30%)
          - Avoid nitrous oxide (supports combustion)
          - Substitute helium to the gas mixture (increases the amount of energy needed to produce combustion)
        - Minimize fuel
          - Use **laser-resistant cuffed tubes**
            - Red rubber wrapping
            - Aluminum wrapping
            - Only all-metal tubes are completely laser proof
          - Carefully place drapes to minimize fire risk and spread
          - Allow sterilizing prep solutions to dry
        - Minimize ignition
          - Use electricity and lasers cautiously and only when necessary
          - Carbon dioxide laser often used for airway surgery
      - Treatment
        - Remove endotracheal tube
        - Stop flow of oxygen
        - Pour saline on field
        - Remove flammable material
        - Consider bronchoscopy
  - Tonsillectomy
    - Indications include obstructive sleep apnea, tonsillitis, abscess, and tumor
      - Adenoidectomy performed for respiratory obstruction
    - Postoperative bleeding is a feared complication
      - Primary bleeds occur within 6 hours of surgery
        - Bleeding can also occur after days
      - Anesthesia should include IV access prior to induction, immediately available blood products, fluid or blood resuscitation, and a rapid sequence intubation

- ➤ Intubation can be challenging due to intraoral swelling and active bleeding
- Anesthetic considerations for ear surgery
  - Middle ear surgery
    - ◆ Avoid nitrous oxide for middle ear surgery due to closed air spaces
      - ➤ Nitrous oxide increases middle pressures
      - ➤ Rapid nitrous oxide absorption following anesthetic may create negative middle ear pressures
    - ◆ Nausea and vomiting
      - ➤ High incidence of nausea and vomiting after ear procedures involving the labyrinth and vestibular nerve
      - ➤ Vomiting and retching can increase venous pressure, ICP, bleeding, and risk dislodgement of devices
  - Myringotomy tubes
    - ◆ Short procedure performed typically in the pediatric population
    - ◆ Often done with mask ventilation without intravenous access
      - ➤ Deep sedation required to prevent movement
- Anesthetic considerations for nasal surgery
  - Nasal vasoconstrictors
    - ◆ Cocaine, phenylephrine, and oxymetolazone can be used to constrict the nasal vessels and decrease blood loss → can also cause systemic effects such as coronary vasoconstriction and hypertension
  - Emergence
    - ◆ Smooth emergence essential to prevent use of face mask or positive pressure ventilation that can damage surgical correction
- Awake Intubation
  - Must block CN IX and X
  - Glossopharyngeal nerve block
    - ◆ At caudal aspect of the posterior tonsillar pillar
    - ◆ Anesthetizes the oropharynx, soft palate, tongue, and epiglottis
  - Sensory and motor supply of the larynx and trachea are via the superior laryngeal nerve (SLN) and recurrent laryngeal nerve (RLN)
  - SLN block
    - ◆ Inferior to the greater cornu of the hyoid bone bilaterally
  - RLN block (aka inferior laryngeal nerve)
    - ◆ Blocks all laryngeal muscles except the cricothyroid (which is innervated by the exterior SLN)
    - ◆ Transtracheal injection
- Awake tracheostomy
  - Just need to block RLN (CN IX and SLN are supraglottic)
- SLN palsy
  - Voice can be hoarse
  - Loss of sensation above the vocal cords (VC)
  - Increased risk of aspiration
- RLN palsy
  - Ipsilateral VC assumes the paramedian position
  - Voice is weak and hoarse
  - Phonation will NOT be possible with bilateral injury
  - Airway obstruction can occur with bilateral injury

QUESTIONS

1. Which of the following is associated with an increase in IOP?

   A. Blinking
   B. Hyperventilation
   C. Head elevation
   D. Diuretic administration

2. Which of the following statements regarding the OCR is most correct?

   A. Traction on medial rectus muscle is unlikely to incite the reflex
   B. The reflex can occur if the globe is enucleated
   C. The reflex is potentiated by repeated stimulation
   D. It is dissipated by direct pressure on the globe

3. Normal IOP is closest to which of the following pressures?

   A. 0–4 mm Hg
   B. 5–9 mm Hg
   C. 10–20 mm Hg
   D. 21–30 mm Hg

4. Which of the following statements is most correct with regard to the management of an airway fire?

   A. The F_{IO_2} should be reduced immediately by adding nitrous oxide to the circuit.
   B. Saline should be poured into the airway to extinguish the fire
   C. The endotracheal tube should remain in place until the fire has been extinguished
   D. Rigid bronchoscopy should be avoided if there is concern for residual debris in the airway

5. A patient with upper airway obstruction requires an awake tracheostomy. Blockade of which of the following nerves is most appropriate to facilitate the procedure?

   A. Superior laryngeal nerve
   B. Recurrent laryngeal nerve
   C. Glossopharyngeal nerve
   D. Trigeminal nerve

LAPAROSCOPY

- Peritoneal space is insufflated with carbon dioxide for surgical visualization
  - Intra-abdominal pressures (IAPs) typically 12 to 15 mm Hg
- Benefits of laparoscopy to open surgery
  - Smaller incision
  - Reduced stress response
  - Reduced postoperative pain
  - Reduced pulmonary dysfunction
  - Reduced postoperative ileus
- Organ system effects of pneumoperitoneum
  - Cerebral effects
    - Increased $Paco_2$ → increased cerebral blood flow
    - Increased intracranial pressure
  - Cardiovascular effects
    - Reduced venous return → mild decrease in cardiac output
    - Increased catecholamines, vasopressin, and angiotensin–renin → increased systemic vascular resistance → increased blood pressure
    - Reflex response to peritoneal stretch → arrhythmias
      - Intense vagal stimulation during insufflation→ severe bradycardia and possible asystole
  - Respiratory effects
    - Decreased lung compliance
    - Decreased functional residual capacity (FRC)
    - Increased minute ventilation necessary to maintain normocarbia
    - Increased $Paco_2$ to $ETco_2$ gradient
  - Renal effects
    - Decreased renal blood flow
    - Increased angiotensin–renin → decreased urine output
- Complications
  - Extraperitoneal insufflation → cutaneous emphysema
  - Insufflation through diaphragmatic defects → pneumothorax or pneumomediastinum
  - Intravascular injection → gas embolism

GENERAL SURGERY CONSIDERATIONS

- **Aspiration precautions**
  - Many patients undergoing urgent or emergent gastrointestinal surgery should be considered full-stomachs regardless of NPO (nil per os; Latin for "nothing by mouth") duration
    - Examples: small bowel obstruction, gastrointestinal bleed, acute appendicitis, bowel perforation
  - Aspiration of >25 cc (and pH <2.5) of gastric acid material can cause destruction of the surfactant-producing cells in the lungs and damage capillary endothelium
  - Aspiration of fecal material carries a high mortality risk
  - Mendelson syndrome
    - Aspiration of gastric acid that leads to pulmonary edema, decreased pulmonary compliance, and pulmonary hypertension

- **Gastroesophageal reflux disease**
  - Weakness of lower esophageal sphincter or increased gastric acid secretion → increased risk of aspiration
  - **Hiatal hernia** is a protrusion of the stomach into the diaphragm → increased aspiration risk
- Anesthetic considerations
  - Continue perioperative H_2-blockers and proton pump inhibitors
  - Consider rapid sequence intubation
  - Sitting, awake intubation may be indicated in cases of high-risk aspiration
- Obesity
  - Classification by body mass index (BMI)
    - BMI 25 to 30: overweight
    - BMI 30 to 40: obese
    - BMI >40: morbid obesity
  - Anesthetic considerations for obesity
    - Increased gastric volumes and decreased gastric emptying → increased aspiration risk
    - Increased redundant airway tissues → increased difficulty mask ventilating
      - Associated with BMI >26
    - Decreased FRC → rapid desaturation
    - Increased closing capacity → increased atelectasis
    - Decreased thoracic compliance secondary to chest wall weight and abdominal fat → increased work of breathing
    - Increased preexisting hypertension, hyperlipidemia, and diabetes → increased cardiovascular complications
    - Increased volume of distribution and lipid reserve → alters drugs dosing and metabolism
  - Associated diseases
    - **Obstructive sleep apnea (OSA)**
      - Repetitive pauses in breathing during sleep despite efforts to breathe
        - Diagnosed by polysomnography
        - 71% of bariatric population with OSA
      - Apnea–Hypopnea index (AHI) used to diagnose OSA
        - AHI = number of apneic, hypopneic episodes per hour
          - Apnea = no ventilation for >10 seconds
          - Hypopnea = 50% decrease in airflow or decrease in O_2 saturation ≥4%
        - Classification of OSA
          - AHI <5 → normal
          - AHI 5 to 15 → mild
          - AHI 15 to 30 → moderate
          - AHI >30 → severe
      - Anesthetic implications
        - OSA patients who mix opioids with alcohol → 3× desaturations
        - OSA associated with pulmonary hypertension and cor pulmonale → right heart failure
        - Increased sensitivity to opioids → increased respiratory depression
        - Recovery
          - Monitor in PACU (postanesthesia care unit) for 3 hours longer
          - Monitor for 7 hours after last episode of airway obstruction
    - Obesity hypoventilation syndrome (Pickwickian syndrome)
      - Sleep-disordered breathing where obesity results in chronically inadequate ventilation
        - Morbid obesity (BMI >30)
        - Chronic hypoventilation ($Paco_2$ >45)
      - Laboratory value findings
        - Respiratory acidosis
        - Metabolic alkalosis (HCO_3 often >30)
        - Hypoxemia
      - Associated with increased mortality
        - Severe pulmonary HTN (hypertension) and right ventricular failure common
    - Metabolic syndrome
      - Disorder of energy utilization and storage

- Diagnosis (3/5 required)
  - Central obesity
  - Hypertension
  - Hyperglycemia
  - Hypertriglyceridemia
  - Low high-density cholesterol
- Associated with coronary artery disease, diabetes, heart failure

■ **Hepatic dysfunction**
- Hepatic anatomy
  - Consists of four lobes (right, left, caudate, quadrate)
  - **Blood flow**
    - Distribution
      - Liver receives 25% of cardiac output
        - Portal vein carries 75% of total hepatic flow (blood is partially deoxygenated)
        - Hepatic artery is 25% of total hepatic flow (blood is oxygenated)
      - Portal vein and hepatic artery each provide 50% of oxygen to the liver
    - Regulation
      - Hepatic arterial buffer response
        - If portal blood flow decreases → hepatic artery dilates
        - If hepatic artery constricts → portal flow increases
      - Hepatic arterial buffer response modulated by adenosine
        - Adenosine is a vasodilator that accumulates during low portal venous flow → increases hepatic artery flow
- **Liver function** (Fig. 10.1)

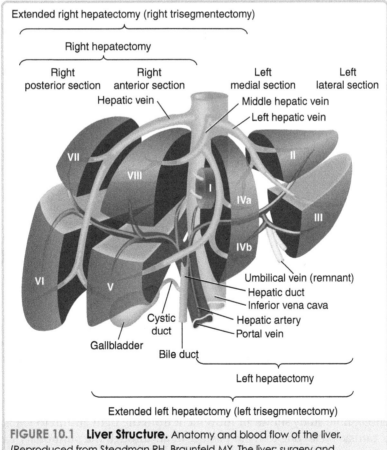

FIGURE 10.1 Liver Structure. Anatomy and blood flow of the liver. (Reproduced from Steadman RH, Braunfeld MY. The liver: surgery and anesthesia. In: Barash PG, Cullen BF, Stoelting RK, et al., eds. *Clinical Anesthesia.* 7th ed. Philadelphia, PA: Wolters Kluwer; 2013:1320.)

- ◆ Glucose homeostasis
- ◆ Fat metabolism
- ◆ Protein synthesis
  - ➤ All proteins are made in the liver EXCEPT gamma globulins
  - ➤ Major protein = albumin (half-life ~23 days)
- ◆ Coagulation
  - ➤ All factors are produced in the liver EXCEPT Factor VIII (RBCs)
- ◆ Cholinesterase
- ◆ Biotransformation of drugs
  - ➤ Many drugs are cleared by hepatic metabolism, and if liver dysfunction is present, their clearance is therefore less effective and drug effects can be prolonged
- ◆ Bilirubin excretion
- ◆ Bile excretion
- ● **Liver disease markers**
  - ◆ Hepatic function: albumin, international normalized ratio (INR)
    - ➤ **Albumin:** marker of protein synthesis
    - ➤ **INR:** marker of coagulation factor synthesis
  - ◆ Hepatocellular integrity: aspartate aminotransferase (AST), alanine aminotransferase (ALT), ammonia, gamma-glutamyl transferase (GGT)
    - ➤ AST: present in liver, heart, muscles, and kidneys
    - ➤ ALT: more specific to liver than AST
    - ➤ Ammonia: marker of hepatocellular damage and disruption of urea synthesis
    - ➤ GGT: elevated in liver disease during alcohol abuse
  - ◆ Excretory function: alkaline phosphatase, bilirubin
    - ➤ Alkaline phosphatase: excreted in bile → reflects patency of biliary tree
    - ➤ Conjugated (direct) bilirubin: reflects hepatocellular dysfunction, intrahepatic cholestasis, and extrahepatic biliary obstruction
    - ➤ Unconjugated (indirect) bilirubin: reflects hemolysis or defects in bilirubin conjugation
    - ➤ Clinical jaundice occurs when total bilirubin > 3
  - ◆ Serum ascites albumin gradient (SAAG): serum albumin—ascitic albumin
    - ➤ Low SAAG: peritonitis, malignancy, nephrotic syndrome, pancreatitis, tuberculosis
    - ➤ High SAAG: cirrhosis, congestive heart failure, myxedema, portal vein thrombosis, Budd–Chiari syndrome
- ● Hemodynamic changes and clinical findings associated with liver disease
  - ◆ Hepatic encephalopathy
  - ◆ High cardiac output
  - ◆ Tachycardia
  - ◆ Low systemic vascular resistance
  - ◆ Increased IAP
- ● Syndromes
  - ◆ Hepatopulmonary syndrome
    - ➤ Triad
      - ❖ Hepatic dysfunction
      - ❖ Increased A-a gradient
      - ❖ Intrapulmonary vasodilation
    - ➤ Mechanism
      - ❖ Inability of liver to clear vasodilating substances → elevated nitric oxide levels → intrapulmonary vasodilation → shunts occur within pulmonary circulation
      - ❖ Reversal of hypoxic pulmonary vasoconstriction → increased V/Q mismatch → hypoxemia
        - › Hypoxemia may be worsened in upright position (orthodeoxia)
    - ➤ Diagnosis
      - ❖ Echo bubble study shows air movement from the right atrium to left atrium in three to six cardiac cycles due to rapid passage of air through the pulmonary vasculature
      - ❖ In patients without hepatopulmonary syndrome, small microbubbles will not pass through the pulmonary capillaries

- ◆ Hepatorenal syndrome
  - ➤ Mechanism
    - ❖ The splanchnic system is severely vasodilated, but the renal arteries are vasoconstricted
      - › Portal hypertension and concomitant renal failure
    - ❖ Pre-renal condition due to decreased intravascular tone → perception of inadequate volume status by the kidneys
  - ➤ Diagnosis is difficult due to multiple causes that may impact renal perfusion
    - ❖ Hepatorenal syndrome is a diagnosis of exclusion
    - ❖ Patients without other modes of renal injury such as shock, sepsis, nephrotoxins
    - ❖ Patients are not fluid responsive
  - ➤ Treatment options
    - ❖ Dialysis
    - ❖ Transjugular intrahepatic portosystemic shunt
    - ❖ Liver transplantation
- ◆ **Portopulmonary hypertension**
  - ➤ Mechanism
    - ❖ Cirrhosis → increased hepatic resistance → increased portal venous pressure → blood shunts from portal to systemic circulation → hyperdynamic circulatory changes
    - ❖ Shunt of blood from portal to systemic circulation → toxins and metabolites reach pulmonary circulation → smooth muscle hypertrophy (increased medial thickness in pulmonary arteries with narrowing of vascular lumen due to fibrosis)→ pulmonary hypertension
  - ➤ Diagnosis
    - ❖ Mean pulmonary artery pressure (PAP) >25 mm Hg and pulmonary artery occlusion pressure (PAOP) <15 mm Hg
    - ❖ Pulmonary vascular resistance >240 dynes $\times$ s $\times$ cm^{-5}
  - ➤ Cause of right-sided heart failure after transplantation
- ● **Anesthetic management in liver disease**
  - ◆ **Altered metabolism** of anesthetic drugs
    - ➤ Opioids, propofol, benzodiazepines, ketamine, and several neuromuscular blockers are metabolized at the liver
  - ◆ Hemodynamic changes
    - ➤ Liver disease may be associated with hypotension that is exacerbated by anesthetics → increased risk of postoperative hepatic dysfunction
    - ➤ Lower central venous pressure during liver operations may be associated with reduced bleeding
  - ◆ Coagulopathy
    - ➤ Increased prothrombin time (PT), partial thromboplastin time (PTT) can occur in liver disease and predispose to increased bleeding
    - ➤ May restrict neuraxial or regional anesthesia use
- ● Causes of postoperative liver dysfunction
  - ◆ Surgical injury or surgical restriction of blood flow
  - ◆ Massive transfusion
  - ◆ Halothane hepatitis
- ■ **Abdominal compartment syndrome** (Fig. 10.2)
  - ● Classification
    - ◆ Normal IAP: 5 to 7 mm Hg
    - ◆ Intra-abdominal hypertension: >12 mm Hg
    - ◆ Abdominal compartment syndrome: IAP >20 mm Hg
      - ➤ Abdominal compartment syndrome requires IAP >20 mm Hg and new organ system dysfunction
      - ➤ Common organ systems affected include renal (decreased urine output), pulmonary (increased pulmonary pressures), and gastrointestinal (mesenteric ischemia)
  - ● IAP pressure influences abdominal perfusion pressure
    - ◆ Abdominal perfusion pressure = mean arterial pressure − intra-abdominal pressure

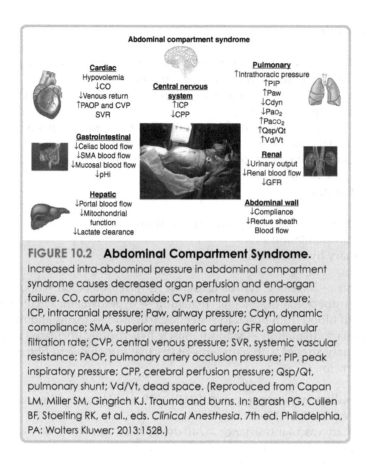

FIGURE 10.2 Abdominal Compartment Syndrome.
Increased intra-abdominal pressure in abdominal compartment syndrome causes decreased organ perfusion and end-organ failure. CO, carbon monoxide; CVP, central venous pressure; ICP, intracranial pressure; Paw, airway pressure; Cdyn, dynamic compliance; SMA, superior mesenteric artery; GFR, glomerular filtration rate; CVP, central venous pressure; SVR, systemic vascular resistance; PAOP, pulmonary artery occlusion pressure; PIP, peak inspiratory pressure; CPP, cerebral perfusion pressure; Qsp/Qt, pulmonary shunt; Vd/Vt, dead space. (Reproduced from Capan LM, Miller SM, Gingrich KJ. Trauma and burns. In: Barash PG, Cullen BF, Stoelting RK, et al., eds. *Clinical Anesthesia*. 7th ed. Philadelphia, PA: Wolters Kluwer; 2013:1528.)

- Factors causing increased abdominal pressure
  - Obesity
  - Pregnancy
  - Burns
  - Massive fluid resuscitation
  - Ascites or hemoperitoneum
  - Abdominal inflammation or edema
  - Postsurgical inflammation
- Treatment
  - Medical options to temporize abdominal compartment syndrome include deep sedation and paralytics
  - Increased blood pressure may aid perfusion, but may also worsen underlying cause (e.g., hemorrhage)
  - Surgical laparotomy and decompression may be required

SPECIFIC GENERAL SURGERIES

- **Bariatric surgery**
  - Preoperative patient risk factors
    - Cardiovascular status
      - Increased risk of coronary artery disease and hyperlipidemia
      - Increased risk of left ventricular hypertrophy
      - Increased risk of essential hypertension
    - Respiratory status
      - Decreased FRC
      - Increased OSA
      - Increased pulmonary hypertension

- Gastrointestinal status
  - Increased gastroesophageal reflux disease
  - Increased risk of liver disease, especially nonalcoholic steatohepatitis (NASH)
- Endocrine status
  - Increased risk of diabetes mellitus type II
  - Increased risk of metabolic syndrome
- Pharmacologic considerations
  - Hydrophilic medications should be dosed by ideal body weight
    - Examples: opioids, nondepolarizing muscle relaxants
  - Lipophilic medications should be dosed by total body weight
    - Example: propofol
  - Succinylcholine should be dosed by total body weight due to increased cholinesterase
- Anesthetic management
  - Preoxygenation
    - Decreased FRC → rapid desaturation
    - Decreased closing capacity → increased atelectasis
    - Do not induce until expired oxygen >80%
    - Consider adding 5 cm H_2O of positive end-expiratory pressure (PEEP) during preoxygenation to prevent atelectasis
  - Intubation
    - Increased Mallampati score is not very sensitive or specific for difficult intubations
    - Increased BMI is not associated with increased difficulty intubating assuming optimal positioning
    - Mask ventilation may be more difficult due to redundant tissue
  - Ventilation
    - Increased PEEP improves oxygenation
    - Increased tidal volumes not associated with improved oxygenation
- Postoperative management
  - Opioids
    - Obesity increases sensitivity to opioids
    - Increased risk of desaturations
  - PACU monitoring
    - Consider increased monitoring in PACU or postoperatively
- **Intestinal obstruction**
  - Causes
    - Ileus
      - Postsurgical (paralytic) ileus is common postoperatively
      - Effect increased with opioids and antimuscarinics
      - Often resolve with time
      - Epidural with local anesthetics may increase parasympathetic tone → decrease ileus
    - Mechanical
      - Masses such as tumors or obstruction caused by adhesions, hernias, volvulus, or intussusception
      - Require operative intervention
    - Vascular
      - Decreased flow or occlusion of the celiac, superior mesenteric, or inferior mesenteric arteries
      - Require reperfusion or operative intervention
  - Physiological changes
    - Vomiting → hypochloremic metabolic alkalosis
    - Mesenteric ischemia → metabolic acidosis
    - Limited oral intake → hypovolemia
    - Abdominal distention → decreased FRC, respiratory distress, increased aspiration risk
  - Anesthetic management
    - Assume full stomach
    - Fluid resuscitate to correct metabolic derangements
    - Avoid nitrous oxide to prevent bowel dilation

- Liposuction
  - Done under local anesthesia or general anesthesia
    - Semitumescent liposuction requires deep sedation or general anesthesia
    - Tumescent liposuction can be done under local anesthesia
  - Local anesthesia involves injecting a large amount of dilute fluid supplemented with lidocaine and epinephrine into the fat to be removed
    - Benefits of local anesthesia with epinephrine include analgesic effects, decrease in blood loss, and increased firmness to facilitate fat removal
    - Maximum dose of lidocaine recommended for liposuction is 55 mg/kg with 0.055 mg/kg of epinephrine
      - 55 mg/kg would be an otherwise toxic dose of lidocaine (typical limit is 7 mg/kg)
      - Toxicity is rare
        - Most lidocaine removed when fat is removed
        - Diffusion into circulation is slow—peak lidocaine levels occur at 8 hours postoperatively
- Thyroidectomy
  - Postoperative concerns
    - Neck hematoma → compression of trachea
      - Requires emergent decompression of hematoma and securing airway
    - Recurrent laryngeal nerve injury → airway obstruction due to inability to abduct the cords
    - Hypocalcemia occurs 24 to 72 hours postoperatively due to hypoparathyroidism → presents with labored breathing, stridor, and laryngospasm
      - Treatment is with calcium repletion

ABDOMINAL ORGAN TRANSPLANTATION

- **Liver transplantation**
  - Candidacy
    - Indicated for end-stage liver disease (ESLD) caused by cirrhosis (alcoholic, hepatitis induced), hemochromatosis, Wilson disease
    - ABO blood type
      - Identical matching associated with improved graft survival
    - Scoring for ESLD and transplant candidacy
      - Model for end-stage liver disease (MELD)
        - Components: INR, bilirubin, and creatinine
        - MELD is scored numerically
        - MELD score is correlated with 3-month mortality
      - Child–Pugh
        - Components: INR, bilirubin, albumin, ascites, hepatic encephalopathy
        - Child–Pugh is scored A through C (C is the worst)
        - Child–Pugh score is correlated with 1- and 2-year mortality
    - Contraindications to liver transplantation
      - Pulmonary hypertension
      - Significant coronary artery disease
      - Sepsis or refractory infection
    - Hyponatremia is associated with increased risk of death prior to transplantation
  - Stages of surgical procedure
    - Dissection
      - Dissection of the native liver and gallbladder
      - Associated with significant fluid losses through ascites and hemorrhage
    - Anhepatic
      - Liver isolated from circulation
        - Removal of the native liver and creation of the new vein anastomoses
        - Circulation can be supported by veno–veno bypass or the piggyback technique during clamp time
      - Associated with decreased venous return, metabolic acidosis, coagulopathy, hyperkalemia, and citrate toxicity/hypocalcemia

- ◆ Reperfusion
  - ➤ Removal of the portal vein clamp
  - ➤ Washout of embolic material, cytokines, and electrolytes → significant hemodynamic instability → including arrhythmias, hypotension, and potential for hyperkalemic cardiac arrest
  - ➤ Hypothermia
  - ➤ Air embolism
  - ➤ Right ventricular (RV) overload
  - ◆ Posthepatic
    - ➤ Reconstruction of hepatic artery, biliary anastomoses, and ensuring adequate hemostasis
- Veno–veno bypass vs. Piggyback for anhepatic stage
  - ◆ Veno–veno bypass
    - ➤ Used in liver transplantation to shunt venous blood from below the liver to the superior vena cava following inferior vena cava clamping
    - ➤ Advantages
      - ❖ Maintenance of cerebral, cardiac, pulmonary, and renal blood flow
      - ❖ Decreased venous congestion
    - ➤ Disadvantages
      - ❖ Increased risk of pulmonary or air emboli
      - ❖ Thrombosis
      - ❖ Vascular access injury
      - ❖ No evidence of improved organ function
      - ❖ Increased cost
  - ◆ Piggyback
    - ➤ Used in liver transplantation to preserve the native inferior vena cava, which is only partially clamped
    - ➤ Advantages
      - ❖ Improved hemodynamic stability
      - ❖ Decreased blood loss
    - ➤ Disadvantages
      - ❖ Increased technical difficulty
- Anesthetic considerations
  - ◆ Majority of these patients will have portal hypertension
    - ➤ Ascites, splenomegaly, collateral venous flow, and arteriovenous shunting
  - ◆ Rapid sequence intubation due to ascites and delayed gastric emptying
  - ◆ Necessary volume access for potential massive intraoperative bleeding
    - ➤ Patients are often coagulopathic secondary to liver disease
    - ➤ Potential for major blood loss given proximity of large vessels
  - ◆ Frequent blood gas and electrolyte checks during anhepatic and reperfusion phases to monitor for coagulopathy, acidosis, and electrolyte abnormalities
  - ◆ Preparation for reperfusion should include 100% oxygen, hyperventilation, increased vasopressors, and calcium

■ **Kidney transplantation**
- Candidacy
  - ◆ ABO blood type and HLA (human leukocyte antigen) capability desired between donor and recipient
  - ◆ Indicated for end-stage renal disease (ESRD)
    - ➤ Patients may be on dialysis or near dialysis
  - ◆ Donor organ can be from living donor, brain-dead donors, or cardiac-death donors
    - ➤ With adequate preservation, cadaveric donor kidneys can last up to 48 hours
  - ◆ Contraindications vary, but include significant preoperative cardiovascular disease, cancer, severe infections, and substance use/abuse
- Surgical procedure
  - ◆ Donor kidneys implanted into the iliac fossa using the external iliac artery and vein for vascular anastomoses
- Anesthetic considerations

- Use of succinylcholine is not contraindicated in ESRD
  - Potassium increases to the same degree as those without ESRD and then normalizes
- Ensure adequate volume status to improve perfusion to kidneys
  - Lactated ringers associated with less hyperkalemia than normal saline
  - Vasopressors may decrease renal blood flow
- Monitor urine output closely
  - Decreased urine output may be a sign of postrenal obstruction or defective anastomoses
- Diuretics may be used to expand urine volume
  - Mannitol may protect kidney from ischemic injury
- Cyclosporine is often used to prevent rejection
  - Inhibits the T cell–mediated response
  - Levels need to be monitored closely as it can cause nephrotoxicity in up to 40% of patients
- **Pancreas transplant**
  - Candidacy
    - ABO, HLA, and crossmatching necessary between donor and recipient
    - Indicated primarily for type I diabetes
  - Surgical procedure
    - Donor pancreas implanted into the abdomen
    - Arterial and venous blood supply can be connected to a variety of vessels based on surgical preference
    - Exocrine pancreatic flow is connected to the small bowel
  - Anesthetic considerations
    - Patients should be assessed for diabetic comorbidities
    - Blood glucose levels should be monitored frequently intraoperatively

SPECIFIC GENITOURINARY PROCEDURES

- **Transurethral resection of the prostate (TURP)**
  - Cystoscope with electrocautery to resect tissue → relieves symptoms of benign prostatic hypertrophy
    - Significant amount of irrigation is used for visualization
  - Anesthetic choice
    - General or spinal
    - Spinal must be at least at level of T8 to block sensation from the bladder, ureters, and renal pelvis
  - Complications
    - Opening of large prostatic venous sinuses → irrigant absorption
      - Can absorb ~20 cc fluid/min and up to 6 to 8 L in prolonged cases
      - Symptoms
        - Water irrigation solutions → can cause severe hyponatremia and electrolyte abnormalities → hemolysis, seizures, cerebral edema
        - Glycine irrigation solutions → glycine metabolized to ammonia → **hyperammonemia** → sedation and temporary blindness
        - Significant volume absorption → hypertension, pulmonary edema, and **congestive heart failure**
        - Electrolyte shifts → arrhythmias
      - Factors increasing irrigant absorption
        - Increased height of irrigant above patient
          - Keep solution <60 cm above level of surgical field to minimize pressure gradient for absorption
        - Decreased peripheral venous pressure
        - Increased surgery duration
        - Increased surface area disrupted during surgery
    - Bladder perforation
      - Extraperitoneal perforation → suprapubic fullness or pain
      - Intraperitoneal perforation → abdominal pain or referred shoulder pain

- **Lithotripsy**
  - Acoustic shock waves → urinary stone fracture
    - First-generation lithotripsy: requires immersion of patient in water bath
    - Second-generation lithotripsy: eliminates water bath and can be done on table
  - Anesthetic
    - General, spinal, or sedation
  - Complications
    - Skin bruising or hematoma at entry site
    - Hematuria due to genitourinary endothelial injury
    - Arrhythmias due to interaction of shock waves on cardiac conduction system
    - Application to lung tissue → alveolar rupture
    - Common peroneal nerve damage from over flexing legs in lithotomy position

QUESTIONS

1. A 50-year-old man develops acute respiratory distress and has an acute oxygen desaturation in the PACU shortly after undergoing total thyroidectomy. On examination, the neck appears firm with moderate enlargement. HR is 135 bpm; BP is 170/80 mm Hg. While preparing for emergent intubation, which of the following is the most appropriate next step for management?

   A. Opening of the neck wound
   B. Administration of IV calcium
   C. Transport to the operating room
   D. Administration of IV labetalol

2. A 45-year-old woman is undergoing preoperative evaluation for abdominoplasty. She has a history of hypertension and smokes 1/2 pack of cigarettes per day. She reports that her husband often complains that she snores at night and has observed her stop breathing during sleep. She denies feeling tired or sleepy during the daytime. On examination, she has a neck circumference of 40 in. and a BMI of 33. On the basis of the STOP-Bang questionnaire, what is her risk for OSA?

   A. None
   B. Low
   C. Moderate
   D. High

3. Which of the following statements regarding use of the MELD score assessing the severity of chronic liver disease is most correct?

   A. The components of the score are INR, bilirubin, and albumin
   B. It is scored A through C
   C. It is most strongly correlated with 1–2-year survival
   D. Scores may increase or decrease for a given individual

4. A 35-year-old woman is stabbed in the liver. She arrives in the emergency department hypotensive, and after an emergent laparotomy and large volume fluid resuscitation, she was admitted to the ICU. Vital signs in the ICU are: T 36.8, HR 105, R 20, BP 100/77, O_2 saturation 98%, and CVP is 6. She is receiving volume control ventilation with TV 400, R16, PEEP 8, and 80% FIO_2. Peak and plateau pressures are 30 and 28. An arterial blood gas on those settings is 7.32/38/92. Lactate is 0.9. Urine output has been 25 cc/hr for the last 2 hours. Bladder pressure is measured and is 20 mm Hg. Which of the following is the next most appropriate step in treatment?

   A. Fluid bolus
   B. Decompressive laparotomy
   C. Paracentesis
   D. Diuresis

5. Which of the following is most consistent with the diagnosis of TURP syndrome?

   A. Hypernatremia
   B. Hypercalcemia
   C. Hypervolemia
   D. Hyperosmolarity

RENAL ANATOMY AND PHYSIOLOGY

- **Fluid compartments**
  - 60% of total body weight is water
    - Two-third of total body weight is intracellular
    - One-third of total body weight is extracellular
      - Three-fourth of extracellular fluid is interstitial
      - One-fourth of extracellular fluid is intravascular
  - **Response to hypovolemia**
    - Renin–angiotensin–aldosterone (RAA) (Fig. 11.1)
      - The juxtaglomerular apparatus releases renin → cleaves angiotensinogen to angiotensin I → angiotensin-converting enzyme (ACE) converts angiotensin I (in lungs)→ stimulates aldosterone release
      - RAA activated by sympathetic stimulation, renal hypoperfusion, and hyponatremia
      - Aldosterone increases reabsorption of sodium
    - Antidiuretic hormone (ADH)
      - Secreted by the posterior pituitary
      - ADH release stimulated by increased osmolality, hypovolemia, and sympathetic stimulation
        - Surgery can increase ADH levels
      - Stimulates the renal tubule to reabsorb water
- Renal anatomy
  - Kidneys are located in the retroperitoneal space (Fig. 11.2)
  - Blood supply
    - Receives 20% of cardiac output
      - Receives blood from renal artery → drains in to renal veins
      - Autoregulation (maintenance of a relatively consistent perfusion/blood flow despite blood pressure changes) is well established for
        - Systolic blood pressure (SBP) ranging from 90 to 200 mm Hg
        - Mean arterial pressure (MAP) ranging from 60 to 160 mm Hg
    - Afferent arterioles
      - Branch of renal artery → diverge into capillaries of the glomerulus → supply the nephrons
    - Efferent arteriole
      - Collection of capillaries draining blood from the glomerulus → supply the efferent arteriole
    - Afferent and efferent arteriole regulate renal blood flow through constriction or dilation
      - Afferent arteriole constricts from sympathetic stimulation, angiotensin II, and endothelin
      - Afferent arteriole dilates from prostaglandin, nitric oxide, atrial natriuretic peptide, dopamine, fenoldopam, and bradykinin
  - Structures
    - Outer renal cortex
    - Inner renal medulla
    - Nephron is a functional unit that spans both the cortex and medulla
  - Pathway of filtrate through kidney
    - Proximal convoluted tubule
      - Reabsorbs sodium, chloride, glucose, amino acids, and bicarbonate
    - Loop of Henle
      - Descending

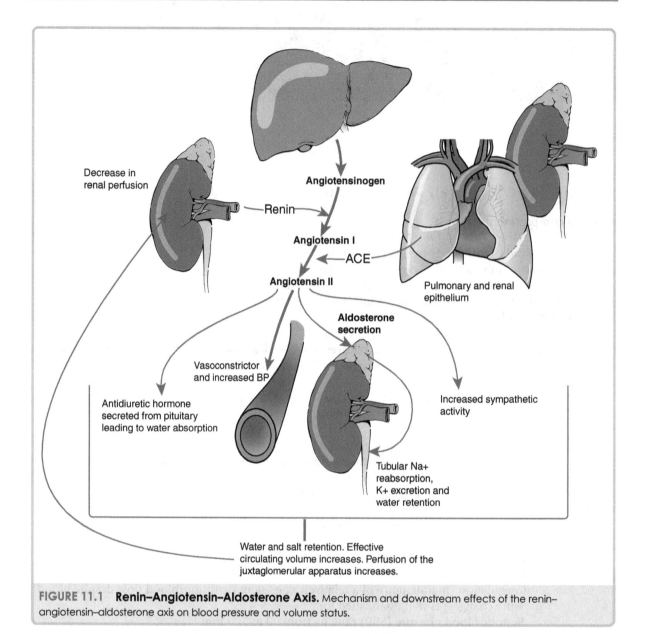

FIGURE 11.1   Renin–Angiotensin–Aldosterone Axis. Mechanism and downstream effects of the renin–angiotensin–aldosterone axis on blood pressure and volume status.

- ❖ Reabsorbs water
  - ➤ Ascending
    - ❖ Impermeable to water
    - ❖ Reabsorbs sodium, potassium, chloride
- ❖ Distal convoluted tubule
  - ➤ Reabsorbs sodium and chloride
- ❖ Collecting tubule
  - ➤ Reabsorbs sodium and water
  - ➤ Excretes potassium and protons
- ■ **Diuretics** (Fig. 11.3)
  - ● **Thiazide**
    - ❖ Function at the distal convoluted tubule
    - ❖ Inhibits the sodium–chloride transporter
      - ➤ Associated with hypokalemia, hyponatremia, hypomagnesia
      - ➤ Associated with hypercalcemia, hyperglycemia, hyperuricemia
    - ❖ Example: hydrochlorothiazide

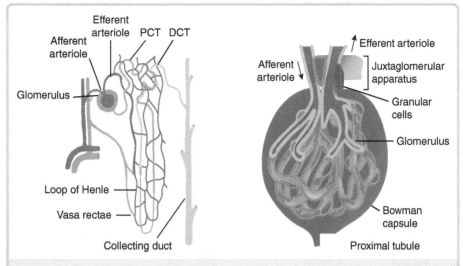

FIGURE 11.2 Kidney Structure. Structure of the kidney and pathway of blood flow. PCT, proximal convoluted tubule; DCT, distal convoluted tubule. (Reproduced from Stafford-Smith M, Shaw A, Sandler A, et al. The renal system and anesthesia for urologic surgery. In: Barash PG, Cullen BF, Stoelting RK, et al., eds. *Clinical Anesthesia*. 7th ed. Philadelphia, PA: Wolters Kluwer; 2013:1402.)

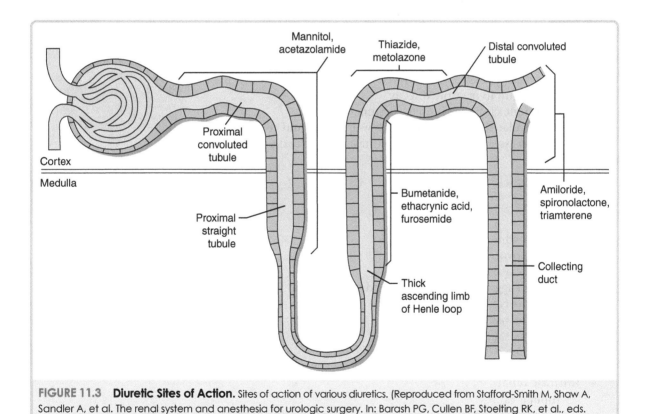

FIGURE 11.3 Diuretic Sites of Action. Sites of action of various diuretics. (Reproduced from Stafford-Smith M, Shaw A, Sandler A, et al. The renal system and anesthesia for urologic surgery. In: Barash PG, Cullen BF, Stoelting RK, et al., eds. *Clinical Anesthesia*. 7th ed. Philadelphia, PA: Wolters Kluwer; 2013:1414.)

- **Loop**
  - Function at ascending loop of Henle
  - Inhibit Na-K-2Cl transporter
  - Examples: furosemide, torsemide

- ◆ Associated with hypokalemia
- ● **Osmotic**
  - ◆ Filtered at the glomerulus, but are not reabsorbed
    - ➤ Increased osmolality in filtrate → increased water elimination
  - ◆ Example: mannitol
- ● **Carbonic anhydrase inhibitor**
  - ◆ Function at the proximal convoluted tubule
  - ◆ Inhibits carbonic anhydrase and promotes bicarbonate excretion
  - ◆ Example: acetazolamide
- ● **Aldosterone antagonists**
  - ◆ Potassium "sparing" diuretics
  - ◆ Function at distal convoluted tubule and collecting duct
  - ◆ Inhibit sodium reabsorption
  - ◆ Examples:
    - ➤ Spironolactone—will only work when aldosterone is present as it is a direct inhibitor
    - ➤ Amiloride and triamterene—will work independent of the presence of aldosterone
- ■ Renal function tests
  - ● Creatinine
    - ◆ Creatinine is a breakdown product from muscle
      - ➤ Produced at a fairly constant rate → eliminated by the kidneys
    - ◆ Elevated creatinine can be a sign of inappropriate elimination and renal damage
  - ● Blood urea nitrogen (BUN)
    - ◆ BUN is a breakdown product of proteins → eliminated by the kidneys
    - ◆ Elevated BUN can be a sign of inappropriate elimination and renal damage
      - ➤ Other causes of elevated BUN include gastrointestinal hemorrhage, increased catabolism, steroid use, and a high protein diet
  - ● Glomerular filtration rate (GFR)
    - ◆ GFR is an estimate of the flow rate of filtered fluid through the kidney
      - ➤ Difficult to measure directly
    - ◆ Creatinine clearance is used to estimate GFR
      - ➤ Calculated value based on age, weight, sex, and creatinine
    - ◆ Used to assess renal function and stage of kidney disease

RENAL DISORDERS

- ■ Classification
  - ● **Pre-renal**
    - ◆ Decreased renal perfusion
      - ➤ Hypovolemia
      - ➤ Decreased blood pressure
    - ◆ Results suggestive of pre-renal conditions include
      - ➤ Urine Na <25
      - ➤ Urine osm >500
      - ➤ FENa <1%
      - ➤ FEurea <35%
      - ➤ BUN: Cr ratio >15
  - ● **Intrinsic renal**
    - ◆ Tubular causes
      - ➤ Ischemic injury from hypotension or nephrotoxic drug
    - ◆ Glomerular causes
      - ➤ Glomerulonephritis or autoimmune renal disease
    - ◆ Interstitial causes
      - ➤ Associated with drug reactions
    - ◆ Vascular causes
      - ➤ Embolic causes
    - ◆ Results suggestive of intrinsic renal conditions include

TABLE 11.1 Urine Analysis

Urinary analysis findings	Suggestive of
1. Proteinuria	Renal parenchymal disease
2. Red blood cells	Trauma, tumor, infection
3. White blood cells +/− bacteria	Infection
4. Fatty casts	Nephrotic syndrome
5. Ketones	Diabetic ketoacidosis, starvation

- ➤ Urine Na >40
- ➤ Urine osm ~200 to 300
- ➤ FENa >3%
- ➤ FEurea >50%
- ➤ Bun:Cr ratio <15
- ● **Postrenal**
  - ◆ Obstruction of urinary flow (Table 11.1)
- ■ Risk, Injury, Failure, Loss, and ESRD (RIFLE) classification
  - ● Risk: creatinine increase 1.5× baseline, GFR decrease of 25%
    - ◆ Urine output <0.5 cc/kg/hr × 6 hours
  - ● Injury: creatinine increase 2× baseline, GFR decrease of 50%
    - ◆ Urine output <0.5 cc/kg/hr × 12 hours
  - ● Failure: creatinine increase 3× baseline, GFR decrease of 75%, or serum creatinine ≥4.0
    - ◆ Urine output <0.3 cc/kg/hr × 24 hours or anuria
  - ● Loss: loss of renal function >4 weeks
  - ● ESRD: loss of renal function >3 months
- ■ Contrast nephropathy
  - ● Definition
    - ◆ Greater than 25% increase in serum creatinine or absolute increase in serum creatinine of 0.5 mg/dL following intravenous contrast use
  - ● Risk factors
    - ◆ Age >75
    - ◆ Preexisting renal disease
    - ◆ Hypotension
    - ◆ Congestive heart failure
    - ◆ Increased use of contrast agent
  - ● Prevention
    - ◆ Hydration with normal saline or sodium bicarbonate
      - ➤ Evidence does not support sodium bicarbonate over normal saline
    - ◆ *N*-acetylcysteine
      - ➤ Theorized that antioxidant and vasodilatory properties of *N*-acetylcysteine ↑ renal blood flow
      - ➤ Studies have not shown reduction in acute renal failure or need for hemodialysis
    - ◆ No evidence to support furosemide or mannitol
- ■ Hemofiltration and dialysis
  - ● **Hemodialysis**
    - ◆ Usage of a semipermeable membrane to remove waste products, eliminate fluid, and restore electrolyte concentrations
    - ◆ Access is through a fistula or large-bore catheter with two lumina
  - ● **Peritoneal dialysis**
    - ◆ Uses the patient's peritoneum as a membrane for fluid and electrolyte exchange
    - ◆ Access is through a peritoneal catheter to the abdomen
    - ◆ Increased risk of infection compared to hemodialysis
  - ● **Continuous renal replacement therapy**
    - ◆ Continuous mode of dialysis that is associated with less hemodynamic instability than hemodialysis

ANESTHETIC CONSIDERATIONS IN RENAL FAILURE

- Preoperative assessment
  - Patients with severe renal disease may be hypervolemic → assess volume status
  - Patients on chronic dialysis → dialysis should occur prior to surgery
    - Consider checking electrolytes and potassium
  - Patients with acute renal injury of undiagnosed etiology should have elective surgery postponed or delayed to allow renal recovery and evaluate possible causes
- **Drug selection**
  - Many anesthetic agents are eliminated by the kidneys and can have prolonged effects in renal failure
  - Some perioperative drugs may cause toxicity in patients with renal disease due to their metabolites and mode of clearance
    - Example: nitroprusside
- **Hemodynamic effects on the kidney**
  - Most anesthetic agents cause hypotension and reduced renal blood flow
  - Patients with chronic hypertension may not autoregulate renal blood flow at normal blood pressures → may require higher intraoperative blood pressures

ACID–BASE DISORDERS

- Framework for understanding acid–base disorders
  - Traditional model
    - Based off the Henderson–Hasselbalch equation that quantifies the relationship between weak acids and conjugate bases
    - Bicarbonate and protons are used in the traditional model to explain changes in pH and calculate base excess and base deficit
  - Stewart model
    - Based off the theory of conservation of charge that quantifies the relationship between strong ions and weak acids
      - Considers the traditional model inferior because it does not consider noncarbonate buffers
    - **Strong ion difference (SID)** is used to assess acidemia, alkalemia, and its underlying cause
    - $SID = [Na^+] + [K^+] + [Ca^{2+}] + [Mg^{2+}] - [Cl^-] - [lactate] - [other strong anions]$
    - Normal SID = 40 mEq/L
      - Acidemia causes a decrease in the SID
      - Alkalemia causes an increase in the SID
- **Buffering systems**
  - Bicarbonate
    - Bicarbonate is an important extracellular buffer that adds protons to form carbonic acid
      - $H^+ + HCO_3^- \leftrightarrow H_2CO_3 \leftrightarrow H_2O + CO_2$
    - Equilibrium is regulated through carbonic anhydrase
      - Bicarbonate is eliminated by the kidneys
      - Carbon dioxide (CO_2) is eliminated by the lungs
  - Hemoglobin
    - Hemoglobin is an intracellular buffer for protons
  - Ventilatory system
    - Response
      - Increased minute ventilation can buffer an acidosis
      - Decreased minute ventilation can buffer an alkalosis
    - Mechanism
      - Acidosis and breathing
        - Intravascular acidosis → sensed at carotid bodies → stimulates ventilation
        - Cerebrospinal acidosis → sensed at medullary chemoreceptors at fourth cerebral ventricle → stimulates ventilation
      - Alkalosis and breathing
        - Metabolic alkalosis is poorly compensated due to minimal ability to hypoventilate

- **Acidosis**
  - Types
    - Metabolic
      - **Anion gap**
        - Definition
          - Anion gap measures unmeasured anions (such as lactate)
          - Anion gap = $[Na^+] - [Cl^-] - [HCO_3^-]$
          - Anion gap is positive if >14
        - Causes
          - Lactic acidosis
          - Ketoacidosis
          - Uremic acidosis
          - Ethanol intoxication
          - Methanol intoxication
          - Ethylene glycol intoxication
          - Aspirin (salicylate) intoxication
      - Nongap
        - Definition
          - Acidemia with anion gap <14
        - Causes
          - Normal saline administration
          - Renal tubular acidosis
          - Gastrointestinal losses (diarrhea)
          - Pancreatic fistula
          - Ureterosigmoidostomy
    - Respiratory
      - Causes
        - Increased CO_2 production
          - Sepsis or inflammation
          - Following CO_2 insufflation from laparoscopic surgery
          - Tourniquet release from an extremity
        - Impaired alveolar ventilation
          - Residual anesthetic agents
          - Effects of opioids or benzodiazepines
          - Residual neuromuscular blockade
          - Splinting
          - Sleep apnea
          - Pneumonia
  - Clinical effects
    - Cerebral
      - Increased cerebral blood flow
      - Increased intracranial pressure
    - Cardiac
      - Decreased cardiac contractility
      - Increased sympathetic surge, but decreased catecholamine response
      - Increased arrhythmias
    - Pulmonary
      - Increased pulmonary vascular resistance
    - Renal
      - Hyperkalemia
      - Increased protein catabolism
- **Alkalosis**
  - Types
    - Metabolic
      - Vomiting
      - Iatrogenic gastric suctioning

- ➤ Diuretic-induced contraction alkalosis
- ➤ Hyperaldosteronism (e.g., Conn syndrome)
  - ◆ Respiratory
    - ➤ Anxiety
    - ➤ Pain
    - ➤ Hypoxemia
- ● Clinical effects
  - ◆ Cerebral
    - ➤ Cerebral vasoconstriction
    - ➤ Decreased cerebral blood flow
    - ➤ Decreased intracranial pressure
  - ◆ Cardiac
    - ➤ Increased arrhythmias
    - ➤ Reduced coronary blood flow
  - ◆ Pulmonary
    - ➤ Decreased pulmonary vascular resistance
  - ◆ Renal
    - ➤ Hypokalemia
    - ➤ Hypomagnesemia
    - ➤ Hypophosphatemia
- ■ Laboratory values and compensation
  - ● Respiratory acidosis
    - ◆ $Pa_{CO_2} \rightarrow$ change in pH
      - ➤ Acute: Pa_{CO_2} increase 1 mm Hg $\rightarrow$ pH decrease 0.008
      - ➤ Chronic: Pa_{CO_2} increase 1 mm Hg $\rightarrow$ pH decrease 0.003
    - ◆ Metabolic compensation
      - ➤ Acute: Pa_{CO_2} increases 10 mm Hg $\rightarrow$ HCO_3^- increases 1 mEq/L
      - ➤ Chronic: Pa_{CO_2} increases 10 mm Hg $\rightarrow$ HCO_3^- increases 5 mEq/L
  - ● Respiratory alkalosis
    - ◆ $Pa_{CO_2} \rightarrow$ change in pH
      - ➤ Acute: Pa_{CO_2} decrease 1 mm Hg $\rightarrow$ pH increase 0.008
      - ➤ Chronic: Pa_{CO_2} decrease 1 mm Hg $\rightarrow$ pH increase 0.003
    - ◆ Metabolic compensation
      - ➤ Acute: Pa_{CO_2} decreases 10 mm Hg $\rightarrow$ HCO_3^- decreases 2 mEq/L
      - ➤ Chronic: Pa_{CO_2} decreases 10 mm Hg $\rightarrow$ HCO_3^- increases 5 mEq/L
  - ● Metabolic acidosis
    - ◆ $HCO_3 \rightarrow$ pH
      - ➤ HCO_3^- decrease 1 mEq/L $\rightarrow$ pH 0.015 decrease
    - ◆ Respiratory compensation
      - ➤ Pa_{CO_2} (mm Hg) = $1.5 \times HCO_3^-$ (mEq/L) + 8
  - ● Metabolic alkalosis
    - ◆ $HCO_3 \rightarrow$ pH
      - ➤ HCO_3^- increase 1 mEq/L $\rightarrow$ pH 0.015 increase
    - ◆ Respiratory compensation
      - ➤ Pa_{CO_2} (mm Hg) = $0.7 \times HCO_3^-$ (mEq/L) + 20
- ■ Delta gap (DG)
  - ● Used to determine if a mixed acid–base disorder exists
    - ◆ Delta gap = (measured anion gap – normal anion gap)/(normal serum bicarbonate – measured serum bicarbonate)
  - ● Interpretation
    - ◆ DG <1: anion-gap acidosis and non–anion-gap acidosis
    - ◆ DG 1–2: pure anion gap acidosis
    - ◆ DG >2: anion gap acidosis and metabolic alkalosis
- ■ Specific acid–base disorders
  - ● Lactic acidosis
    - ◆ Marker of circulatory failure due to hypoperfusion

- Etiology can be septic, hypovolemic, cardiogenic, or obstructive
  - Treatment must be directed at cause
- Treated lactic acidosis resolves quickly as lactate is converted to bicarbonate
- Timing of lactate resolution correlates well with survival
- Aspirin intoxication
  - Intoxication of greater than 300 mg/kg often needed to cause significant morbidity
  - Physiological effects
    - Salicylate inhibits the Krebs cycle and mitochondrial oxidative phosphorylation → metabolic acidosis
    - Salicylate is a direct respiratory stimulant → respiratory alkalosis
  - Treatment
    - Activated charcoal
    - Intravenous fluids
    - Alkalinization of urine

ELECTROLYTE DISORDERS

- Sodium balance
  - Hypernatremia
    - Hypovolemic hypernatremia
      - Cause: loss of both sodium and water, but water losses > sodium losses
      - Presentation: hypotensive, decreased skin turgor, dry mucous membranes
      - Diagnosis
        - Urine Na >20 mmol/L = renal losses
        - Urine Na <20 mmol/L = extrarenal losses (skin, respiratory)
      - Treatment: fluid repletion
    - Isovolemic hypernatremia
      - Cause: central diabetes insipidus
        - Decreased vasopressin secretion
        - Presentation: constant need for water, nocturia
        - Diagnosis
          - Serum osm >295
          - Test vasopressin levels and monitor response to water deprivation test
        - Treatment
          - Vasopressin short term, desmopressin (DDAVP) long term, hypotonic solutions
      - Cause: nephrogenic diabetes insipidus
        - Defective vasopressin receptors
        - Presentation: often diagnosed at infancy
        - Treatment: hypotonic solutions (isotonic solutions worsen condition)
      - Cause: primary polydipsia
        - Due to compulsive water drinking
        - Diagnosis: serum osm <270
        - Treatment: slowly correct electrolyte disturbances
    - Hypervolemic hypernatremia
      - Causes: hypertonic resuscitation, ingestion of table salts, loop diuretic use
      - Presentation: altered mental status, lethargy, seizures, irritability, nausea, vomiting, thirst
      - Treatment: loop diuretics and water repletion
  - Hyponatremia
    - Hypovolemic hyponatremia
      - Causes: high gastrointestinal/renal losses and intake of hypotonic fluids
        - Mechanism: hypovolemia → increased vasopressin release → increased water reabsorption (but not as much sodium reabsorbed)
      - Presentation: hypotension, tachycardia, dry mucous membranes
      - Diagnosis: Urine Na <10 (from volume contraction by kidney)
      - Treatment: volume resuscitation
    - Isovolemic hyponatremia

- ➤ Cause: syndrome of inappropriate ADH secretion (SIADH)
- ➤ Diagnosis
  - ❖ Impaired vasopressin suppression
  - ❖ Plasma osm <270
  - ❖ Urine osm >100
  - ❖ Isovolemic
  - ❖ Elevated urine sodium concentration
- ➤ Treatment
  - ❖ Free water restriction
  - ❖ Demeclocycline
  - ❖ Salt tabs (2 to 3 g/d)
  - ❖ Loop diuretics
- ❖ Hypervolemic hyponatremia
  - ➤ Causes: congestive heart failure, cirrhosis, nephrotic syndrome, renal failure
    - ❖ Decreased arterial blood volume → vasopressin release
  - ➤ Treatment
    - ❖ Loop diuretics
- ❖ Correction of hyponatremia
  - ➤ Rapid overcorrection can lead to osmotic demyelination syndrome
    - ❖ More common in patients with severe hyponatremia (Na <120, but usually <115) whose serum sodium concentration was raised by more than 10 to 12 mEq/L within 24 hours
    - ❖ In the past, the goal Na level was >120 mEq/L
      - ⟩ This did not improve the prognosis of severe hyponatremia
  - ➤ In an attempt to avoid overcorrection, target an increase of 4 to 6 (<8) mEq/L in 24 hours
- ● Osmolality
  - ❖ Serum osmolality is primarily determined by sodium
    - ➤ Expected serum osmolality = 2 × sodium + BUN/2.8 + glucose/18
  - ❖ When expected serum osmolality does not match the laboratory value, suspect toxins, electrolytes, or metabolic derangements that may be causing the osmolality gap
- ■ Potassium balance
  - ● Hypokalemia
    - ❖ Causes
      - ➤ Potassium deficit through gastrointestinal or renal losses
      - ➤ Intracellular shifts through alkalosis or drug effects (insulin)
    - ❖ ECG findings
      - ➤ Increased PR intervals, U waves, flattened T waves
    - ❖ Treatment
      - ➤ Potassium repletion
  - ● Hyperkalemia
    - ❖ Causes
      - ➤ Lack of appropriate potassium elimination (renal failure)
      - ➤ Extracellular shifts through acidosis
      - ➤ Inappropriate potassium release (tumor lysis)
    - ❖ ECG findings
      - ➤ Increased PR intervals, QRS widening, peaked T waves
    - ❖ Treatment
      - ➤ Treat underlying cause
      - ➤ Calcium to stabilize myocardium
      - ➤ Insulin and glucose
      - ➤ Hyperventilation/bicarbonate
      - ➤ Albuterol
      - ➤ Potassium-wasting diuretics
      - ➤ Sodium polystyrene sulfonate
      - ➤ Hemodialysis
- ■ Calcium balance

- Hypocalcemia
  - Causes
    - Hypoparathyroidism
    - Vitamin D deficiency
    - Renal disease
      - Decreased Ca absorption, decreased Vitamin D synthesis, and uremia causes bone resistance to PTH
    - Pancreatitis
  - Presentation
    - Fatigue, cramps, facial nerve irritability, laryngospasm/stridor, mental status changes, seizures, Chvostek and Trousseau signs positive
  - ECG
    - Decreased PR, narrowed QRS, T-wave flattening
  - Treatment
    - Calcium repletion
    - Vitamin D supplementation
- Hypercalcemia
  - Causes
    - Hyperparathyroidism
    - Cancer
      - Especially breast, lung, multiple myeloma
    - Immobility
    - Thyrotoxicosis
    - Vitamin D intoxication
    - Thiazide diuretics
    - Milk–alkali syndrome
    - Sarcoidosis
    - Infections
      - TB, coccidiomycosis
  - Presentation
    - Altered mental status, seizures, psychosis, dehydration, abdominal pain, nausea
  - ECG
    - Widened QRS, peaked T waves
  - Treatment
    - Hydration
    - Furosemide
    - Bisphosphonates

QUESTIONS

1. A 67-year-old man develops acute kidney injury (AKI) after undergoing open repair of an abdominal aortic aneurysm. His creatinine increases from 0.5 to 1.0 and his urine output has been 20 to 25 cc/hr for the last 12 hours. According to the RIFLE Criteria, his AKI is categorized as:

   A. Risk
   B. Injury
   C. Failure
   D. Loss

2. A 67-year-old woman with nephrolithiasis develops urosepsis after undergoing ureteroscopy and stone removal. Broad spectrum antibiotics, fluids, and vasopressor support are administered. Blood gas analysis early in the resuscitation reveals a metabolic acidosis with pH 7.23. As she clinically improves, the strong ion difference will be expected to:

   A. Increase
   B. Decrease
   C. Remain unchanged
   D. Exceed 50 mEg/mL

3. Which of the following is the most characteristic ECG finding in a patient with hypercalcemia?

   A. QT prolongation
   B. PR shortening
   C. U wave
   D. Osborn wave

4. An 87-year-old man with CKD is scheduled to undergo an abdominal CT scan with PO and IV contrast. Pretreatment with which of the following is most effective for decreasing the development of contrast-induced nephropathy?

   A. Normal saline
   B. Mannitol
   C. *N*-acetylcysteine
   D. Fenoldopam

5. Which of the following features is most characteristic of acute tubular necrosis (ATN) rather than a prerenal cause of acute kidney injury?

   A. Urine osmolarity >350
   B. Hyaline casts
   C. Muddy-brown granular casts
   D. FENa tends to be less than 1%

CHAPTER 12 | Hematologic System

BLOOD DISORDERS

- Red blood cell (RBC) disorders
  - **Anemia**
    - Anemia is characterized by low hemoglobin (Hb) concentration
      - Defined as Hb <12 g/dL in adult women and Hb <13 g/dL in adult men
      - Defined as Hb <11 g/dL in pregnancy
    - Mechanism of anemia
      - Decreased production
        - Iron deficiency: lack of Hb synthesis
        - Megaloblastic anemia: B_{12} or folic acid deficiency
        - Thalassemias: deficient Hb synthesis
        - Aplastic anemia: deficient production across all blood cell lines
        - Renal failure: decreased erythropoietin
        - Myelodysplastic syndrome: disorder of stem cells in bone marrow
      - Increased destruction
        - Hemolytic anemia: due to variety of conditions including infections, autoimmune diseases, hypersplenism, hereditary spherocytosis, and glucose-6-phosphate dehydrogenase deficiency
      - Blood loss/hemorrhage
    - Laboratory values
      - Mean corpuscular volume (MCV)
        - MCV <80: microcytic anemia
          - Common with iron deficiency, chronic blood loss, and thalassemia
        - MCV = 80 to 100: normocytic anemia
          - Common with acute blood loss, hemolytic anemia
        - MCV >100: macrocytic anemia
          - Common with B_{12} or folate deficiency, alcoholism, hypothyroidism, and postgastric bypass surgery
      - Reticulocyte count
        - Low count → inappropriate response to anemia (e.g., defect in heme synthesis)
        - Elevated count → appropriate response to anemia (e.g., chronic blood loss)
      - RBC destruction products
        - Indirect bilirubin and lactate dehydrogenase are elevated in hemolytic anemia
    - **Mechanisms to compensate for anemia**
      - Increased cardiac output
        - Decreased Hb → decreased blood viscosity → increased blood flow
        - Hypovolemia → increase in heart rate and decrease in systemic vascular resistance → increased blood flow
      - Decrease oxygen–Hb affinity
        - The oxyhemoglobin dissociation curve shifts to the right → improved oxygen delivery to tissues
      - Increased oxygen extraction at tissues
      - Redistribution of blood flow
        - Blood flow preferentially directed to brain, heart, and other vital organs

- **Polycythemias**
  - Polycythemia is defined as an abnormally high Hb concentration
    - Defined as Hb >16.5 g/dL in adult women and Hb >18.5 g/dL in adult men
  - Mechanism of polycythemia
    - Bone marrow defect
      - Polycythemia vera: myeloproliferative disorder resulting in overproduction of all cell lines
    - Physiological response to increased erythropoietin
      - Hypoxic conditions such as chronic obstructive pulmonary disease (COPD), congenital heart disease, and elevated altitudes
- Hematological disorders and anesthetic implications
  - **Sickle-cell disease**
    - Mechanism
      - Sickle-cell patients possess a mutation at position 6 of the Hb β-chain → referred to as hemoglobin S (HbS)
        - Mutated HbS possesses a glutamate at position 6
        - Normal Hb possesses a valine at position 6
      - Infants with sickle cell are protected due to presence of fetal Hb
      - Deoxygenated HbS can aggregate and form an insoluble gelatinous network → capable of polymerizing and restricting flow → tissue infarcts
    - Presentation
      - About ten percentage of African-Americans have sickle trait, 0.2% have sickle disease
      - Sickling occurs at a higher oxygen saturation in sickle-cell disease (So_2 <80%) compared to sickle-cell trait (So_2 <40%)
      - Sickle-cell exacerbation presents with pain, ischemia, jaundice, cholelithiasis, leg ulcers, and organ microinfarction
    - Conditions associated with sickle-cell disease
      - Aplastic crisis
        - Sickle cells are removed in 10 to 20 days by reticuloendothelial system (compared to 120 days for normal RBCs)
        - Increased destruction → stresses bone marrow to produce enough RBCs to compensate for anemia → additional insult to RBC production can halt RBC production
          - Folate deficiency or parvovirus that interferes with erythropoiesis → aplastic crisis
        - Treatment is with supportive care and transfusions until reticulocyte count improves
      - Acute chest syndrome
        - Local inflammation at lung tissue of sickle-cell patients → decreased oxygen saturation → increased sickling → vaso-occlusive crisis in the pulmonary vasculature
          - Causes include infections, pulmonary infarction, fat embolism, and hypoventilation
        - Commonly present with new infiltrate on CXR (chest x-ray)
        - Treatment includes supportive care, antibiotics, blood transfusion, and analgesics
    - Long-term treatments
      - Folic acid repletion
      - Hydroxyurea → increases fetal Hb
      - Supportive care, transfusions, and analgesics during acute attacks
    - Anesthetic implications
      - Avoid hypotension, hypovolemia, venous stasis, hypothermia, dehydration, acidosis, and hypoxia
      - Avoid hyperviscosity
        - Splenic sequestration crisis due to blood accumulation at spleen → leads to splenic infarct
      - Tourniquet use increases sickling and should be avoided
      - Neuraxial anesthetic technique is acceptable
      - Goal oxygenation saturation >95%
      - Hb transfusion threshold
        - Preoperative Transfusion in Sickle-cell Disease Study Group found no benefit of exchange transfusion (HbSS <30%) over a target Hb of 10
  - **Thalassemias**

- Genetic disorder of abnormal Hb production of either α or β chain
  - ➤ Minor: asymptomatic hypochromic, microcytic anemia
    - ❖ No problems with oxygen delivery
  - ➤ Intermediate: decreased 2,3 DPG
    - ❖ Left shift of oxyhemoglobin curve
  - ➤ Major: aka Cooley anemia; severe
    - ❖ Presents in infancy as failure to thrive
- Inherited in autosomal recessive pattern
- Hb has shorter life span due to defect
- May increase need for transfusions
- Porphyrias
  - Disorder of enzymes that produce Hb
    - ➤ Inducible porphyrias
      - ❖ Acute intermittent porphyria, variegate porphyria, hereditary coproporphyria
      - ❖ Anesthetic implications
        - ⟩ Avoid barbiturates, thiopental, and etomidate → can precipitate an acute attack
        - ⟩ Avoid hyponatremia, minimize stress response, and prevent dehydration
        - ⟩ Carbohydrate source may prevent porphyrin synthesis
          - ▸ 10% glucose in saline may be beneficial while NPO
        - ⟩ Decrease fasting period as much as possible
    - ➤ Noninducible porphyrias
      - ❖ Porphyria cutanea tarda
      - ❖ Anesthetic implications
        - ⟩ Unlike inducible porphyrias, not affected by drugs
        - ⟩ No alternations in anesthetic plan needed
        - ⟩ Barbiturates, etomidate, and ketamine have been implicated with triggering of a porphyric crisis
        - ⟩ Propofol is considered safe
- Osler–Weber–Rendu syndrome (hereditary hemorrhagic telangiectasia)
  - Vascular dysplasia affecting pulmonary, cerebral, gastrointestinal, and spinal vasculature
    - ➤ Disorder where no small capillaries connect the arteries and veins
    - ➤ Patients possess many arteriovenous malformations (AVMs)
      - ❖ Increased risk of rupture
      - ❖ Large AVMs → right-to-left shunt and heart failure
    - ➤ Need screening for pulmonary AVMs due to increased risk of pulmonary hemorrhage
    - ➤ AVMs enlarge with pregnancy
  - Anesthetic implications
    - ➤ Avoid nasal intubation
    - ➤ Minimize use of NG/OG tube
    - ➤ Avoid excessive positive pressure ventilation
    - ➤ Avoid excessive hypertension
    - ➤ Airway manipulation has potential for bleeding
    - ➤ Several cases of paralysis and spinal cord compression following neuraxial anesthesia
      - ❖ Recommend MRI prior to procedure to scan for AVMs

COAGULATION DISORDERS

- **von Willebrand Disease (vWD)**
  - von Willebrand factor (vWF) is an adhesion protein that protects factor VIII from inactivation and helps divert platelets to injury locations
    - vWD can be due to defective or insufficient vWF
      - ➤ Prolonged bleeding times
      - ➤ Reduced factor VIII
    - Prothrombin time (PT)/Partial thromboplastin time (PTT) times unchanged
  - Subtypes
    - I: quantitative decrease in vWF
    - II: qualitative deficiency of vWF

- IIA: qualitative defect with an absence of intermediate and large molecular weight multimers
- IIB: qualitative abnormality with increased affinity of vWF for its platelet receptor (associated with thrombocytopenia)
  - DDAVP can be counterproductive and worsen thrombocytopenia
  - III: no vWF and low factor VIII levels
- Treatment
  - DDAVP (releases vWF)
    - Administer 1 to 2 hours prior to surgery for Type I subtype
    - Peaks after 30 minutes, lasts 6 to 8 hours
    - DDAVP also works in bleeding for uremic patients in renal failure (0.3 µg/kg)
  - Humate-P is vWF/factor VIII concentrates
    - Risks: viral transmission, prion transmission, and thrombosis
  - Blood products with factor VIII and vWF (cryoprecipitate, fresh frozen plasma [FFP])
    - Do not use recombinant factor VIII alone because it lacks vWF
- Hemophilia
  - Hemophilia A
    - Lack of functional clotting factor VIII → increased bleeding risk
      - X-linked recessive: 1 to 2/10K
    - Classification by functional factor VIII levels
      - Mild: 6% to 40% of factor VIII level (frequently undiagnosed)
      - Moderate: 1% to 5% (prolonged bleeding, occasional spontaneous hemorrhage)
      - Severe: <1% (common spontaneous hemorrhage)
    - Goal of surgery is to get level to 50% to 100% of normal factor VIII levels, then maintain >40% factor VIII levels for 7 days
      - Factor VIII at 50 U/kg will deliver 100% of normal factor VIII levels
      - DDAVP works for hemophilia A, but not B
  - Hemophilia B
    - Lack of functional clotting factor IX → increased bleeding risk
      - X-linked recessive: 1/20K
    - Consider factor IX concentrates prior to surgery or FFP
- **Disseminated intravascular coagulation**
  - Diffuse bleeding disorder due to consumption of coagulation factors and platelets
    - Excessive fibrin deposition and impaired degradation
    - Increased coagulation → formation of clots
    - Overall depletion of platelets and factors (mainly V and VIII)
  - Causes include trauma, sepsis, incompatible blood transfusions, and malignancy
    - Treatment must target underlying cause
  - Laboratory values
    - Decreased platelets
    - Decreased fibrinogen
    - Increased PT
    - Increased PTT
    - Increased fibrinogen split products

PLATELET DISORDERS

- **Thrombocytopenia**
  - Disorder of low platelets in blood
    - Normal platelet count is 150K to 450K
  - Causes
    - Decreased production
      - Sepsis
      - Liver failure
      - Myelodysplastic syndrome
      - Congenital genetic conditions
    - Increased destruction
      - Idiopathic thrombocytopenia purpura (ITP)

- ➤ Thrombotic thrombocytopenia purpura (TTP)
- ➤ Disseminated intravascular coagulation (DIC)
- ➤ Hemolytic uremic syndrome (HUS)
- ➤ Systemic lupus erythematosus (SLE)
  - ◆ Medication side effects
- ■ Specific platelet conditions
  - ● ITP
    - ◆ Mechanism
      - ➤ Patient possesses IgG antibodies (Abs) toward platelet antigens → platelet destruction
    - ◆ Treatment
      - ➤ Remove IgG Abs via plasmapheresis or IVIG therapy
      - ➤ Steroids and immunosuppressants
      - ➤ Splenectomy
    - ◆ Anesthetic implications
      - ➤ Target platelet count of 100K for major surgery
      - ➤ Platelet transfusion generally not effective because autoimmune disease destroys transfused platelets
  - ● TTP
    - ◆ Mechanism
      - ➤ Spontaneous aggregation of platelets and coagulation activation → platelet and coagulation factor consumption → microthrombi formation → shearing of red cells → microangio-pathic hemolytic anemia
      - ➤ Five clinical signs that traditionally characterize TTP include thrombocytopenia, anemia, fevers, renal failure, and altered mental status
    - ◆ Treatment
      - ➤ Plasmapheresis
      - ➤ Immunosuppressants
    - ◆ Anesthetic implications
      - ➤ Postpone elective surgery until remission
      - ➤ Check platelet and coagulation factors prior to considering neuraxial or regional anesthesia
      - ➤ Mental status changes may reduce anesthetic requirements
      - ➤ Consider steroids or stress dose steroids if on immunosuppression
      - ➤ Consider antiplatelet drugs to decrease thrombi
      - ➤ Platelet transfusions will increase risk of microthrombi
  - ● Heparin-induced thrombocytopenia (HIT)
    - ◆ Heparin can induce the formation of abnormal antibodies that bind and inhibit platelets
      - ➤ Onset is at 5 to 14 days after heparin exposure
      - ➤ Despite thrombocytopenia, patients remain at risk for venous thrombosis due to platelet activation
    - ◆ Types
      - ➤ Nonimmune (Type I)
        - ✦ Transient and clinically insignificant
        - ✦ Heparin binds to platelets with modest decrease in platelet count
      - ➤ Immune (Type II)
        - ✦ IgG antibodies are formed that bind to heparin and platelet protein factor 4
        - ✦ Results in 50% decrease in platelets and venous/arterial thrombosis
    - ◆ If a patient has HIT and needs anticoagulation → use a direct thrombin inhibitor
      - ➤ Director thrombin inhibitors: hirudin, kepirudin, bivalirudin, or argatroban
      - ➤ Avoid warfarin → causes necrosis
        - ✦ HIT is thrombogenic and warfarin is initially thrombogenic via protein C inhibition → risk of gangrene necrosis

TRANSFUSION MEDICINE

- ■ **Blood product storage**
  - ● Packed RBCs (PRBCs)
    - ◆ RBCs cooled and stored at 4 °C to decrease metabolism

- ◆ CPDA-1 is added as a preservative and anticoagulant
  - ➤ Citrate: anticoagulation
  - ➤ Phosphate: energy formation
  - ➤ Dextrose: energy source
  - ➤ Adenine: ATP formation
- ◆ Storage time
  - ➤ CPD (citrate phosphate dextrose): 35 days
  - ➤ Adding adsol, nutricel, optisol extends storage time to 42 days
    - ❖ Additives include adenine, glucose, and saline (removing plasma removed these components)
  - ➤ Frozen RBCs can be stored up to 10 years
    - ❖ Uses glycerol as a cryoprotective agent
- ◆ Changes in blood with time
  - ➤ Decreased pH
  - ➤ Increased potassium
  - ➤ Decreased 2 to 3 DPG
- ● **Fresh frozen plasma**
  - ◆ Plasma is separated from blood and frozen
  - ◆ Depending on the temperature of freezing, FFP can be stored for 1 to 7 years
  - ◆ Must be thawed prior to use
    - ➤ Shelf life of 24 hours after thawing
- ● **Platelets**
  - ◆ Stored at room temperature
    - ➤ Increased risk of infection and bacteremia due to room temperature storage
  - ◆ Shelf life is approximately 5 days
  - ◆ Pooled platelets expose patients to multiple donors and therefore increased risk of exposure to antigens
    - ➤ Single donor platelets are preferred
- ● **Albumin**
  - ◆ Heat treated at 60°C to inactivate viruses
  - ◆ Stored at room temperature
- ■ RBC transfusion
  - ● **Calculating blood loss**
    - ◆ Total blood volumes can be predicted based on weight
      - ➤ Preterm newborn is 100 to 120 mL/kg
      - ➤ Newborn is 90 mL/kg
      - ➤ Infant is 80 mL/kg
      - ➤ Child is 70 mL/kg
      - ➤ Adult is 65 mL/kg
    - ◆ Volume to transfuse
      - ➤ [(Hct desired − Hct present) × blood volume/Hct transfused blood]
  - ● Transfusion threshold
    - ◆ Hb goals should be individually targeted to the patient, surgery, and degree of active bleeding
    - ◆ In a nonactively bleeding patient, the Transfusion Requirements in Critical Care (TRICC) trial suggests that targeting a Hb of 7 to 9 g/dL may be superior to targeting a Hb of 10 to 12 g/dL
  - ● **Blood filters**
    - ◆ Blood filters should be used during transfusions to remove debris
    - ◆ Standard blood filters are approximately 170 µm and can be used for all blood components
    - ◆ Microaggregate filters are approximately 40 µm and can be used for leukocyte reduction
  - ● **Blood matching**
    - ◆ **Type and screen**: patient's sample tested for blood type and antibodies
      - ➤ Recipient's RBCs mixed with serum containing anti-A and anti-B
      - ➤ Recipient's serum then mixed with RBCs with known A and B antigen
      - ➤ Recipient's cells mixed with anti-D Abs
      - ➤ Recipient's serum mixed with Rh-positive RBC

- ➤ A screen tests common antigens such as Kell, Duffy, and Lutheran with the recipient's blood
  - ◆ **Type and cross:** patient's blood and donor blood tested for compatibility
- Release of donor blood
  - ◆ Crossmatched blood
    - ➤ Ideally, the blood bank will have time to crossmatch donor units with the recipient's blood
    - ➤ Crossmatched blood has the least risk of a transfusion reaction
  - ◆ **Uncrossmatched blood**
    - ➤ Release of blood that is typed, but not crossmatched with the recipient
    - ➤ ABO compatible, but may risk antibody-mediated reaction
    - ➤ Used in cases of emergency when time or resources do not permit time for crossmatching
  - ◆ Emergency release
    - ➤ In cases of emergencies when blood typing is not done, O^- blood can be transfused
    - ➤ Packed RBCs preferable to whole blood during emergency release
      - ❖ Whole blood has anti-A and anti-B antibodies
      - ❖ If whole blood transfused, continue transfusing O^- blood until determining anti-A and anti-B levels
    - ➤ O^+ blood can be given to men and women greater than childbearing age in emergencies
      - ❖ For women of childbearing age, Rh-positive blood risks erythroblastosis fetalis if she is Rh-negative
- **Autologous blood**
  - ◆ Patient donation of blood prior to elective surgery
    - ➤ Blood can be stored for 42 days, so donation must be done within 42 days of surgery
  - ◆ **Intraoperative autotransfusion (cell saver)**
    - ➤ Blood collected from the surgical field is filtered, centrifuged, and washed → transfused intraoperatively
      - ❖ Deficient in plasma and platelets
      - ❖ Avoided in oncological surgery and when a patient has an active infection
    - ➤ Advantages of autotransfusion
      - ❖ Decreased risk of transmitted diseases, normal DPG, removal of inflammatory clotting factors, and removal of inflammatory cytokines
    - ➤ Disadvantages of autotransfusion
      - ❖ Need to recover a minimum amount of blood prior to cell saver processing, bacterial contamination, lysis of red cells, risk of fat embolism, and removal of platelets and clotting factors
- **Synthetic and recombinant Hb**
  - ◆ Synthetic Hb and synthetic oxygen carriers have been developed, but none are currently FDA approved for use
- Jehovah Witnesses
  - Due to religious reasons, Jehovah Witnesses may not accept blood transfusions
  - **Strategies to prevent the need for RBC transfusion**
    - ◆ Strategies to increase preoperative RBCs
      - ➤ Erythropoietin
        - ❖ Hormone from the kidney that stimulates erythropoiesis
        - ❖ Patient must have adequate iron stores
        - ❖ Must be started 1 to 3 weeks prior to surgery to allow adequate time to work
          - › One unit of blood can be made over 7 days of therapy
          - › Five units of blood can be made over 28 days of therapy
        - ❖ Increased RBC mass can lead to hypertension, increased viscosity of blood, and congestive heart failure
      - ➤ Iron, folate, and B_{12} supplementation
    - ◆ Strategy to increase intraoperative RBCs
      - ➤ Autologous donation (controversial for some)
        - ❖ Requires predonation Hb >11 g/dL and donation >3 days prior to surgery to allow restoration of intravascular volume
        - ❖ Donation should not be more than 10.5 cc/kg

➤ Acute normovolemic hemodilution at start of case and then transfusion back to patient when necessary during the case

➤ Autotransfusion (cell saver intraoperatively)

✦ Strategies to reduce bleeding

➤ Recombinant factor VIIa

✦ Improves platelet adhesiveness

✦ Improves activation of extrinsic coagulation pathway

✦ Improves activation of intrinsic coagulation pathway based on use in hemophilia A and B populations

✦ Reduces clot lysis and bleeding

➤ Antifibrinolytic drugs

✦ Aprotinin (bovine)

› Aprotinin prevents kallikrein activity → decreases activation of plasminogen to plasmin → prevents clot lysis

› Increases platelet adhesiveness through factor XII

› High risk of anaphylaxis

✦ Aminocaproic acid and transexamic acid

› Bind plasminogen and prevent conversion to plasmin → prevents clot lysis

› Will reduce bleeding if patient can generate blood clots

› Will not assist clot formation with abnormal platelets

› Useful in cardiac surgery due to the fibrinolysis caused by cardiac bypass

➤ Desmopressin improves platelet function and adhesiveness

✦ Tachyphylaxis can occur with repeated dosing

✦ Mainly used in bleeding in a uremic patient

NON-RBC TRANSFUSION

■ **Clotting factors and pathways**

● Intrinsic and extrinsic pathways

✦ PT tests factor VII in the extrinsic pathway

✦ aPTT tests VIII and IX in the intrinsic pathway

✦ **Activated clotting time (ACT)** tests the intrinsic clotting system

✦ Factors I, II, V, X are common to both pathways

✦ Factors II, VII, IX, X are "vitamin K dependent"

➤ Vitamin K is responsible for the production of γ-carboxyglutamic acid, which is required for the proper functioning of these factors

➤ Vitamin K is synthesized in the gut with the help of intestinal flora and is then absorbed with the help of bile acids

➤ IV Vitamin K takes ~3 to 6 hours to begin to reverse the coagulopathy and decrease the INR

● Factor half-life

✦ Factor VII has the shortest $t_{1/2}$ of 4 to 6 hours

➤ First factor depleted in liver failure, Coumadin use, and vitamin K deficiency

✦ Factor IX is at 24 hours

✦ Factor X is at 25 to 50 hours

✦ Factor II is at 50 to 80 hours

● Factor III, IV (ionized calcium), and VIII are not made by the liver

✦ Factor VIII is synthesized by vascular endothelial cells and megakaryocytes

➤ Factor VIII has a half-life of 12 hours

✦ Factor III is made at the endothelium

● Plasminogen is an inactive protein made by the liver and found in plasma

✦ Plasminogen incorporated into fibrin cross-links

✦ Tissue plasminogen activator (tPA) is released by endothelial damage and activates plasminogen into plasmin → degrades fibrin → releases D-dimers

✦ Plasmin counteracts the clotting cascade (Fig. 12.1)

■ FFP

● One unit of FFP is one unit of whole blood without RBCs, leukocytes, or platelets

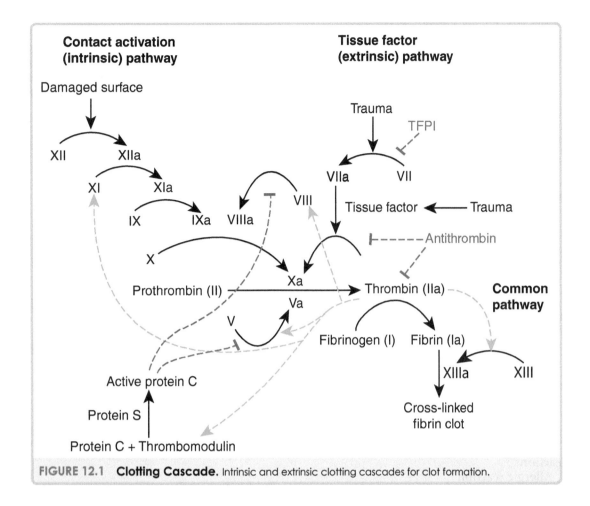

Contact activation (intrinsic) pathway

Damaged surface

XII → XIIa

XI → XIa

IX → IXa   VIIIa   VIII

X

Prothrombin (II)

V

Active protein C

Protein S

Protein C + Thrombomodulin

Tissue factor (extrinsic) pathway

Trauma   TFPI

VIIa   VII

Tissue factor ← Trauma

Antithrombin

Xa → Thrombin (IIa)   **Common pathway**

Va

Fibrinogen (I)   Fibrin (Ia)

XIIIa   XIII

Cross-linked fibrin clot

FIGURE 12.1   Clotting Cascade. Intrinsic and extrinsic clotting cascades for clot formation.

- ◆ Each unit of FFP increases coagulation factors by 3% to 6% in the absence of ongoing consumption
- ◆ Contains all coagulation factors at normal concentrations
- ◆ AB is the universal donor for plasma because no antibodies are present
- ● FFP contains increased citrate (for anticoagulation) compared to RBCs
- ● American Society of Anesthesiologists indications for FFP transfusion
  - ◆ Correction of microvascular bleeding with INR >2.0, PT > 1.5× normal, or aPTT >2× normal
  - ◆ Correction of microvascular bleeding in patient transfused >1 blood volume and coagulation factors cannot be obtained
  - ◆ Urgent reversal of warfarin
  - ◆ Correction of known coagulation factor deficiencies
  - ◆ Heparin resistance (ATIII deficiency) in a patient requiring heparin
- ● Effect of FFP
  - ◆ PT or PTT must be at >1.5× normal to reflect a clinically significant decrease in clotting factors
  - ◆ FFP has mild effect on correcting mild-to-moderate PT elevations (<2× normal)
- ■ Platelets
  - ● ASA 2006 Task Force Practice Guidelines for Perioperative Blood Transfusion recommends platelet transfusion for count <50K in the setting of active bleeding
    - ◆ One unit of platelets typically increases platelet count by 5K to 10K in a 70-kg patient
    - ◆ Platelets survive in circulation for ~10 days
    - ◆ Platelets do not require ABO compatibility
      - ➤ ABO compatibility is preferred because platelets survive better
      - ➤ Rh-negative females should only get Rh-negative platelets
    - ◆ Spontaneous bleeding risk increases at platelet count of 5K to 10K

- Platelet plug mechanism
  - Vessel injury → vWF binds to exposed collagen → GP1b of platelets adheres to endothelium via vWF-GP1b interaction → platelet adherence causes exposure of GIIb/IIIa receptors → granules release thromboxane A_2 and platelet-activating factor → platelet aggregation and vasoconstriction → formation of thrombin by coagulation factors and platelets aggregate with each other via fibrinogen
- Cryoprecipitate
  - White insoluble precipitate that is removed from FFP as it is thawing
    - Contains factor VIII, XIII, fibrinogen, vWF, and fibronectin
    - Does not contain donor antibodies
      - ABO compatibility is not needed
  - Indicated for hypofibrinogenemia, vWD, and hemophilia A
    - 70 to 100 mg/dL of fibrinogen needed for hemostasis
    - One unit of cryoprecipitate/10 kg increases plasma fibrinogen by 50 to 70 mg/dL
- Prothrombin complex concentrates (PCC)
  - Contains vitamin K–dependent factors II, VII, IX, and X from pooled plasma
    - Reverses Coumadin → risks thrombosis
  - Effective in as little as 10 minutes
- Dextran
  - Polysaccharide used as antithrombotic or volume expander
    - Interacts with platelets, factor VIII, and endothelial cells to decrease platelet aggregation and blood viscosity
  - Side effects
    - Anaphylaxis, renal failure, coagulopathy, and interference in crossmatching blood

BLOOD PRODUCT REACTIONS AND COMPLICATIONS

- **Reactions**
  - **Allergic reaction**
    - Antibody–allergen interaction between donor and recipient → histamine release
    - Urticarial/puritic
    - Presents with itching, redness, stable vitals
      - 1% to 3% of transfusions; most common
    - Treatment
      - Stop transfusion, supportive care with antihistamines, ranitidine, and/or steroids
      - Can resume transfusion if patient is stable
  - **Nonhemolytic febrile reaction**
    - Recipient's allo-antibodies interact with antigens on donor leukocytes
      - Increase in body temperature by >1 °C
      - Leukocyte reduction filtration decreases the risk nonhemolytic febrile reactions
      - Likelihood of reaction increases with increased transfusion history
    - Presents with fever, chills, nausea, headaches, myalgias, and possibly hypotension
    - Treatment
      - Stop transfusion, assess for hemolytic transfusion reaction
      - Consider acetaminophen and leukocyte reduction for further transfusions
  - **Hemolytic reactions**
    - **Acute**
      - Mechanism
        - ABO-incompatible blood transfused → recipient antibodies attach to donor RBCs → activates complement system → intravascular RBC hemolysis
        - Bradykinin release and mast cell activation → hypotension, DIC
        - RBC lysis and Hb precipitation → renal failure
      - Presents with fever, hypotension, hemoglobinuria, bleeding, dyspnea
      - Risk
        - No.1 cause is clerical error
        - 1/1K if type and screened

- ❖ 1/10K if crossmatched
  - ➢ Treatment
    - ❖ Stop transfusion, support hemodynamics, intravenous fluids, consider mannitol, and/or furosemide to support kidneys
    - ❖ If blood is acutely needed, transfuse O-RBCs and AB FFP until tests are clarified
- ◆ **Delayed**
  - ➢ Minor antigen incompatibility (e.g., kidd, kell, duffy) → delayed hemolytic reaction
    - ❖ Removal of antigen–antibody complexes by reticuloendothelial system → extravascular hemolysis → delayed anemia, increased bilirubin levels, and jaundice
    - ❖ Occurs in <1/2,000 transfusions
  - ➢ Diagnosis
    - ❖ Positive direct antiglobulin test, elevated bilirubin levels, hemosiderinuria
  - ➢ Treatment
    - ❖ Supportive care, correct anemia
- IgA deficiency
  - ◆ Patients with hereditary IgA deficiency can develop anti-IgA antibodies following a transfusion
    - ➢ Second exposure to IgA → anaphylactic reaction
  - ◆ Prevention
    - ➢ Use washed RBCs or transfuse red cells from IgA deficient patients
- Graft vs. host disease
  - ◆ Rare, but potentially fatal complication where donor lymphocytes attack the host's lymphoid tissue
    - ➢ Immunocompetent patients are able to destroy donated lymphocytes
    - ➢ Immunosuppressed patients may not be able to destroy donated lymphocytes
  - ◆ Presentation
    - ➢ Fever, rash, fatigue, abdominal pain
    - ➢ Diagnosis is by skin biopsy
  - ◆ Risk
    - ➢ RBCs and platelets have lymphocytes
    - ➢ FFP and cryoprecipitate do not have lymphocytes
  - ◆ Prevention
    - ➢ Use irradiated products
- ■ Complications
  - ● **Infectious transmission**
    - ◆ Routine blood testing includes HIV, hepatitis B and C, human T-cell lymphotropic virus (HTLV), and West Nile virus
    - ◆ Risks of specific infectious agents during transfusions
      - ➢ CMV: <1% (prevented through leukocyte-depleted blood)
      - ➢ Bacterial contamination: 1/25K
      - ➢ Hepatitis B: 1/200K
      - ➢ Hepatitis C: 1/600K
      - ➢ HTLV: 1/641K
      - ➢ HIV: 1/800K
      - ➢ West Nile virus: 1/1M
  - ● **Immunosuppression**
    - ◆ Blood products are associated with increased perioperative infections
    - ◆ Mechanism is unclear
  - ● Metabolic and electrolyte effects
    - ◆ **Citrate toxicity**
      - ➢ Citrate is an anticoagulant added to donor blood → binds ionized calcium
        - ❖ Citrate metabolized at liver into bicarbonate → metabolic alkalosis
        - ❖ Citrate levels can become elevated with significant blood transfusions
          - › More likely with FFP than PRBCs
      - ➢ Clinical effects of elevated citrate levels
        - ❖ Decreased myocardial contractility, elevated central venous pressure, and arterial hypotension

- ❖ ECG (electrocardiogram) changes: QT prolongation, flattened T waves
  - ➤ Treatment: calcium replacement
- ❖ **Hyperkalemia**
  - ➤ Prolonged RBC storage → increased extracellular potassium
  - ➤ Effects are only significant in cases of massive transfusion or renal failure
- ❖ **Acidosis**
  - ➤ Transfused RBCs are acidotic due to RBC metabolites
  - ➤ Effects are rarely clinically significant
- ● **Transfusion-related acute lung injury (TRALI)**
  - ❖ Mechanism
    - ➤ Not understood—could be two-hit model
      - ❖ Initial vascular insult and neutrophil release of cytokines and proteases
    - ➤ Involves neutrophil priming, activation, endothelial injury, and capillary leak
      - ❖ Could be mediated through leukocyte antibodies
  - ❖ Presentation
    - ➤ Occurs 1 to 4 hours after transfusion
    - ➤ Presents with fever, shortness of breath, hypoxia, noncardiogenic pulmonary edema, and leukopenia
    - ➤ No.1 cause of blood related mortality at 51%
      - ❖ 5% to 10% mortality in actual cases
  - ❖ Risk
    - ➤ Risk is greater with platelet and FFP transfusions than PRBCs
    - ➤ Most cases linked to female donors who have been previously pregnant and developed anti-HLA antibodies
  - ❖ Treatment
    - ➤ Supportive care
- ● **Transfusion associated circulatory overload (TACO)**
  - ❖ Mechanism
    - ➤ Rapid transfusion in patients at risk of cardiac or pulmonary failure
  - ❖ Presentation
    - ➤ Shortness of breath, hypertension, pulmonary edema
  - ❖ Treatment
    - ➤ Supportive care, diuresis
- ● Massive transfusion
  - ❖ Defined as greater than 10 U of PRBCs or one blood volume in a 24-hour period
  - ❖ Transfusion of PRBCs without FFP can cause significant **coagulopathy**
    - ➤ Consider matching PRBCs with FFP and platelets
- ● **Hypothermia**
  - ❖ Since blood is cooled for storage, significant transfusions can cause hypothermia
  - ❖ Consider a fluid warmer or method to prevent hypothermia

ANTICOAGULANTS

- ■ Heparin
  - ● Unfractionated heparin
    - ❖ Highly negatively charged and acidic glycosaminoglycan that activates antithrombin III → inactivates thrombin and factor Xa
      - ➤ Acts indirectly via a cofactor (antithrombin III) which neutralizes factors IX, X, XI, and inactivates thrombin → preventing its action on fibrinogen
    - ❖ Effect is monitored through PTT or activated clotting time (ACT)
    - ❖ Half-life is ~1 hour
    - ❖ Inactivated in the liver and kidney
  - ● Low-molecular-weight heparin
    - ❖ Target antifactor Xa instead of antithrombin
    - ❖ Reduced risk of heparin-induced thrombocytopenia

- ◆ Effect is monitored through anti-Xa levels
- ■ Direct thrombin inhibitors
  - ● Mechanism
    - ◆ Inhibit thrombin (factor II)
    - ◆ Examples: bivalirudin, lepirudin, argatroban, dabigatran
  - ● Use
    - ◆ Used in cases where heparin is contraindicated (heparin-induced thrombocytopenia)
    - ◆ Useful in long-term anticoagulation
  - ● Contraindications
    - ◆ Effect cannot be pharmacologically reversed
- ■ Protamine
  - ● Heparin antagonist isolated from sperm of fish species
  - ● Mechanism
    - ◆ Large amount of arginine → alkaline and positive
    - ◆ Binds to negatively charged and acidic heparin → complex removed by reticuloendothelial system
    - ◆ If patient has not received heparin, or too much protamine is administered, it can bind platelets and coagulation factors → anticoagulant effect
  - ● Dosing
    - ◆ 1.3 mg/100 U heparin
  - ● Side effects
    - ◆ Can induce allergic reactions (anaphylactoid) → histamine release → hypotension (usually seen with rapid administration) and bronchoconstriction
      - ➤ Protamine reactions: 3 types
        - ❖ Type I: hypotension
        - ❖ Type II: anaphylactic and anaphylactoid
        - ❖ Type III: pulmonary hypertension crisis
    - ◆ Catastrophic pulmonary hypertension
    - ◆ Patients at risk of allergic reactions include
      - ➤ Patients exposed to protamine (diabetics on NPH)
      - ➤ Men with vasectomy due to development of antibodies against sperm antigens
      - ➤ Patients with seafood allergies
    - ◆ Prevention
      - ➤ Pretreat with histamine blockers and steroids
      - ➤ Administer protamine over 3 to 10 minutes
    - ◆ Treatment
      - ➤ Mainly supportive
        - ❖ Epinephrine and IV fluids

ANTIPLATELETS

- ■ Aspirin
  - ● Antiplatelet agent that irreversibly inhibits cyclooxygenase-1 and cycloxygenase-2 → inhibits conversion of arachidonic acid to thromboxane A_2 → decreases platelet aggregation
- ■ Thienopyridine
  - ● Class of antiplatelet agents that irreversibly inhibit adenosine diphosphate (ADP) receptor on platelet cell membranes → decreases platelet activation and cross-linking
  - ● Example: clopidogrel and ticlopidine
- ■ Glycoprotein IIb/IIIa inhibitors
  - ● Class of antiplatelet agents that inhibits the glycoprotein IIb/IIIa receptors on the surface of platelets
  - ● Example: eptifibatide, abciximab
- ■ Dipyridamole
  - ● Antiplatelet agent that inhibits platelet cyclic adenosine monophosphate (cAMP)-phosphodiesterase and adenosine uptake → inhibits platelet response to ADP → decreases platelet activation

THROMBOELASTOGRAPHY (FIG. 12.2)

- Method of testing coagulation status, although it is now less commonly used
  - Blood is placed in a device that assesses the speed and strength of clot formation
  - Measures the visceroelastic properties of blood
- Measurements
  - *R* (reaction time): time from beginning of test to clot formation
  - *K* (clot formation): time from start of clot formation to 20-mm clot amplitude
  - Alpha-angle: angle of acceleration of fibrin formation
  - Max amplitude (MA): highest point on thromboelastography (TEG) curve
  - A60: amplitude 60 minutes after test, reflects clot destruction
  - LY30: difference between MA and A30 (30 minutes later)
- Pattern can indicate disease or coagulation deficiency (Fig. 12.3)
  - Anticoagulants or factor deficiency: prolonged *R* and *K*, decreased alpha-angle, and MA
  - Antiplatelet agents: prolonged *K*, decreased MA
  - Fibrinolysis: increased LY30, decreased A60
  - Hypercoagulation: decreased *R* and *K*, increased alpha-angle and MA
  - DIC: decreased *R* and *K*, increased LY30

INFECTIOUS DISORDERS

- HIV
  - Transmitted through blood or bodily fluids
    - Intravenous drug use, sexual contact
  - Disease course
    - Initial infection may cause flu-like symptoms such as fever, fatigue, and swollen lymph nodes
    - Without treatment, HIV can progress to AIDS and severe immunodeficiency
  - Diagnosis
    - ELISA to test for antibodies to HIV-1
    - Confirmation through Western blot
  - Needlestick injury
    - Rate of seroconversion following needlestick injury is 0.3%
      - Risk increased with hollow needles, advanced HIV patient, deep puncture, and visible blood on surface of needle or scalpel
    - If exposure is severe or if source is higher risk HIV group → initiate 3-drug regimen
      - Two nucleoside reverse transcriptase inhibitors plus a protease inhibitor as a third drug
      - Continue regimen for 28 days or until HIV status of source is known
      - Check for seroconversion at 6 weeks, 3 months, 6 months

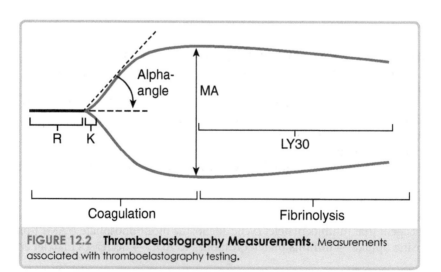

FIGURE 12.2 Thromboelastography Measurements. Measurements associated with thromboelastography testing.

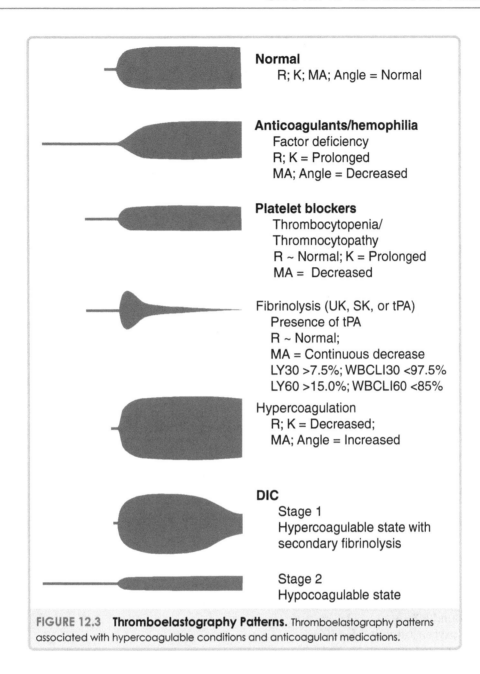

FIGURE 12.3 **Thromboelastography Patterns.** Thromboelastography patterns associated with hypercoagulable conditions and anticoagulant medications.

  ◆ If injury is less severe and source is asymptomatic → 2-drug regimen
■ Hepatitis B
  ● Transmitted through blood or bodily fluids
    ◆ Intravenous drug use, sexual transmission, transmission from childbirth
  ● Disease course
    ◆ Initial infection may not result in any symptoms
    ◆ Acute presentation includes jaundice, loss of appetite, nausea, and vomiting
    ◆ Chronic infection may lead to cirrhosis and hepatocellular carcinoma
  ● Vaccine provides lifelong immunity in 90% to 95%
  ● Needlestick injury
    ◆ Ratio of seroconversion following needlestick injury is as high as 20% to 30%
    ◆ If unvaccinated
      ➤ Hepatitis B vaccine series and hepatitis B immunoglobin
    ◆ If vaccinated

- ➤ Nonresponders to vaccine should be treated with hepatitis B immunoglobin and revaccinated
    - ➤ Responders to vaccine require no treatment
- ■ Hepatitis C
    - ● Transmitted through blood-to-blood contact
        - ◆ Intravenous drug use is most common form of transmission
    - ● Disease course
        - ◆ Initial infection only results in symptoms in a small percentage of patients
        - ◆ Symptoms include generalized fatigue, decreased appetite, and weight loss
        - ◆ Chronic infection may lead to cirrhosis and hepatocellular carcinoma
    - ● Diagnosis
        - ◆ HCV RNA detectable at 1 to 2 weeks
        - ◆ Seroconversion takes 2 to 6 months, so anti-HCV is less reliable for acute diagnosis
            - ➤ Enzyme immunoassay (EIA) screens for antibody to HCV
            - ➤ RIBA (recombinant immunoblot assay) used to confirm HCV infection
        - ◆ Elevated liver enzymes 2 to 8 weeks after exposure
            - ➤ ALT can be 10× to 20× normal in acute infection
    - ● **Needlestick injury**
        - ◆ Rate of seroconversion following needlestick injury is 1.8%
        - ◆ No postexposure prophylaxis is available

ACUTE NORMOVOLEMIC HEMODILUTION

- ■ Not commonly practiced
- ■ Thought is to decrease blood viscosity → increase tissue perfusion → decrease intraoperative blood loss
- ■ This actually decreases the arterial oxygen content
- ■ Can lead to tachycardia → increased cardiac output → increased myocardial oxygen consumption → myocardial ischemia

METHEMOGLOBINEMIA

- ■ Ferric form cannot bind oxygen
- ■ Leftward shift of the Hb-O_2 curve
    - ● Decreased amount of oxygen is unloaded to the tissues
- ■ Will see cyanosis with 10% Meth-Hb, cerebral ischemia 15% to 20%, and death when the percentage reaches around 60%
- ■ Decreased oxygen saturation (~85%)
- ■ Chocolate-colored urine and blood
- ■ Treatment
    - ● Methylene blue 1 to 2 mg/kg over 5 minutes
    - ● Vitamin C has been tried as well
    - ● If supplemental oxygen and methylene blue are unsuccessful, can attempt to perform an exchange transfusion
- ■ Congenital vs. acquired (priolocaine, benzocaine, phenacetin, large doses of nitroglycerin)

CARBOXYHEMOGLOBINEMIA

- ■ Carbon monoxide (CO) competes with O_2 for Hb (~250 times stronger)
- ■ Symptoms include: headache, nausea, dizziness, and confusion
- ■ Commonly seen in house fires
- ■ PaO_2 is not affected so the O_2 saturation will appear normal
    - ● Need a co-oximeter to distinguish the difference
- ■ CO elimination is dependent upon minute ventilation, duration of exposure, and FIO_2
    - ● Half-life of CO is
        - ◆ Approximately 4 to 6 hours when breathing room air

- ◆ Approximately 1 hour when breathing 100% oxygen
- ◆ Approximately 15 to 30 minutes if placed in a hyperbaric oxygen chamber
- Hyperbaric indications are controversial
  - Recommended if patient
    - ◆ is comatose
    - ◆ has suffered any loss of consciousness assumed to be caused by hypoxia
    - ◆ is pregnant and CO levels are >15%
    - ◆ has CO-Hb levels >40%
    - ◆ shows signs of cardiac ischemia
    - ◆ has symptoms that do not resolve after receiving 100% supplemental oxygen for 4 to 6 hours

GLUCOSE-6-PHOSPHATE DEFICIENCY (G6PD)

- Decreased half-life of RBCs
- Most common of the four types of Heinz Body Anemias
  - Microscopic denaturation and precipitation of the Hb chains into aggregates
- X-Linked
- Approximately 1% of African-Americans are affected
- G6PD is a necessary component of the RBCs defense system (glutathione dependent) against oxidative damage by infections and drugs
  - Viral pneumonia, malaria, sepsis
  - ASA, INH, phenacetin, chloramphenicol
- Sodium nitroprusside and prilocaine are contraindicated in these patients
- Methylene blue can stimulate hemolysis in this patient population
- Hemolytic reactions usually occur within 48 to 72 hours of exposure to the offending agent
  - Present with abdominal pain, jaundice, and hemoglobinuria
  - Will see Heinz bodies in the blood
  - Hemolysis tends to be self-limiting

QUESTIONS

1. A 70-year-old man develops thrombocyto-penia and is diagnosed with a pulmonary embolism 6 days after undergoing aortic valve replacement with a mechanical valve. Admin-istration of which of the following anticoagu-lants is most appropriate for treatment?

   A. Heparin
   B. Low-molecular-weight heparin
   C. Coumadin
   D. Fondaparinux
   E. Bivalirudin

2. Thromboelastography is performed in a trauma patient for diagnosis of coagulopathy. Which of the following is most closely associ-ated with the diagnosis of DIC?

   A. Decreased LY30
   B. Increased LY30
   C. Decreased MA
   D. Increased MA

3. Transfusion of which of the following blood products is associated with the greatest risk of bacterial sepsis?

   A. PRBCs
   B. Fresh frozen plasma
   C. Albumin
   D. Platelets
   E. Cryoprecipitate

4. Which of the following laboratory indicators is most useful for differentiating between TRALI and TACO?

   A. Leukocytosis
   B. Leukopenia
   C. Thrombocytopenia
   D. Thrombocytosis

5. A 36-year-old man with sickle-cell anemia is scheduled to undergo under colectomy for a newly diagnosed colonic mass. He has a his-tory of numerous hospitalizations in the past for sickle-related crises including acute chest syndrome. He has been taking hydroxyurea for his sickle-cell disease. His CBC reveals WBC 6, Hb 8.0, hematocrit 26, platelets 420. What is the most appropriate preoperative therapy to reduce his risk of perioperative complications?

   A. Phlebotomy
   B. Transfusion
   C. Erythropoietin
   D. No transfusion

ANATOMY AND FUNCTION

- **Organs**
  - Endocrine system is composed of the hypothalamus, pituitary, thyroid, parathyroid, adrenals, pancreas, and reproductive organs
  - Complex feedback between endocrine organs and their targets regulate hormone release
- **Hypothalamus**
  - Located between the thalamus and the brainstem
    - Connected to the pituitary gland via the infundibular stem
  - Secreted hormones
    - Thyrotropin-releasing hormone (TRH) → stimulates thyroid-stimulating hormone (TSH) release from the anterior pituitary
    - Growth hormone–releasing hormone (GHRH) → stimulates growth hormone (GH) release from the anterior pituitary
    - Gonadotropin-releasing hormone (GRH) → stimulates follicle-stimulating hormone (FSH) and luteinizing hormone (LH) release from the anterior pituitary
    - Corticotrophin-releasing hormone (CRH) → stimulates adrenocorticotrophic hormone (ACTH) release from the anterior pituitary
    - Antidiuretic hormone (ADH) → stimulates water reabsorption in the distal convoluted tubule and collecting duct of the kidney
- **Pituitary**
  - Located at the base of the brain in the sella turcica
  - Pituitary hormones
    - Anterior pituitary
      - GH → stimulates insulin-like growth factor release from the liver
      - TSH → stimulates thyroxine and triiodothyronine synthesis and release from the thyroid
      - ACTH → stimulates mineralocorticoid and glucocorticoid synthesis and release from the adrenal glands
      - FSH → stimulates maturation of the follicles in females and stimulates spermatogenesis in males
      - LH → stimulates ovulation in females and stimulates testosterone synthesis in males
      - Prolactin → stimulates milk synthesis at mammary glands
    - Posterior pituitary
      - Stores hormones (does not secrete hormones)
      - Antidiuretic hormone (vasopressin) → water reabsorption
      - Oxytocin → stimulates uterine contraction and lactation
- **Thyroid**
  - Thyroxine and triiodothyronine regulate metabolism, basal metabolic rate, and interact with nearly every organ system
  - Produces calcitonin that decreases calcium release from the bone
- **Parathyroid**
  - Parathyroid hormone stimulates calcium and phosphate release from bone
- **Liver**
  - Insulin-like growth factor regulates cell growth
- **Adrenals**
  - Cortex secretes glucocorticoids and mineralocorticoids

- ◆ Glucocorticoids stimulates gluconeogenesis and inhibits protein synthesis
  - ➤ Glucocorticoids have anti-inflammatory and immunosuppressive effects
  - ➤ Normal daily glucocorticoid production is equivalent to 10 mg of hydrocortisone
    - ❖ An equivalent of 100 mg of hydrocortisone can be produced during times of stress
    - ❖ Patients on chronic steroids may have a suppressed glucocorticoid response to stress
  - ➤ Steroid conversion
    - ❖ 7.5 mg dexamethasone = 50 mg of prednisone = 200 mg hydrocortisone
    - ❖ Hydrocortisone contains mineralocorticoid activity
    - ❖ Prednisone has minimal mineralocorticoid activity
    - ❖ Dexamethasone does not contain mineralocorticoid activity
  - ◆ Mineralocorticoids stimulate sodium reabsorption
    - ➤ Mineralocorticoid production is equivalent to fludrocortisones 0.125 mg daily
  - ● Medulla secretes catecholamines
    - ◆ Epinephrine, norepinephrine, and dopamine secreted by the chromaffin cells as part of the fight-or-flight response
- ▪ **Pancreas**
  - ● Insulin is secreted by β-islet cells to utilize blood glucose
  - ● Glucagon is secreted by α-islet cells to release blood glucose
- ▪ Reproductive organs
  - ● Testosterone secreted by Leydig cells to stimulate anabolic effects and virilization
  - ● Progesterone secreted by granulosa and theca cells to support pregnancy
  - ● Estrogen secreted by granulosa cells support multiple homeostatic functions

PITUITARY DISORDERS

- ▪ **Defects in ADH secretion**
  - ● **Central diabetes insipidus (DI)**
    - ◆ Absence of ADH due to posterior pituitary destruction (tumor, mass) or failure of the renal tubules to respond to ADH
    - ◆ Head trauma, brain injury resulting in inadequate levels of ADH
      - ➤ May actually not present itself until several days postinjury
    - ◆ Presents with polydipsia and polyuria → isovolemic hypernatremia
    - ◆ Treat with vasopressin, desmopressin (DDAVP)
      - ➤ Nephrogenic DI will NOT respond to DDAVP
  - ● "Postprocedure" DI
    - ◆ Intraoperative DI should resolve within ~24 hours after the surgical procedure
    - ◆ Can be seen after the pituitary is removed secondary to acromegaly, Cushing disease, or cancer
    - ◆ Treat with D5 ¼ NS and an infusion of vasopressin
  - ● **Syndrome of inappropriate ADH (SIADH) secretion**
    - ◆ Brain injury or mass resulting in impaired ADH suppression
    - ◆ Can be secondary to lung cancer, surgery, porphyrias
    - ◆ Presents with isovolemic hyponatremia
    - ◆ Na <110 → seizures, cerebral edema, and brain damage
    - ◆ Treat with fluid restriction, salt repletion, diuretics, or demeclocycline (antagonizes the effect of ADH on the renal tubules to inhibit H_2O reabsorption)
      - ➤ Do NOT increase serum Na >0.5 mEq/hr
      - ➤ Correcting Na too quickly → central pontine myelinolysis
      - ➤ Urine osm > serum osm
- ▪ **Acromegaly**
  - ● Adenoma at adenohypophysis that secretes growth hormone
  - ● Anesthetic implications
    - ◆ Increased difficulty intubating and ventilating (see Chapter 8)
    - ◆ Thick mandible, large tongue and epiglottis, extraneous pharyngeal tissue all can increase risk for airway obstruction
    - ◆ Decreased tracheal subglottic diameter
    - ◆ These patients are at increased risk for HTN, CAD, V/Q mismatch

THYROID AND PARATHYROID DISORDERS

- Thyroid disorders
  - **Hypothyroidism**
    - Causes: previous thyroid surgery or radiation, Hashimoto thyroiditis, iodine deficiency, or drug side effects
      - Most common cause is over treating hyperthyroidism
    - **Presentation:** fatigue, cold intolerance, weight gain, impaired mentation, and depression
    - **Myxedema coma** is extreme hypothyroidism → medical emergency
      - Manifested as altered mental status, hypothermia, bradycardia, hypotension, hypoventilation, hyponatremia, and hypoglycemia
      - Treatment involves stress dose steroids, thyroid hormone repletion, and supportive care
    - **Anesthetic implications**
      - Patients with an enlarged tongue or goiter may have difficult airway
      - Delayed gastric emptying → increased aspiration risk
      - Increased conduction abnormalities → bradycardia and arrhythmias
      - Cardiomyopathy → decreased cardiac function
      - Hypovolemic with increased SVR → increased hypotension
      - Increased sensitivity to sedatives → delayed emergence
    - Treatment: synthroid half-life is ~7 days)
      - T_3 works in ~6 hours
      - T_4 works in ~10 days
  - **Hyperthyroidism**
    - Causes: Graves disease, toxic multinodular goiter
    - Presentation: hypermetabolic state, sweating, heat intolerance, fatigue, weight loss, diarrhea, tremors, and palpitations
    - Can also see dysrhythmias and congestive heart failure
    - **Thyroid storm** is a medical emergency due to severe thyrotoxicosis
      - Precipitants: sepsis, stress, excess iodine, infection, trauma, toxemia, diabetic ketoacidosis (DKA)
      - Signs and symptoms
        - Hyperthermia, tachycardia, arrhythmias, shock
      - Presentation may mimic malignant hyperthermia
        - Unlike malignant hyperthermia, creatine kinase levels are normal
      - Treatment
        - Inhibition of thyroid hormone
          - Dexamethasone → inhibits synthesis, release, and conversion of T_4 to T_3
          - Propylthiouracil → inhibits thyroid hormone production
          - Propranolol → decreases tachycardia and inhibits T_4 to T_3 conversion
          - Sodium iodine → inhibits release of thyroid hormone
            - Use last because it may initiate synthesis of thyroid hormone in autoimmune thyroiditis
        - Supportive care
          - Acetaminophen
          - Reduction of body temperature
          - Intravenous fluids
    - **Anesthetic implications**
      - Goiter or thyroid mass → increased airway difficulty
      - Sympathetic stimulation → exaggerated hemodynamic response
      - Rapid metabolism → need for increased drug dosing
    - If elective surgery is planned, the patient should be symptom free
      - A combination of soidum-iodide and propranolol usually can render the patient symptom free/euthyroid in ~10 days
  - Postoperative complications of a thyroidectomy
    - RLN (most common) and/or SLN injury
    - Inadvertent removal of the parathyroid gland(s)

- ➤ Hypocalcemia, laryngospasm
- ➤ Tracheal compression, tracheomalacia
- ➤ Hypothyroidism
- ■ Parathyroid disorders
  - ● **Hypoparathyroid**
  - ● Ca <4.5
    - ◆ Causes: removal or damage to parathyroid gland
    - ◆ Presentation
      - ➤ Weakness, muscle cramps, facial nerve irritability, stridor, laryngospasm, and hypotension
      - ➤ Hypocalcemia and hyperphosphatemia
      - ➤ ECG (electrocardiogram) with prolonged QT interval
    - ◆ Anesthetic implications
      - ➤ Correct calcium preoperatively
      - ➤ Avoid alkalosis and hypothermia that can worsen hypocalcemia
      - ➤ Increased risk of cardiac conduction abnormalities
  - ● **Hyperparathyroid**
    - ◆ Causes: parathyroid adenoma, parathyroid carcinoma
    - ◆ Presentation
      - ➤ Nausea, dehydration, altered mental status, abdominal pain
      - ➤ Hypercalcemia and hypophosphatemia
      - ➤ ECG: prolonged PR, short QT, wide QRS
    - ◆ Anesthetic implications
      - ➤ Correct hypercalcemia preoperatively with intravascular fluid
        - ◆ Calcium <12: minimal symptoms
        - ◆ Calcium 14 to 16: kidney stones, seizures, nausea, weakness, depression, psychosis, coma
      - ➤ Replete phosphate
        - ◆ Hypophosphatemia presents with muscle weakness, increased sensitivity to neuromuscular blockade, confusion, and seizures
      - ➤ Avoid acidosis, which increases calcium levels
      - ➤ Hypercalcemic crisis can manifest with vasodilation under anesthesia and cause autonomic dysfunction
      - ➤ Increased calcium causes unpredictable effects on neuromuscular blockade
      - ➤ Increased arrhythmias

PANCREATIC DISORDERS

- ■ Diabetes
  - ● Classification
    - ◆ **Type I:** caused by autoimmune destruction of β-islet cells → insulin deficiency → treated with insulin
    - ◆ **Type II:** caused by insulin resistance → treated with oral agents and insulin
  - ● Emergent conditions
    - ◆ **Diabetic ketoacidosis (DKA)**
      - ➤ Ketoacidosis = metabolic acidosis + hyperglycemia
        - ◆ Usually in the setting of infection
        - ◆ The metabolic acidosis masks the presence of decreased total body K (serum levels may be normal)
      - ➤ Mechanism
        - ◆ Lack of insulin and/or acute illness in a type 1 diabetic → ketoacidosis, hyperosmolarity, and volume depletion
      - ➤ Presentation
        - ◆ Presents with polyuria, polydipsia, weakness, and altered mental status
      - ➤ Diagnosis
        - ◆ Anion-gap acidosis
        - ◆ Elevated plasma glucose
        - ◆ Ketones in serum or urine

- ➤ Treatment
  - ❖ Volume resuscitation
  - ❖ Insulin to correct anion gap
  - ❖ Potassium and phosphate repletion after correction of acidosis
  - ❖ Can consider HCO_3^- if severely acidotic (pH < 7.1) without a concurrent respiratory acidosis
- ◆ Patients tend to have an underlying
  - ➤ Autonomic neuropathy
    - ❖ Abnormal responsiveness to hypotension
    - ❖ These patients tend to suffer from orthostatic hypotension
  - ➤ Peripheral neuropathy
  - ➤ Gastroparesis
    - ❖ Assume "full stomach"
  - ➤ Nephropathy
    - ❖ Increased risk for perioperative renal failure
  - ➤ Myocardial infarction (MI) is the most common cause of death in long-standing diabetics
- ◆ **Hyperglycemic hyperosmolar syndrome (HHS)**
  - ➤ Mechanism
    - ❖ Insulin resistance → extreme hyperglycemia (levels as high as 1,000 mg/dL)
    - ❖ Patient's insulin is enough to prevent ketoacidosis, but not enough to prevent hyperglycemia
  - ➤ Presentation
    - ❖ Altered mental status (more profound than DKA), polyuria, polydipsia
  - ➤ Diagnosis
    - ❖ Hyperglycemia (usually >600)
      - ⟩ Higher vs. DKA patients
    - ❖ Hyperosmolarity (usually >300 to 350)
    - ❖ No anion-gap acidosis and no ketones
      - ⟩ pH tends to be >7.3
      - ⟩ Can be lower/more acidotic if there is a concurrent lactic acidosis
  - ➤ Treatment
    - ❖ Volume resuscitation
    - ❖ Insulin to correct osmolarity
    - ❖ Electrolyte repletion
      - ⟩ In hyperglycemic states, sodium is underestimated
      - ⟩ For every 100 mg/dL increase in glucose → sodium decreases 1.6 mEq/dL (pseudohyponatremia)
- ● Anesthetic considerations
  - ◆ Preoperative glucose management
    - ➤ Type 1 diabetics should receive insulin perioperatively
      - ❖ Insulin should never be stopped → risks DKA
      - ❖ Perioperative management of insulin prior to surgery should be in consultation with an endocrinologist or the patient's primary care physician
    - ➤ Type 2 diabetics on oral agents should hold metformin and sulfonylureas on the day of surgery
      - ❖ Metformin is associated with lactic acidosis
      - ❖ Sulfonylureas can cause hypoglycemia
      - ❖ Type 2 diabetics on insulin should receive approximately half their insulin dose on the night before or morning of surgery
  - ◆ Intraoperative glucose management
    - ➤ Maintain intraoperative glucose between 120 and 180 mg/dL
      - ❖ Hypoglycemia → cerebral injury
      - ❖ Hyperglycemia → increases infections, worsens wound healing
    - ➤ Management of glucose intraoperatively is best done with an IV insulin infusion
      - ❖ Subcutaneous absorption may be unreliable under anesthesia
  - ◆ Comorbid risks

- ➤ Diabetics are predisposed to macrovascular and microvascular disease
- ➤ Macrovascular disease
  - ❖ Coronary artery disease
    - › Increased diastolic dysfunction
  - ❖ Cerebrovascular disease
  - ❖ Peripheral vascular disease
- ➤ Microvascular disease
  - ❖ Retinopathy
  - ❖ Nephropathy
  - ❖ Neuropathy
- Insulinoma
  - Neuroendocrine β-cell tumor that secretes excess insulin
  - Presents with hypoglycemia and elevated insulin levels
  - Anesthetic considerations
    - ❖ Frequent glucose monitoring intraoperatively
    - ❖ Insulinoma manipulation may cause rapidly fluctuating glucose levels

ADRENAL DISORDERS

- **Cushing disease** (excess glucocorticoid)
  - Causes
    - ❖ Iatrogenic glucocorticoid medications
    - ❖ ACTH secreting tumor
      - ➤ Pituitary
      - ➤ Lung
      - ➤ Testes, prostate
      - ➤ Pancreas
  - Clinical features
    - ❖ Truncal obesity, moon facies, hypertension, hypernatremia, hypervolemia, osteoporosis, poor wound healing, and hypercoagulation
    - ❖ Can also see hypokalemia, metabolic alkalosis, polyuria
  - Anesthetic considerations
    - ❖ Chronic steroid use or steroid exposure → suppression of the hypothalamic–pituitary–adrenal axis
      - ➤ May require stress dose steroids if daily dose is >5 mg prednisone daily (or equivalent)
    - ❖ Truncal obesity and moon faces → difficult airway
    - ❖ Hypervolemia and hypertension → difficult to manage blood pressure
    - ❖ Increased risk of coronary artery disease
    - ❖ Increased sensitivity to muscle relaxants
    - ❖ May require potassium repletion
- Conn (excess aldosterone)
  - Aldosterone increases Na reabsorption and H_2O is the distal convoluted tubule and collecting duct
  - Causes
    - ❖ Adrenal adenoma or hyperplasia producing excess aldosterone
    - ❖ Renin coverts angiotensinogen → angiotensin 1 (in the blood) → angiotensin 2 (in the lungs) → secretion of aldosterone
  - Clinical features
    - ❖ Hypertension, hypervolemia, myalgias, and weakness
  - Anesthetic considerations
    - ❖ Increased refractory hypertension
    - ❖ May be on aldosterone antagonists preoperatively
      - ➤ Spironolactone will only work if aldosterone is present as it competes with at the receptor sites; can cause hyperkalemia
      - ➤ Amiloride and triamterene work independent of aldosterone
- **Adrenal insufficiency**
  - Causes

- ◆ Idiopathic, autoimmune, surgical removal
- ◆ Primary adrenal insufficiency is **Addison disease**
- ◆ Secondary adrenal insufficiency is caused by low ACTH secretion
- Clinical features
  - ◆ Hypotension, weight loss, abdominal pain
  - ◆ Hyponatremia, hyperkalemia, hypoglycemia
- Anesthetic considerations
  - ◆ Increased sensitivity to sedatives and anesthetics
  - ◆ Increased hypovolemia → may require volume resuscitation
  - ◆ Avoid etomidate that may worsen adrenal insufficiency
  - ◆ Stress of surgery may cause profound hypotension or death → consider stress dose steroids

NEUROENDOCRINE TUMORS

- ■ **Pheochromocytoma**
  - 70% chromaffin tissue is in the adrenal medulla; 30% in the sympathetic chain
  - Mechanism
    - ◆ Neuroendocrine tumor that secretes significant amounts of epinephrine, norepinephrine, and dopamine
  - Presentation
    - ◆ Hypertension, tachycardia, palpitations, diaphoresis, headaches, weight loss, and hyperglycemia
  - **Diagnosis**
    - ◆ 24-hour urine or serum catecholamine levels
    - ◆ Elevated urine metanephrines (or normetanephrines)
      - ➤ If test is positive, get a CT scan
    - ◆ Vanillylmandelic acid (VMA) is an OLD test
      - ➤ False elevations seen in patients taking methyl-dopa and bronchodilators
    - ◆ Associated with MEN IIa and MEN IIb, neurofibromatosis, tuberous sclerosis, and von Hippel–Lindau
    - ◆ 90%–10% rule
      - ➤ 90% found at adrenal medulla
      - ➤ 10% bilateral, 10% extra-adrenal, 10% malignant
  - **Anesthetic considerations**
    - ◆ Preoperative α-blockade to block hypertensive effects of pheochromocytoma
      - ➤ Goal BP <160/90 prior to surgery
        - ❖ Phenoxybenzamine is a noncompetitive α-blocker that is uptitrated preoperatively
        - ❖ Phentolamine is a reversible α-blocker that can be titrated as an infusion
      - ➤ β-block only after α-blockade to prevent unopposed α-blockade → hypertensive crisis
    - ◆ Preoperative volume resuscitation following α-blockade
      - ➤ Patient should be orthostatic, but BP should be >80/45
    - ◆ Preoperative ECG
      - ➤ No more than one premature ventricular contraction every 5 minutes
      - ➤ No ST changes for at least 1 week
    - ◆ Intraoperative goals
      - ➤ Avoid sympathomimetic or vagolytic drugs prior to tumor removal
      - ➤ Ability to treat hypertensive crisis prior to tumor removal
      - ➤ Ability to treat severe hypotension with intravenous fluids and vasopressors after tumor removal
    - ◆ Postoperative care
      - ➤ Hypotension → may require vasopressors
      - ➤ Insulin increases → hypoglycemia
      - ➤ Patients often somnolent due to loss of catecholamines
- ■ **Carcinoid tumor**
  - Mechanism
    - ◆ Neuroendocrine tumor that releases a variety of hormones including serotonin, histamine, tachykinins, and prostaglandin

- Presentation
  - Location
    - Tumor typically located at the small intestine and appendix
      - 70% in intestines (50% in appendix, 25% at ileum, and 20% at rectum)
      - 20% in the lungs
    - Hormone release from intestinal carcinoid is inactivated by the liver → patients asymptomatic
      - When metastases reaches the liver → hormones enter systemic circulation → carcinoid syndrome
    - Hormone release from pulmonary carcinoid can cause systemic symptoms
  - Carcinoid syndrome
    - Flushing, bronchospasm, diarrhea
  - Half of patients with right-sided cardiac lesions, including pulmonic stenosis and tricuspid regurgitation
- Diagnosis
  - 5-hydroxyindoleacetic acid, a serotonin metabolite, in blood and urine
- Anesthetic considerations
  - Preoperative assessment
    - Correct hypovolemia and electrolyte disturbances
    - Assess for valvular abnormalities
  - Serotonin suppression
    - Somatostatin suppresses serotonin and other substances from carcinoid tumor
      - Dosed by infusion because half-life of somatostatin is 3 minutes
    - Octreotide is an synthetic somatostatin analog with 2.5 hours of activity that can be dosed subcutaneously or intravenously
      - Started 24 to 48 hours prior to surgery to decrease risk of serotonin crisis
    - Ondansetron treats serotonin-induced diarrhea
  - Prevention of vasoactive release
    - Vasopressors such as ephedrine, norepinephrine, epinephrine, and dopamine can trigger release of vasoactive hormones from tumor and worsen hypotension
    - Anesthetic drugs such as succinylcholine, atracurium, and thiopental can increase hormone release
    - Fluid load and provide analgesics to prevent catecholamine release
  - Endocrinological response to surgery
    - Increased
      - ACTH
      - ADH
      - Aldosterone
      - Catecholamines
      - Glucagon
      - Cortisol
      - Thyroid hormone
    - Can see a relative hyponatremia postoperatively
      - Secondary to a relatively higher increase in ADH as compared to aldosterone
    - Hyperglycemia is common secondary to an increase of all of the hormones listed above

QUESTIONS

1. Which of the following corticosteroids does not have mineralocorticoid activity?

   A. Prednisone
   B. Hydrocortisone
   C. Fludrocortisone
   D. Dexamethasone

2. A 36-year-old woman develops severe hypertension and tachycardia during an exploratory laparotomy for an abdominal mass. A pheochromocytoma is suspected. Administration of which of the following treatments is most appropriate in this setting?

   A. Magnesium
   B. Metoprolol
   C. Ketamine
   D. Phenoxybenzamine

3. A 25-year-old woman develops an acute onset of hypotension during resection of a carcinoid tumor. In addition to a fluid bolus administration of which of the following drugs is most appropriate?

   A. Ephedrine
   B. Phenylephrine
   C. Norepinephrine
   D. Octreotide

4. A 40-year-old woman with a history of Graves disease develops thyroid storm 6 hours after undergoing appendectomy. Which of the following medications is most effective for blocking the release of thyroid hormones?

   A. Iodine
   B. Propylthiouracil
   C. Propranolol
   D. Corticosteroid

5. A healthy 42-year-old woman, gravida 2 para 1, presents to the emergency department with a 2-day history of weakness, dizziness, and fatigue. A finger stick glucose was 70, and IV fluids with dextrose were administered. Ten days earlier, she had undergone a cesarean section complicated by severe postpartum bleeding and was taken back to the operating room for an emergent hysterectomy. During hysterectomy she was hypotensive and coagulopathic and received numerous units of blood, platelets, and fresh frozen plasma. Which of the following is the most appropriate initial therapy for this patient?

   A. Hydrocortisone
   B. Thyroxine
   C. Estrogen
   D. DDAVP

CHAPTER 14 Neuromuscular and Musculoskeletal System

NEUROPATHIC DISEASES

- **Multiple sclerosis (MS)**
  - Mechanism and presentation
    - Inflammatory autoimmune disorder that destroys the myelin sheath of neurons
      - Disease course can be progressive or relapsing-remitting
      - Exacerbated by stress, infections, and hyperthermia
    - Presents with a variety of possible neurological defects, including optic neuritis, autonomic instability, and muscle weakness
    - Treatment options include steroids, monoclonal antibodies, and immunosuppressants
  - Perioperative implications
    - Avoid hyperthermia intraoperatively
    - General anesthesia
      - Succinylcholine has potential to cause worsened hyperkalemia due to denervation
      - Patients may have increased sensitivity to nondepolarizing neuromuscular blockers
      - Patients with pharyngeal weakness may be at increased risk of postoperative respiratory failure
    - Spinal anesthesia
      - May exacerbate MS due to the neurotoxic effects of local anesthetics
    - Epidural and regional anesthesia
      - Case studies have reported successful use without exacerbation
- **Guillain–Barré syndrome**
  - Mechanism and presentation
    - Antecedent viral illness → ascending symmetrical weakness over 2 to 4 weeks
      - Cell-mediated immunologic reaction against peripheral nerves → demyelination
    - Pathophysiological implications
      - 90% with pain
      - 75% with hypotension due to baroreceptor impairment
      - 50% with syndrome of inappropriate ADH (antidiuretic hormone) secretion
      - 25% with respiratory failure requiring mechanical ventilation
        - Risk high if vital capacity <15 cc/kg
    - Treatment
      - Plasmapheresis or intravenous immunoglobulin (IVIG)
  - Perioperative implications
    - Neuraxial not contraindicated, but could worsen condition
      - Cerebrospinal fluid in Guillain–Barré patients contains substances with sodium channel blocking effects
        - Local anesthetics may worsen muscle weakness
    - Succinylcholine contraindicated due to upregulation of acetylcholine receptors
    - Increased sensitivity to nondepolarizing muscle relaxants
    - Hemodynamics
      - Autonomic dysfunction and hypotension common
      - α-agonists → exaggerated response
- **Charcot–Marie–Tooth disease**
  - Mechanism and presentation
    - Inherited motor and sensory neuropathy due to defect in nerve axon or myelin sheath

- Presents with weakness (often lower extremity), loss of sensation, dyspnea, vision changes
    - Treatment is focused on supportive care, including physical and occupational therapy
  - Perioperative implications
    - Avoid succinylcholine → risk for hyperkalemic arrest
    - Avoid nitrous oxide → potential to worsen neuropathy
    - Unpredictable response to non-depolarizing muscle relaxants
    - Patients with kyphoscoliosis may have decreased respiratory reserve
- **Amyotrophic lateral sclerosis (ALS)**
  - Mechanism and presentation
    - Progressive neurodegenerative disease affecting upper and lower motor neurons in the brain and spine
    - Presents with weakness and muscle wasting that eventually results in difficulty breathing and swallowing
    - Treatment is supportive, including mechanical ventilation and enteral access for feeding
  - Perioperative implications
    - Avoid succinylcholine → risk for hyperkalemic arrest
    - Increased sensitivity to nondepolarizing muscle relaxants
    - Respiratory muscle weakness → may require prolonged or continued ventilator support
    - Neuraxial relatively contraindicated due to potential of worsening ALS
- **Spinobulbar muscular atrophy**
  - Mechanism and presentation
    - Progressive neurodegenerative disorder of motor neurons in the brain and spinal cord
      - X-linked inheritance due to mutation on androgen receptor
    - Presents with muscle cramps and weakness as well as gynecomastia and testicular atrophy due to androgen receptor defect
    - Treatment is supportive
  - Perioperative implications
    - Avoid succinylcholine → risk for hyperkalemic arrest
    - Respiratory muscle weakness → may require prolonged ventilator support
- **Hereditary spastic paraplegia**
  - Mechanism and presentation
    - Neurodegenerative disorder characterized by axonal degeneration
    - Presents with spasticity and developmental impairment
  - Perioperative implications
    - Avoid succinylcholine → risk for hyperkalemic arrest
    - Spinal anesthesia reported safe in several case reports

MUSCULAR DYSTROPHIES

- Definition
  - Group of muscular diseases that are characterized by mutations on the dystrophin gene
    - Dystrophin links actin and dystroglycans of the sarcolemma
  - Diagnosed by muscle biopsy and electromyography
- Types of muscular dystrophies
  - Duchenne muscular dystrophy
    - Most common childhood muscular dystrophy
    - Absent or severely limited amount of dystrophin
    - X-linked recessive inheritance
    - Painless muscle atrophy with pseudohypertrophy due to fatty infiltration of skeletal muscles
  - Becker muscular dystrophy
    - Dystrophin is partially functional
    - Less severe clinical implications compared to Duchenne
    - X-linked recessive inheritance
  - Limb-girdle muscular dystrophy
    - Muscle weakness affecting arms and legs
    - Autosomal recessive inheritance
  - Congenital muscular dystrophy

- ◆ Diagnosed at birth due to severe joint deformity and possible brain malformation
- ◆ Autosomal recessive inheritance
- ● Myotonic muscular dystrophy
  - ◆ Characterized by muscle wasting, fibrosis, and fatty degeneration at tissues
  - ◆ Autosomal dominant inheritance
- ■ Perioperative implications
  - ● Associated diseases
    - ◆ Many patients with muscular dystrophies have heart defects such as dilated cardiomyopathy and papillary muscle dysfunction → require cardiology evaluation and testing preoperatively
    - ◆ Many patients with conduction abnormalities → may require pacing
    - ◆ Increased restrictive lung disease → respiratory complications
  - ● Anesthetic issues
    - ◆ Increased sensitivity to anesthetic medications
    - ◆ Avoid succinylcholine for potential to cause profound hyperkalemia
    - ◆ In myotonic dystrophy, avoid drugs (etomidate) and conditions (shivering) that cause muscle contraction
    - ◆ Regional anesthesia does not relax tonic muscles because the disease is at the muscles, not the neuromuscular junction

MYOPATHIES

- ■ **Mitochondrial myopathies**
  - ● Definition
    - ◆ Group of diseases characterized by mitochondrial dysfunction
      - ➢ Kearns–Sayre syndrome, myoclonic epilepsy, mitochondrial encephalomyopathy
    - ◆ Presents with muscle weakness, heart failure, arrhythmias, movement disorders, neurological deficits, and seizures
  - ● Perioperative implications
    - ◆ Many anesthetic agents have negative effects on mitochondrial function, but short-term and long-term effects are unclear
      - ➢ Propofol has been implicated as harmful to mitochondria due to the effects on the electron transport chain
    - ◆ Avoid stressors like long periods of fasting
    - ◆ Support the patient with a dextrose containing IV fluid
    - ◆ Consider avoiding Lactated Ringer's solution
    - ◆ Consider avoiding succinylcholine
    - ◆ Increased risk of cardiac conduction abnormalities
    - ◆ Increased risk of respiratory complications
- ■ **Ion channel myopathies**
  - ● Hyperexcitable ion channel myopathies
    - ◆ **Neuromyotonia**
      - ➢ Autoimmune disorder due to antibodies against the potassium channels on motor nerves → hyperexcitable neurons
    - ◆ **Myotonia congenita**
      - ➢ Genetic defect in chloride channel on motor nerve → prevents contraction from terminating → hyperexcitable neurons
    - ◆ Anesthetic implications
      - ➢ Chronic downregulation of acetylcholine → increases susceptibility to neuromuscular blockers
  - ● Periodic paralysis
    - ◆ **Hyperkalemic periodic paralysis**
      - ➢ Autosomal dominant disorder with muscle weakness associated with hyperkalemia due to defect of sodium channels
      - ➢ Triggers include potassium-rich foods, stress, vigorous exercise, and fasting
      - ➢ Perioperative considerations
        - ✧ Avoid hyperkalemia
          - › Avoid acidosis

> Avoid hypoventilation
> Avoid succinylcholine
- Maintain glucose >100 mg/dL
- Prevent shivering
- **Hypokalemic periodic paralysis**
  - Autosomal dominant disorder with muscle weakness associated with hypokalemia due to defect at calcium channel
  - Triggers include vigorous exercise and rest, hypernatremia, hypothermia, and stress
  - Perioperative considerations
    - Avoid hypokalemia
      > Use lactated Ringer's or potassium-supplemented intravenous fluid
    - Avoid alkalosis
    - Avoid hyperventilation
    - Prevent hypothermia
- **Myasthenia gravis**
  - Mechanism and presentation
    - Autoimmune condition caused by IgG antibodies against ACh receptors in skeletal muscle
    - Presents with muscle weakness, easy fatigability, and ocular symptoms
    - Treated with pyridostigmine, steroids, and thymectomy
      > Myasthenic crisis is treated with neostigmine
      > Thymectomy is usually performed when patients are resistant to drug therapy
        - 75% improve after this procedure
  - Perioperative considerations
    - Continue anticholinesterase therapy perioperatively
    - More resistant to succinylcholine
    - Increased sensitivity to nondepolarizing muscle relaxants
    - Cardiomyopathy and conduction block common
    - Pharyngeal and laryngeal muscles often involved → aspiration risk
    - Increased risk of postoperative mechanical ventilation
      > Risk factors
        - Disease >6 years
        - Daily pyridostigmine dose >750 mg
        - Vital capacity <2.9 L
        - Pulmonary disease unrelated to myasthenia
      > Often present similarly to patients with residual neuromuscular blockade
  - Pregnancy
    - Continue anticholinesterase therapy throughout pregnancy
    - Can see neonatal myasthenia in ~30% of births
      > Characterized by general weakness
      > Increased risk of development of respiratory insufficiency in the newborn period
      > Treatment with anticholinesterases for up to 1 month
- **Lambert–Eaton syndrome**
  - Mechanism and presentation
    - Autoimmune disorder caused by IgG antibodies against presynaptic voltage-gated calcium channels at the neuromuscular junction
    - Presents with weakness, especially proximal muscles, and ocular symptoms
    - Improved muscle strength with exercise
    - Associated with certain cancers
      > Particularly small cell lung cancer
  - Perioperative considerations
    - Increased sensitivity to succinylcholine and non-depolarizing muscle relaxants
    - Increased gastroparesis → risks aspiration

RHEUMATOID CONDITIONS

- Ankylosing spondylitis
  - Mechanism and presentation

- ◆ A spondyloarthropathy that affects the axial skeleton and sacroiliac joint
  - ◆ Begins in the second decade of life → advanced form may result in complete fusion of the spine
    - ➤ Appearance of "bamboo spine" on imaging
  - ● Perioperative considerations
    - ◆ Cervical neck is stenotic and rigid, but not unstable → difficult airway
    - ◆ Intervertebral spaces limited and ossified → neuraxial difficult and increased risk of epidural hematoma
- ■ **Rheumatoid arthritis**
  - ● Mechanism and presentation
    - ◆ Inflammatory disorder of the synovium → fibrosis of joints
    - ◆ Can affect lungs and pleura → restrictive physiology
    - ◆ Increased propensity to develop atherosclerosis and fibrosis → increased coronary artery disease, conduction block, and pericarditis
  - ● Perioperative considerations
    - ◆ 25% incidence of atlantoaxial instability due to ligamentous and bony changes → unstable airway
      - ➤ C-spine films recommended for patients with neck symptoms
    - ◆ Careful cardiovascular and pulmonary history necessary to assess comorbidities
- ■ **Lupus**
  - ● Mechanism and presentation
    - ◆ Collection of autoimmune diseases that can manifest with symptoms in almost every organ system
    - ◆ Treatment regimens include antimalarial drugs, cyclophosphamide, steroids, methotrexate, mycophenolate, and azathioprine
  - ● Perioperative considerations
    - ◆ Increased risk of atlantoaxial subluxation
    - ◆ Prone to laryngeal complications, including subglottic stenosis, vocal cord paralysis, postextubation edema
    - ◆ Increased risk of autoimmune thrombocytopenia
    - ◆ 50% with asymptomatic pericarditis
    - ◆ 5% to 10% with symptomatic myocarditis
    - ◆ 40% with antiphospholipid antibodies → increased thrombosis risk
    - ◆ May have prolonged aPTT on laboratory testing (not accurate)
      - ➤ Due to a laboratory artifact caused by the antibody affecting the assay
      - ➤ Patients are not at increased risk of bleeding → no need to avoid neuraxial or regional

ORTHOPEDIC CONDITIONS

- ■ **Compartment syndrome (extremity)**
  - ● Elevated local pressures in the extremities impair perfusion to muscle and nerves → hypoxic edema
    - ◆ Causes include bleeding, edema, trauma, reperfusion injury, and burns
  - ● Six Ps
    - ◆ Pain, paresthesias, pallor, paralysis, pulselessness, and poikilothermia
    - ◆ Paresthesias and pain are an early sign
    - ◆ Pulselessness is a late sign
  - ● Acute compartment syndrome requires emergent surgical decompression and fasciotomy
- ■ Methyl methacrylate
  - ● Used as cement for orthopedic surgery
    - ◆ Typically hip and knee arthroplasty
  - ● Anesthetic implications
    - ◆ Methyl methacrylate can cause cytokine release → hypotension
    - ◆ Cement and reaming → fat emboli
- ■ Fat emboli
  - ● Complication following long bone fractures and reaming during orthopedic surgery
  - ● Presents with tachypnea, hypoxemia, tachycardia, and a petechial rash
  - ● Treatment is supportive

QUESTIONS

1. Which of the following statements regarding the perioperative pharmacologic management of a patient's hyperkalemic periodic paralysis is the most correct?

   A. Glucose containing fluids should be administered
   B. Volatile anesthetic agents should be avoided
   C. Potassium-containing fluids should be administered
   D. Nondepolarizing neuromuscular blocking agents should be avoided

2. Which of the following best describes the sensitivity of patients with myasthenia gravis to depolarizing neuromuscular blocking agents (D) and nondepolarizing neuromuscular blocking agents (N)?

   A. $\Downarrow$D,$\Uparrow$N
   B. $\Uparrow$D,$\Downarrow$N
   C. $\Uparrow$D,$\Uparrow$N
   D. $\Downarrow$D,$\Downarrow$N

3. A 24-year-old, 60-kg woman presents with a 4-day history of progressive weakness in her extremities. She has been healthy except for an upper respiratory tract infection 10 days ago. Her temperature is 37.8°C, BP is 130/80 mm Hg, Pulse 94 bpm, respiration rate is 28, and oxygen saturation is 97%. Forced vital capacity is 2.2 L. Which of the following is the most appropriate next step in management?

   A. High flow oxygen
   B. Endotracheal intubation
   C. Noninvasive ventilation
   D. Observation

4. Which of the following statements regarding anesthetic management of a patient with MS is most correct?

   A. Corticosteroids should be discontinued 24 hours before surgery
   B. Nondepolarizing neuromuscular blocking agents should be avoided
   C. Epidural anesthesia is not associated with exacerbations
   D. Mild hyperthermia should be maintained during general anesthesia

5. A 20-year-old man sustains a tibia–fibula fracture in a motor vehicle accident. He has experience significant swelling and pain in his leg since the injury. Which of the following is an early sign of compartment syndrome?

   A. Pallor
   B. Pulselessness
   C. Paresthesias
   D. Intracompartmental pressure of 20 mm Hg

PEDIATRIC ANESTHESIA SETUP AND ANESTHESIA TYPE

- Operating room setup
  - **Anesthetic circuits and equipment**
    - **Circuits**
      - Circle system with rebreathing ("semi-closed")
        - Need a gas reservoir bag, corrugated tubing, two unidirectional valves, an overflow valve, and a CO_2 absorber
        - Advantages
          - **Improved humidity**
          - **Thermal control**
          - **Conservation of humidity**
        - Disadvantages
          - Large compression volume losses
          - Longer equilibration time for anesthetics
          - Increased respiratory effort to open one-way valves
          - Increased resistance to spontaneous ventilation
          - Increased dead space
          - Valve malfunction
        - Low flow rates will NOT cause CO_2 retention UNLESS the CO_2 absorber is exhausted
      - Open circuits
        - Advantages
          - No rebreathing
          - Shorter equilibration times
          - Decreased influence of circuit on volumes and pressures
          - Decreased work of breathing due to lack of one-way valves
        - Disadvantages
          - Increased waste
          - Heat loss
      - Mapleson circuits ("semi-open")
        - Advantages
          - Small resistance to spontaneous ventilation
          - Decreased dead space
          - Easy to use (not bulky)
          - No valves
        - Disadvantages
          - Loss of heat
          - Loss of humidity
          - Poor scavenging ability
          - Need high gas flows to prevent rebreathing
      - Closed
        - Advantages
          - Maximum conservation of heat and humidity
          - Decreased pollution
        - Disadvantages
          - Uncertain delivery of anesthetics

> ⟩ Cannot rapidly change anesthetic concentration
> ⟩ Depends entirely on rebreathing
- ➤ Difference between "semi-open" and "semi-closed"
  - ❖ "Semi-closed" systems permit partial rebreathing of CO_2 and without a CO_2 absorber, CO_2 will build up
  - ❖ Need a reservoir bag as fresh gas flows have to equal the patient's minute ventilation
- ◆ Infant airway (Fig. 15.1)
  - ➤ Funnel shaped
    - ❖ Adults: cylinder shaped
  - ➤ Narrowest at the level of the cricoid cartilage
    - ❖ Adults: narrowest at the glottic opening
  - ➤ Infant glottis is narrower and more cephalad (C3-C4)
    - ❖ Adults: C5-C6
  - ➤ Tendency to develop subglottic edema when there is no leaking around the endotracheal tube (ETT)
- ◆ **ETT selection**
  - ➤ Cuffed vs. uncuffed
    - ❖ Cuffed tubes are commonly used due to improved airway security and control of ventilation
      - ⟩ Cuff pressure should be between 15 and 25 cm H_2O
      - ⟩ Increased cuff pressures → postextubation croup
      - ⟩ Prolonged high cuff pressures can cause tracheal pathology (e.g., stenosis)
    - ❖ Uncuffed tubes are commonly reserved for neonates
      - ⟩ Improved design of cuffed tubes has decreased the risk of tracheal stenosis → decreased use of uncuffed tubes
      - ⟩ If used, ideal uncuffed tube should allow a small air leak at 20- to 30-cm H_2O
        - ▸ If leak is significant → change to larger tube
        - ▸ If no leak at 30-cm H_2O → change to smaller tube

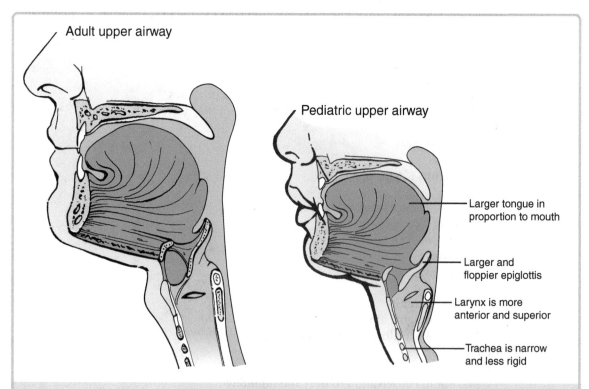

FIGURE 15.1   Pediatrics vs. Adult Airway Anatomy. Compared to the adult airway, the pediatric airway has a larger tongue, a larger and floppier epiglottis, a more anterior and superior larynx, and is narrowest at the level of the cricoid.

- ➤ Tube size
  - ❖ Cuffed tube size can be selected based on age
    - › Size = age/4 + 3
  - ❖ Depth of tube at teeth/gums = ETT size × 3
- ● **Temperature control**
  - ❖ Warm operating room to 80°F
  - ❖ Place warm blankets or radiant warmer on patient
  - ❖ Use fluid warmers
- ■ General anesthesia
  - ● **Premedication**
    - ❖ Need
      - ➤ Rarely needed for infant <6 months
      - ➤ Helpful when children develop separation anxiety at >9 months
    - ❖ **Medications**
      - ➤ Oral midazolam at 0.25 to 0.5 mg/kg
      - ➤ IM ketamine at 10 mg/kg
        - ❖ Consider atropine in addition to ketamine to avoid bradycardia
    - ❖ **Parent presence**
      - ➤ May be helpful in avoiding premedication
      - ➤ Not needed until stranger anxiety develops
  - ● Anesthetic induction
    - ❖ Induction technique
      - ➤ **Intravenous induction**
        - ❖ EMLA (eutectic mixture of local anesthetics [LA]) 2.5% lidocaine, 2.5% prilocaine
          - › Blunt pain from intravenous needle
          - › Apply to dry skin for 1 hour for depth of 5 mm for LA effect
          - › Prilocaine can cause methemoglobinemia
        - ❖ Induction doses
          - › Hypnotics
            - ▶ 2 to 3 mg/kg propofol
            - ▶ 1 to 2 mg/kg methohexital
            - ▶ 1 to 2 mg/kg ketamine
            - ▶ 0.2 to 0.3 mg/kg etomidate
          - › Opioids titrated to effect or based on specific surgery
          - › Neuromuscular blockers
            - ▶ 1 to 2 mg/kg succinylcholine (higher doses for infants)
              - ◌ Do not use routinely due to concerns of undiagnosed muscular dystrophy
              - ◌ May cause bradyarrhythmias and require atropine
              - ◌ Infants and neonates rarely fasciculate
            - ▶ Nondepolarizing muscle relaxant doses are similar to adults
      - ➤ **Inhalational induction**
        - ❖ Single breath
          - › Prime circuit with 8% sevoflurane and 60% nitrous oxide
          - › One tidal volume breath that is held is sufficient for induction
        - ❖ Gradual breathe down
          - › Increase sevoflurane gradually every few breaths until induced
          - › Nitrous oxide can be used to blunt smell of sevoflurane and increase induction speed
        - ❖ 100% oxygen should be administered after induction and prior to airway manipulation
    - ❖ Minimum alveolar concentration (MAC) (Fig. 15.2)
      - ➤ Greatest at 3 months (except for sevoflurane)
      - ➤ Lower in preterm neonates
        - ❖ May be due to elevated progesterone levels
        - ❖ Progesterone levels fall at 3 months
    - ❖ **Stages of anesthesia**
      - ➤ I: analgesia: respond to verbal stimulation, intact lid reflex, normal respiratory patterns, intact airway reflexes, some analgesia

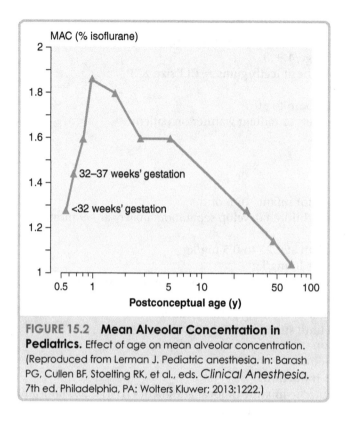

FIGURE 15.2   Mean Alveolar Concentration in Pediatrics. Effect of age on mean alveolar concentration. (Reproduced from Lerman J. Pediatric anesthesia. In: Barash PG, Cullen BF, Stoelting RK, et al., eds. *Clinical Anesthesia.* 7th ed. Philadelphia, PA: Wolters Kluwer; 2013:1222.)

- ➤ II: delirium or excitement: unconsciousness, irregular and unpredictable respiratory patterns, nonpurposeful muscle movements
- ➤ III: surgical anesthesia: return to periodic respirations, achievement of MAC
- ➤ IV: respiratory paralysis; respiratory and cardiovascular arrest
  - ◆ Laryngospasm
    - ➤ Characterized by involuntary vocal cord closure
    - ➤ Often occurs following extubation due to light plane of anesthesia and vocal cord stimulation
    - ➤ Treat with positive pressure ventilation, deepening anesthetic, or muscle relaxation
- ● Drug metabolism and doses
  - ◆ Undeveloped renal and hepatic function in neonates → prolonged effects of drugs requiring metabolism and renal clearance
- ● Complications of general anesthesia
  - ◆ **Postoperative nausea and vomiting**
    - ➤ Common after ear and eye procedures
    - ➤ Variety of medications can be used prophylactically (Chapter 5)
  - ◆ **Apnea of prematurity**
    - ➤ Presentation
      - ◆ Breath holding >20 seconds with accompanied bradycardia/cyanosis
      - ◆ Occurs primarily in <60 weeks postconceptual age after general anesthesia
      - ◆ Can be due to both central and/or obstructive cause
    - ➤ Risk factors
      - ◆ Preexisting apnea and bradycardia spells
      - ◆ Infants <44 weeks postconceptual age are at the highest risk
      - ◆ Anemia (Hct <30)
        - › No evidence that transfusion is helpful
      - ◆ Ketamine and prostaglandin E_1 (for ductal closure) associated with apnea
    - ➤ Treatment and monitoring options

- Admit to hospital for 12 to 24 hours prior to discharge
- IV caffeine
  - Mechanisms
    - Stimulation of central respiratory drive
    - Enhanced chemoreceptor sensitivity to CO_2
    - Increased skeletal muscle contraction
  - Side effects
    - Sinus tachycardia, supraventricular tachycardias, tachypnea, hyperthermia, seizures, irritability, and feeding intolerance
- Theophylline and aminophylline may reduce postoperative apnea
- Emergence delirium
  - Presentation
    - Patients inconsolable, hyperexcited, uncooperative, disoriented, and combative upon emerging from anesthesia
    - Do not recognize parents or follow commands
    - Commonly lasts 10 to 15 minutes, may last up to 45 minutes
  - Risk factors
    - Most common in preschool age children
    - Increases with head, eyes, ear, nose, and throat (HEENT) procedures
    - Increases with use of volatile over propofol
  - Treatment and prevention
    - Midazolam, opioids, toradol, clonidine, propofol, and dexmedetomidine reduce emergence agitation
- **Propofol-related infusion syndrome (PRIS)**
  - Etiology unclear, but could be due to uncoupling of cellular respiration at the mitochondria
    - Propofol inhibits carnitine palmitoyltransferase
  - Risk factors
    - Propofol infusion >48 hours at an infusion rate >5 mg/kg/hr
    - Sepsis
    - Steroid supplementation
  - Presentation
    - Lactic acidosis, acute renal failure, pancreatitis, hepatomegaly, rhabdomyolysis, treatment-resistant asystole (resistant to pacing and catecholamines)
    - Laboratory values
      - Lipidemic serum
      - Severe metabolic acidosis
      - Elevated creatine phosphokinase
      - Hyperkalemia
      - Elevated liver enzymes
      - Hypertriglyceridemia
  - Treatment
    - Depending on severity, supportive care such as extracorporeal membrane oxygenation and hemodialysis
    - Carbohydrate diet may be beneficial
- Neuraxial anesthesia
  - Spinal
    - **Anatomy**
      - Spinal cord ends at L3 in the neonate (adults at L1)
      - Cerebrospinal fluid (CSF) volume in infants is 4 cc/kg (adults have 2 cc/kg)
    - Indications
      - Procedures below the umbilicus in infants prone to postoperative apnea
    - Drugs and dosing
      - Effects of increased CSF volume
        - Infants need larger dose (per kg) of LA than adults
        - Spinal has a shorter duration than adults
      - Higher concentrations provide shorter duration of analgesia

- ◆ Complications
  - ➤ High spinal typically presents with apnea and hypoxia (not bradycardia and hypotension)
  - ➤ Increased risk of LA toxicity due to decreased albumin, decreased drug metabolism, and increased concentrations used
- ● Epidural
  - ◆ **Anatomy**
    - ➤ Epidural space
      - ❖ Between the foramen magnum and the sacral hiatus
      - ❖ Between the posterior longitudinal ligament and the ligamentum flavum
    - ➤ Due to more subtle loss of resistance, do loss of resistance to saline (not air) to avoid air embolism
    - ➤ Medications can be injected or a catheter can be threaded into the epidural space
  - ◆ Indications
    - ➤ Postoperative pain control for all major abdominal, pelvic, and thoracic surgeries
  - ◆ Drugs and dosing
    - ➤ Similar drug concentrations to adults, but infusion rates should be adjusted to weight of patient
- ● Caudal
  - ◆ **Anatomy** (Fig. 15.3)
    - ➤ Target the sacral hiatus
      - ❖ Between the fusion of the fourth and fifth sacral vertebral arches
      - ❖ Between the sacral cornua laterally
      - ❖ Covered by the sacrococcygeal membrane
    - ➤ Advance needle at 30° to 45° cephalad until loss of resistance
      - ❖ Inject medications or thread catheter into sacral epidural space
  - ◆ Indications
    - ➤ Surgical procedures below the umbilicus
    - ➤ Capable of reaching thoracic levels with higher doses, but less reliable and risks spread above T4
  - ◆ Drugs and dosing
    - ➤ Single shot technique often used, but catheters can be placed
    - ➤ Dermatome reached is based on volume of LA injected

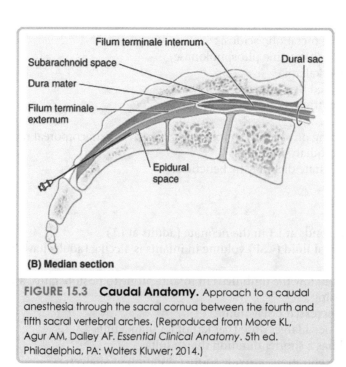

FIGURE 15.3 **Caudal Anatomy.** Approach to a caudal anesthesia through the sacral cornua between the fourth and fifth sacral vertebral arches. (Reproduced from Moore KL, Agur AM, Dalley AF. *Essential Clinical Anatomy*. 5th ed. Philadelphia, PA: Wolters Kluwer; 2014.)

❖ 0.5 cc/kg → sacral dermatomes
❖ 1.0 cc/kg → lumbar dermatomes
❖ 1.25 cc/kg → midthoracic dermatomes

NEONATAL ANATOMY AND PHYSIOLOGY

■ In utero development
  ● First 8 weeks: organogenesis
  ● Second trimester: organ development
  ● Third trimester: muscle and fat addition
■ Organ system development
  ● **Cardiovascular**
    ❖ Shunts bypass lungs and liver
      ➤ Foramen ovale: right atrium → left atrium
      ➤ Ductus arteriosus: pulmonary artery → aorta
      ➤ Ductus venosus: umbilical vein → inferior vena cava
    ❖ **Changes to circulation after birth**
      ➤ Vascular resistance
        ❖ Increase in systemic vascular resistance (SVR)
        ❖ Decrease in pulmonary vascular resistance (PVR)
      ➤ Closure of shunts
        ❖ Foramen ovale closes when left atrial pressure > right atrial pressure
        ❖ Ductus arteriosus closes a few days after birth, but complete closure is at 2 to 3 weeks after birth
        ❖ Ductus venosus closes after birth when portal pressure decreases, but complete closure is at ~1 week after birth
      ➤ Fetal stress such as infections or acidosis can increase pulmonary pressures → revert to fetal circulation
    ❖ Newborn heart
      ➤ Left ventricle is thin and less compliant
      ➤ Heart rate (HR) dependent on filling
      ➤ Cardiac output is HR dependent
      ➤ Increased oxygen consumption (~6 cc/kg vs. 3 cc/kg in adults)
  ● **Pulmonary**
    ❖ Respiration is less efficient in newborns
      ➤ Smaller airway diameter → increased resistance
      ➤ More compliant chest walls → increased work of breathing
      ➤ Less compliant lung tissue → increased work of breathing
      ➤ Less type 1 muscle fibers → easier fatigue
      ➤ Increased atelectasis
        ❖ Decreased number of alveoli
        ❖ Decreased FRC (functional residual capacity)
      ➤ Hypoxemia develops more rapidly
        ❖ Increased minute volume (MV)/FRC
        ❖ Increased metabolic rate drives the increased MV
    ❖ **Airway differences between newborns and adults**
      ➤ Larger tongue
      ➤ Larynx is more cephalic
      ➤ Epiglottis is omega shaped and angled over larynx
      ➤ Larynx narrows at the cricoid
      ➤ Cricoid is at C3-4 at birth (C4-5 in adults)
    ❖ Functional residual capacity (FRC)
      ➤ Equal to adults on a cc/kg basis
      ➤ FRC is dynamically maintained in infants by laryngeal breaking
    ❖ Infants are preferential nasal breathers, but can breathe orally if obstructed
  ● **Renal**

- Kidney maturation occurs after birth until 2 years of age
- The glomerular filtration rate is low at birth and triples over the first 3 months
- Decreased ability to concentrate urine
- Decreased ability to handle large solute loads
- Increased urinary losses
- Total body water (TBW) increased as compared to adults
  - Prone to "overhydration" → cerebral edema and seizures
- **Liver**
  - Enzyme systems are present, but develop after birth
  - Minimal glycogen stores → hypoglycemia
- **Temperature regulation**
  - Infants have a large surface area to weight ratio → increased heat loss
  - Lose heat easily and it is more difficult for them to generate it
    - Do not have the ability to "shiver"
  - Methods to increase temperature
    - Nonshivering thermogenesis
      - Brown fat
      - Less effective at generating heat as compared to shivering
    - Cutaneous vasoconstriction
    - Crying and irritability
- Body distribution
  - Infants are 75% water → replaced by muscle and fat with age
  - Water-soluble drugs have larger volume of distribution → require larger doses
  - Lipid-soluble drugs have less redistribution → prolonged effect with bolus dosing
- Neonatal vitals and laboratory values
  - Vitals
    - HR: 120 to 160
      - Mean HR goes up at 30 days to 160
    - Blood pressure (BP): 65 to 85/45 to 55 mm Hg
      - Systolic BP trends up with age
      - Diastolic BP drops at 1 to 2 months, then increases
      - Systolic BP of ~60 at birth → increases to 80 at 1 year
    - Respiratory rate: 40 to 60
      - Oxygen consumption for a neonate is 2× greater than for an adult (6 to 8 cc/kg vs. 3 to 4 cc/kg)
      - Alveolar ventilation (cc/kg) for a neonate is 2× greater than for an adult
    - Oxygen saturation: 88% to 95%
  - Signs of dehydration
    - Mild: decreased urine output
    - Moderate: dry mucous membranes, decreased skin turgor
    - Severe: extreme thirst, irritability, sunken fontanelles, no urine output
  - Pre-ductal monitoring
    - Used for patients at risk for right-to-left shunting
    - Monitors should be placed on the right side
      - Use right radial or temporal arteries for monitoring
  - Fetal labs
    - **Hemoglobin (Hb)**
      - At birth Hb is 15 to 20 g/dL → **decreases to 10 to 12 g/dL at 2 to 3 months** → Hb increases at 6 to 9 months
      - Decrease due to fetal Hb with shorter life than adult Hb (60 days compared to 120 days) and suppressed erythropoiesis
    - **Glucose**
      - Fetal hypoglycemia definition
        - Glucose <30 mg/dL within first 24 hours of life
        - Glucose <45 mg/dL after 24 hours of life
    - Hypocalcemia

- ➤ Preterm infants susceptible to hypocalcemia due to limited calcium reserves
- ➤ Presents with irritability, twitching, hypotension, bradycardia, and seizures

NEONATAL CONDITIONS

- ■ **Disorders of prematurity**
  - ● Transient tachypnea of newborn
    - ◆ Short-term need for respiratory support or supplemental oxygen due to delayed absorption of fetal lung fluid
    - ◆ Risk factors: maternal diabetes, maternal asthma, C-section delivery
    - ◆ Chest x-ray (CXR) shows increased interstitial fluid markings
    - ◆ Improves rapidly
      - ➤ **Neonatal respiratory distress syndrome**
    - ◆ Mechanism
      - ➤ Insufficient surfactant production and lung immaturity → increased surface tension → increased airspace collapse
      - ➤ Lung is composed of collapsed and hyperinflated areas → hyaline membranes form over time
    - ◆ Complications
      - ➤ Pneumothorax
      - ➤ Pneumomediastinum
      - ➤ Bronchopulmonary dysplasia
    - ◆ Diagnosis
      - ➤ Lecithin–sphingomyelin ratio in amniotic fluid
        - ❖ 2: fetal lung surfactant sufficient
        - ❖ <1.5: fetal lung surfactant insufficient
    - ◆ Treatment
      - ➤ Parturients going into preterm labor prior to 34 weeks gestation are treated with betamethasone
        - ❖ Betamethasone increases hyperglycemia in mother, hypoglycemia in neonate
      - ➤ Infants may require continuous positive airway pressure (CPAP) or mechanical ventilation
        - ❖ Exogenous surfactant can be administered through the ETT
      - ➤ Severe cases may require extracorporeal membrane oxygenation (ECMO) or high frequency oscillation
  - ● **Bronchopulmonary dysplasia**
    - ◆ Chronic form of respiratory distress syndrome in infants due to lung inflammation and scarring
      - ➤ Diagnosed after 28 days of life
      - ➤ Develops after long periods of mechanical ventilation, barotrauma, high oxygen, and infection
    - ◆ Infants are prone to tracheal stenosis, decreased lung compliance, respiratory infections, and airway reactivity
    - ◆ Can see hypoxia, hypercarbia, pulmonary hypertension, and cor pulmonale
    - ◆ Treatment
      - ➤ Supportive care, diuretics, and pulmonary vasodilators
  - ● **Intraventricular hemorrhage**
    - ◆ Affects premature infants due to immature blood–brain barrier and minimally developed cerebral autoregulation
    - ◆ High cerebral blood flow through germinal matrix can lead to bleeding and intraventricular hemorrhage
      - ➤ Germinal matrix regresses at term births → risk decreases
  - ● **Retinopathy of prematurity (ROP)**
    - ◆ Retinal vasculature develops between 16th and 44th week of postconceptual age
      - ➤ ROP risk negligible risk if postconceptional age >44 weeks
    - ◆ ROP is an abnormal proliferation of immature retinal vessels due to exposure at high oxygen concentrations

        - Neovascularization with development of fibrous tissue → hemorrhage, retinal tears, or detachment
        - Likely a two-hit mechanism because patients with congenital heart disease can develop ROP
    - Risk factors
        - Pa_{O_2} >80 or 90 for prolonged periods
        - Hypoxia, hypercarbia, hypocarbia, sepsis, apnea
    - Most ROP regress, but 10% lead to visual impairment, including blindness
- **Necrotizing enterocolitis (NEC)**
    - Bacterial infection of the intestines that commonly affects premature infants
    - Risk factors
        - Low birth weight (<2,500 g)
        - History of umbilical artery catheterization
        - Bacterial infection
        - Gram-negative endotoxemia
    - NEC is associated with acidosis, hypoxemia, and shock
    - Infants may be coagulopathic and acidotic

- **Congenital heart disease**
    - Defect in structure of the heart or great vessels
        - Degree of defect can cause minimal symptoms or be severe enough to warrant neonatal cardiac surgery
        - The most severe congenital heart defects often have two or more lesions
            - The second lesion is often necessary for survival (e.g., ventricular septal defect [VSD] in transposition of the great vessels allows communication between otherwise parallel circulations)
        - May be associated with other congenital diseases (VACTERL)
            - V: vertebral abnormalities
            - A: anal atresia
            - C: congenital heart disease
            - T: tracheoesophageal fistula
            - E: esophageal atresia
            - R: renal abnormalities
            - L: limb defects
    - **Classifications**
        - Shunt lesions
            - Left to right
                - Pulmonary blood flow ~3× that of systemic blood flow
                    - Leads to pulmonary hypertension and heart failure
                - VSD, Atrial septal defect (ASD), and patent ductus arteriosus (PDA)
                    - PDA
                        - Placement of an arterial catheter should be "preductal"
                            - Place in the right upper extremity
                        - Can attempt to close the PDA with indomethacin
                        - Complication of surgical repair is possible injury to the left recurrent laryngeal nerve
                - Want to decrease SVR and increase PVR
                    - Positive pressure ventilation increases PVR and decreases shunting
            - Right to left
                - Infants are cyanotic
                    - Cyanosis is NOT improved with increasing the concentration of F_I
                - Avoid decreasing SVR and increasing PVR
                    - Avoid crying, which increases PVR
                - Tetralogy of Fallot, Eisenmenger syndrome, Ebstein anomaly, pulmonary atresia, tricuspid atresia
        - Mixing lesion (mixing of blood from systemic and pulmonary circulation)
            - Transposition of the great vessels with a VSD
            - Tetralogy of Fallot (Fig. 15.4)

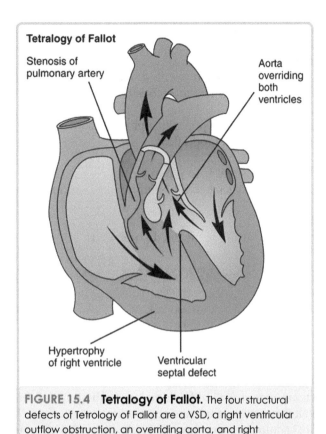

FIGURE 15.4 Tetralogy of Fallot. The four structural defects of Tetrology of Fallot are a VSD, a right ventricular outflow obstruction, an overriding aorta, and right ventricular hypertrophy. (Reproduced from Rosdahl CB, Kowalski MT. *Textbook of Basic Nursing.* 10th ed. Philadelphia, PA: Lippincott Williams & Wilkins; 2011.)

> ➤ Tricuspid atresia
> ➤ Univentricular heart
- ◆ Obstructive lesion
  > ➤ Pulmonic stenosis
  > ➤ Aortic stenosis
  > ➤ Coarctation of the aorta
  > ➤ Hypoplastic left heart
- ◆ Structural defect
  > ➤ Hypoplasia (hypoplastic left heart)
  > ➤ Obstruction defect (outflow tract obstruction)
  > ➤ Septal defect (ASD, VSD)
  > ➤ Cyanotic disease (truncus arteriosus, tetralogy of Fallot, transposition of the great vessels, tricuspid atresia)
- ● **Diseases**
  - ◆ Tetralogy of Fallot
    > ➤ Disease comprising four structural defects
    >   - ❖ VSD, right ventricular outflow tract (RVOT) obstruction, overriding aorta, right ventricular hypertrophy
    > ➤ RVOT obstruction and VSD → mixing of right- and left-sided blood → cyanotic heart defect
    > ➤ Avoid decreases in SVR
    >   - ❖ Increases right-to-left shunt → worsens cyanosis
    >   - ❖ Increases risk of Tet spell, a hypercyanotic attack due to spasm of the infundibular cardiac muscle
    >   - › Treat with phenylephrine (increases SVR) and esmolol (reduces infundibular spasm)
  - ◆ Truncus arteriosus

➢ Failure of truncus arteriosus to divide into pulmonary and aortic trunk → single trunk providing mixed blood to pulmonary arteries and systemic circulation
- Transposition of the great vessels
  ➢ Defect in arrangement of the great vessels → creation of two isolated circulations in parallel
  ➢ Requires defect in septum to mix blood for survival
- Tricuspid atresia
  ➢ Absence of tricuspid valve → hypoplastic right ventricle
  ➢ Requires an ASD to maintain blood flow
- Hypoplastic left heart
  ➢ Hypoplastic left ventricle unable to pump blood
  ➢ Requires ASD to shunt oxygenated blood to right side and PDA to eject into the systemic circulation
- Coarctation of the aorta
  ➢ Narrowing of the aorta at site of the ductus arteriosus

Shunt type/effect	Left to right	Right to left
IV induction	Slower	Faster
INHALATIONAL induction	Normal CO: no change Decreased CO: faster	Slower

- Pediatric cardiac surgery
  - **Palliative surgery**
    ➢ Procedure to temporize structural heart disease until more definitive surgery can take place
      - Goal is to alter structure of heart to sustain life
      - May require creating or worsening certain lesions in an effort to deliver oxygenated blood to the circulation (e.g., creating an ASD to mix blood from the right and left atrium)
    ➢ Commonly performed in infants with lesions not compatible with life due to missing heart components
      - Tricuspid atresia: absent right ventricle and tricuspid valve
      - Hypoplastic left heart: aortic atresia and hypoplastic left ventricle
      - Univentricular heart: absent ventricle
    ➢ Goals of palliative surgery depend on nature of lesions
      - Increase pulmonary blood flow in certain defects with Blalock–Taussig shunt, Glenn shunt, or VSD enlargement
      - Decrease pulmonary blood flow in certain defects with pulmonary artery banding or PDA ligation
      - Increase mixing in certain defects with atrial septostomy
  - **Corrective surgery**
    ➢ Improved surgical techniques has led to increased definitive surgeries being performed in infancy for congenital heart disease
      - Transposition of great arteries: arterial switch
      - Tetralogy of Fallot: VSD closure and RVOT patch
      - Truncus arteriosus: right ventricle to pulmonary artery conduit and VSD closure
- **Noncardiac surgery and chronic disease in adulthood**
  - Due to improved surgical techniques, congenital heart disease patients are surviving longer and necessitating surgeries into adulthood
  - Preoperative conditions
    ➢ Preoperative evaluation should target understanding the surgical procedures performed and their associated physiologic changes
    ➢ Understanding each patient's anatomy, path of blood flow, and cardiac reserve is critical
  - **Anesthetic induction and maintenance**
    ➢ Inhalational induction
      - Selection of inhalational induction depends on tolerance for hypoventilation and potential for shunting
      - Left-to-right shunts have more rapid inhalational induction

- ❖ Right-to-left shunts have slower inhalational induction due to diversion of blood from lungs
  - ➤ IV induction is more rapid due to bypass of pulmonary circulation
    - ❖ Opioid–muscle relaxant combination used for those with little cardiac reserve due to hemodynamic stability
    - ❖ Ketamine is used if maintaining SVR is a high priority
    - ❖ Propofol can be used in those with increased cardiac reserve
  - ➤ Monitoring
    - ❖ Location of monitoring (right vs. left side, upper extremity vs. lower extremity) is important in congenital heart disease depending on the location of the lesion
    - ❖ Specialized monitoring may include an arterial line, central line, pulmonary artery catheter, and echocardiography
- ■ Neonatal conditions and anesthetic considerations
  - ● **Congenital diaphragmatic hernia**
    - ❖ Abdominal viscera protrudes into the chest cavity through a diaphragmatic defect, usually on left side
    - ❖ Scaphoid abdomen and bowel sounds can be auscultated in the chest
    - ❖ Ipsilateral lung is hypoplastic and has a reduced number of alveoli
      - ➤ Contralateral lung is often affected as well
    - ❖ Approximately 25% will have associated cardiac abnormalities
    - ❖ Approximately 30% will have polyhydramnios
    - ❖ Associated GI problems
      - ➤ Incomplete rotation of the cecum
      - ➤ Umbilical defects
      - ➤ Presence of duodenal constricting bands
    - ❖ Can see dehydration and severe metabolic acidosis
    - ❖ Anesthetic considerations
      - ➤ Immediate intubation and stomach decompression needed
        - ❖ Minimize positive pressure ventilation to minimize tidal volumes and pulmonary pressures
        - ❖ Ventilation of lungs with mask and bag may increase stomach distention and worsen respiratory state
      - ➤ Goal of O_2 saturation should be >90 with airway pressures <35 cm H_2O
        - ❖ Accept permissive hypoventilation due to hypoplastic lungs
        - ❖ Do not expand the lungs to normal size due to hypoplastic state → increased risk of rupture
        - ❖ If saturation drops, suspect tension pneumothorax → place chest tube
      - ➤ Avoid nitrous oxide for causing bowel and stomach distention → worsens respiratory status
  - ● **Tracheoesophageal fistula/Esophageal atresia** (Fig. 15.5)

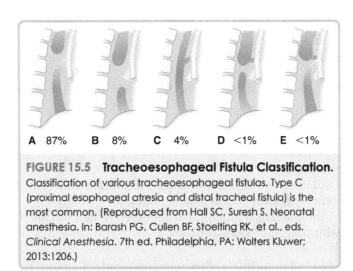

A 87%   **B** 8%   **C** 4%   **D** <1%   **E** <1%

FIGURE 15.5 Tracheoesophageal Fistula Classification.
Classification of various tracheoesophageal fistulas. Type C
(proximal esophageal atresia and distal tracheal fistula) is the
most common. (Reproduced from Hall SC, Suresh S. Neonatal
anesthesia. In: Barash PG, Cullen BF, Stoelting RK, et al., eds.
Clinical Anesthesia. 7th ed. Philadelphia, PA: Wolters Kluwer;
2013:1206.)

- Collection of disorders characterized by an abnormal connection between the esophagus and the trachea
- Approximately 50% of these infants will have other associated congenital abnormalities
- Most common is Type C
  - Proximal esophageal atresia ending in a blind pouch
  - Distal tracheal fistula with esophagus
- Presents with respiratory distress, regurgitation, and increased oral secretions
  - Confirmed with inability to pass suction catheter into stomach
  - Absence of bowel gas on an XRay of the abdomen; kidneys, ureters, bladder (KUB)
- Prone to dehydration and aspiration
- Anesthetic considerations
  - Minimize positive pressure ventilation during induction → stomach inflates
  - Location and size of fistula may make ventilation difficult
    - A secured airway needs to be distal to the lesion for effective ventilation
  - Often associated with VACTERL diseases

- **Neonatal lobar emphysema**
  - Developmental disorder of the bronchopulmonary tract manifested by lobar hyperinflation
  - Presents with respiratory distress
  - May require a lobectomy
  - Anesthetic considerations
    - Minimize assisted ventilation due to potential to worsen hyperinflation and gas trapping
    - May require mainstem ETT to isolate the defective lobe

- **Pyloric stenosis**
  - Narrowing of the duodenum due to muscle hypertrophy surrounding the pylorus
  - Presents with nonbilious projectile vomiting
    - Incidence is $4\times$ more likely in males than females
    - Diagnosed by ultrasound
  - Medical emergency (not surgical emergency)
    - Protracted vomiting → dehydration, hypokalemia, and metabolic alkalosis
    - Correct metabolic derangements and volume resuscitate prior to surgery
      - Na > 130, K > 3, Cl > 85, and UO 1 to 2 cc/kg
  - Anesthetic considerations
    - Gastric decompression prior to operating room
    - Rapid sequence intubation
    - Minimize opioids
      - Hypochloremic metabolic alkalosis from vomiting decreases respiratory drive
      - Additional opioids will worsen respiratory status

- Abdominal wall defects
  - **Omphalocele**
    - Midline defect where the intestinal viscera herniate into the base of the umbilical cord
    - Intestinal contents are covered by a membranous sac
    - Frequency of associated congenital defects are $2\times$ greater
    - Incidence is ~1/6,000
  - **Gastroschisis**
    - Defect of abdominal wall lateral to umbilicus due to occlusion of omphalomesenteric artery during gestation
    - Abdominal contents unprotected and exposed
      - Hypovolemia more severe
    - Incidence ~1/30,000
  - Anesthetic considerations
    - Third space and dehydration losses → require significant fluid resuscitation
    - Exposed viscera → significant heat loss
    - May require multiple-staged procedure if abdomen cannot be closed
    - Associated with congenital cardiac disease

- **Myelomeningocele**
  - Most serious version of spina bifida where meninges and spinal cord protrude through a defect in the vertebral column

- ◆ Anesthetic considerations
  - ➤ Surgical positioning for airway management may be challenging
  - ➤ Risk for significant blood loss
  - ➤ Potential for brainstem herniation

PEDIATRIC DISEASES AND CONDITIONS

- ■ Respiratory and airway infections
  - ● **Upper respiratory tract infection**
    - ◆ Common in children and can increase airway reactivity
      - ➤ Reactive airway can persist for 4 to 6 weeks after upper respiratory infection
      - ➤ Examples: rhinitis, sinusitis, pharyngitis, laryngotracheitis
    - ◆ Anesthetic risks
      - ➤ Irritable airway → increased risk of laryngospasm, bronchospasm, and desaturation
      - ➤ Children often get sick again before the 4 to 6 weeks necessary for airway reactivity to diminish → consider proceeding with surgery if symptoms are mild
      - ➤ Criteria for canceling or postponing elective surgery
        - ❖ Productive cough, fevers, wheezing, nasal congestion, and worsening symptoms
  - ● Specific airway infections
    - ◆ **Croup** (laryngotracheobronchitis)
      - ➤ Presents with difficulty breathing, inspiratory stridor, hoarseness, and barking cough
        - ❖ CXR with steeple sign
      - ➤ Commonly caused by parainfluenza virus
      - ➤ Airway obstruction is rare
      - ➤ Usually affects infants up to ~3 months old
        - ❖ Can see in children up to 3 years old
      - ➤ Treat with supplemental oxygen, nebulized epinephrine, and steroids to decrease airway edema
    - ◆ **Epiglottitis**
      - ➤ Presents with fever, difficulty swallowing, inspiratory stridor, drooling, respiratory distress, and propensity to sit up and lean forward
        - ❖ "Thumb" sign on lateral CXR
      - ➤ Commonly caused by a bacterial infection
        - ❖ H. flu
        - ❖ *Streptococcus pneumonia*
        - ❖ Staph
      - ➤ Usually affects children from ~2 to 6 years old
      - ➤ Treatment
        - ❖ Antibiotics
        - ❖ Secure airway
          - › Secure airway in operating room with surgeon available
          - › Inhalational induction advised to maintain spontaneous respirations
          - › Patient may not tolerate multiple intubation attempts due to profound airway swelling
    - ◆ **Peritonsillar abscess**
      - ➤ Pus collection in the peritonsillar space due to tonsillitis
      - ➤ Presents with sore throat, fevers, and voice changers
        - ❖ Can obstruct the glottic opening
      - ➤ Treatment is with antibiotics and surgical drainage
  - ● **Airway obstruction**
    - ◆ Extrathoracic lesions (inspiratory airway obstruction)
      - ➤ Laryngomalacia, tracheomalacia, laryngeal polyps, epiglottitis
    - ◆ Intrathoracic lesions (expiratory airway obstruction)
      - ➤ Mediastinal mass, obstructive sleep apnea
- ■ Altered airway anatomy
  - ● **Pierre Robin syndrome:** micrognathia, glossoptosis, cleft palate
  - ● **Beckwith–Wiedemann syndrome:** large tongue

- **Klippel–Feil syndrome:** micrognathia, short neck, fused cervical vertebrae, kyphoscoliosis
- **Treacher Collins syndrome:** micrognathia, cleft palate
- **Crouzon syndrome:** underdeveloped upper jaw, cleft palate
- **Goldenhar syndrome:** one-sided facial deformity, micrognathia, vertebral defects
- **Hurler syndrome:** narrow nasal passage, large tongue, short neck, hypoplastic mandible
- Developmental disorders
  - **Cerebral palsy**
    - Neurological disorder that manifests with motor and sensory deficits as well as cognitive impairment
    - Presents with lack of muscle coordination, low muscle tone, spasticity, and developmental impairment
    - Anesthetic implications
      - Decreased MAC
      - Increased sensitivity to succinylcholine and opioids
      - Resistance to nondepolarizing neuromuscular blocks
      - Increased intraoperative hypotension due to hypothalamic dysfunction
      - No hyperkalemic risk to succinylcholine because muscles were never denervated
  - **Trisomy 21 (Down syndrome)**
    - Associated with characteristic facial features, intellectual disability, and impaired growth
    - Anesthetic implications
      - Increased macroglossia
      - Large tonsils
      - Narrow nasopharynx
      - Increased risk of atlantoaxial joint instability
      - Increased congenital heart defects, including endocardial cushion defects
        - AV canal defects, PDA, VSD
      - Predisposition to bradyarrhythmias
      - Increased airway obstruction
      - Problems with appropriate alveolar development
        - Can lead to hypoxemia and pulmonary hypertension
      - Congenital duodenal atresia
      - Increased gastroesophageal reflux
- Musculoskeletal disorders
  - **Osteogenesis imperfecta**
    - Connective tissue disease due to collagen defect → brittle and fragile bones
    - Anesthetic implications
      - Risk of bone fractures with positioning
      - Consider minimal airway manipulation
  - **Marfan syndrome**
    - Connective tissue disorder due to a glycoprotein defect
    - Anesthetic implications
      - Increased risk of cystic medial degeneration of cardiac valves
      - Increased risk of aortic aneurysm and dissection
      - Increased risk of pneumothorax
  - **Achondroplasia**
    - Genetic disorder affecting cartilage formation manifested by short stature
    - Anesthetic implications
      - Abnormal spine curvature may inhibit lung expansion
      - Altered vertebral anatomy and possible C-spine instability → increased intubation difficulty
  - **Juvenile rheumatoid arthritis**
    - Autoimmune disease affecting the joints in children
    - Anesthetic implications
      - Increased airway difficulty if cervical spine involved
      - Lumbar lordosis may limit neuraxial use
      - Assess impact of immunosuppressants on organ systems perioperatively

ANESTHETIC ISSUES FOR SPECIFIC SURGERIES

- Otolaryngology
  - **Myringotomy**
    - Brief procedure that can be accomplished with an inhalational anesthetic and rarely requires IV access
    - Fentanyl can be administered intranasally
    - Postop nausea and vomiting is common postoperative issue
  - **Tonsillectomy and adenoidectomy**
    - Postoperative bleeding occurs in up to 8% of cases
      - 67% at tonsillar fossa, 27% at nasopharynx
      - Most fatal cases occur in the first 6 hours (75% cases); therefore, most patients kept and monitored up to 8 hours
    - Take-back to operating room for bleeding should have IV access for resuscitation
      - Rapid sequence induction should be performed given bleeding near airway and need for hemodynamic support
  - **Cleft lip/palate**
    - Assess for other genetic disorders
    - Tend to have feeding difficulties, increased risk of reflux, aspiration
    - Lip can be repaired ~1 month old
    - Palate is usually repaired ~1 year old
    - Increased difficult laryngoscopy
    - Increased risk of airway obstruction
- Neurosurgery
  - **Craniotomies**
    - **Tumors**
      - Most pediatric brain tumors are infratentorial
        - Medulloblastomas, cerebellar astrocytomas, brainstem gliomas, and ependymomas
        - Infratentorial tumors can obstruct CSF flow → increased intracranial pressure (ICP)
        - Surgical positioning can be challenging and require prone or sitting position
      - Supratentorial tumors are rare
        - Craniopharyngiomas, optic gliomas, pituitary adenomas, and hypothalamic tumors
    - **Vascular malformations**
      - Arteriovenous malformations may present with intracerebral hemorrhage, stroke or seizure
      - Anesthetic considerations include sufficient intravenous access and brain relaxation to improve visualization
    - **Hydrocephalus**
      - Types
        - Primary hydrocephalus is due to excess CSF production
        - Secondary hydrocephalus is from obstruction of CSF flow or absorption
      - Anesthetic plan should minimize increases in ICP
        - Avoid hypoventilation
        - Consider rapid sequence intubation
        - Avoidance of ketamine and other drugs that increase ICP
  - **Craniofacial procedures**
    - Craniosynostosis
      - Cranial sutures close prematurely
      - Patients may have challenging airways due to craniofacial distortion
      - Significant potential for blood loss due to surface area and extensive vascularization of scalp
  - **Tethered cord**
    - Group of disorders where spinal cord is tethered to base of spinal canal
    - Requires prone positioning
    - May require intraoperative evoked potential monitoring
  - **Halo placement**
    - Halo provides stabilization of cervical spine injuries by immobilizing the neck

- Intubation of patients in halos may be incredibly challenging due to inability to extend the neck and physical obstruction of the airway
- Thoracic surgery
  - **Pectus excavatum**
    - Correction of chest wall deformity using a bar that is passed under the sternum and flipped to lift the sternum anteriorly
    - Painful procedure that may require an epidural catheter
  - **Mediastinal mass**
    - Masses in the mediastinum often represent thymomas, lymphomas, teratomas, or neurogenic tumors
    - May cause airway and superior vena cava compression
    - Maintain spontaneous respirations until airway is secured due to possibility of airway collapse under anesthesia or neuromuscular blockade
- General surgery
  - **Intussusception**
    - Telescoping of bowel, often at the ileocolic junction
    - Presents with abdominal pain, currant jelly stools, and palpable abdominal mass in 50%
    - Treated with enema or surgical reduction
      - Enema has 5% to 10% recurrence rate
  - **Neuroblastomas**
    - Neuroendocrine tumors that commonly occur in children
    - Tumor can be located in the spine, abdomen, chest, or bone
    - May be associated with intraoperative hypertension or airway difficulties depending on tumor location and associated hormones
  - **Wilms tumor**
    - Nephroblastoma that is often diagnosed at ages 1 to 3
    - Presents with abdominal pain, nausea, hematuria, and hypertension
    - Preoperative chemotherapy may affect organ function and anesthetic selection
    - Intraoperative considerations include possible hemorrhage and inferior vena cava compression
  - **Circumcision**
    - Anesthesia can be offered through a variety of methods, including EMLA cream, parental opioids, acetaminophen, dorsal nerve penile block, subcutaneous ring block, or caudal anesthesia
- Orthopedic surgery
  - **Congenital hip dysplasia**
    - Misalignment of the hip diagnosed with the Ortolani and Barlow maneuver
    - Treatment is with casts and traction
      - Surgery may be necessary
  - **Scoliosis**
    - Cobb angles >65° associated with decreased lung volumes
      - Restrictive lung disease can cause pulmonary hypertension
      - May also have cardiac disease
      - Vital capacity <40% normal predicts need for postoperative ventilation
    - May be associated with significant intraoperative hemorrhage
    - Neuromonitoring can be done with evoked potentials or a wake-up test
- Burn surgery
  - Skin burns
    - **Degrees**
      - Superficial (1st degree)
      - Partial thickness (2nd degree)
      - Full thickness (3rd degree)
    - **Rule of 9s**
      - Used to estimate percentage of body burned
      - In pediatrics, head may occupy 18% instead of 9% of body surface area
    - **Treatment**
      - Burns → vascular compartment becomes hyperpermeable to plasma proteins → translocate intravascular fluid into the extravascular third space
      - **Resuscitation formula** (Parkland)

- ❖ 4 cc/kg × percentage burned in first 24 hours
  - › Administer two-third of overall fluid in first 8 hours
  - › Administer one-third of overall fluid in last 16 hours
- ❖ After 24 hours, titrate to urine output and tissue perfusion
- ➤ Maintain normothermia or even mild hyperthermia due to reset **thermoregulation**
- ➤ Feed within 24 hours to improve nitrogen balance, albumin concentration, thyroid hormone levels
  - ❖ Secretion of catecholamines and insulin are reduced when feeding is begun within 24 hours
  - ❖ Benefits of feeding are significant and consideration should be given to decrease NPO time prior to surgery
- ❖ Inhalational injury
  - ➤ Presents with carbonaceous sputum, singed hair in nasal passages, and inflammation or soot seen on bronchoscopy
  - ➤ Indication for immediate intubation due to concern for airway edema and high risk for acute respiratory distress syndrome

ANESTHETIC PLANNING

- ■ **Outpatient surgery**
  - ● >45 weeks old for a term infant; >60 weeks postconceptual age for a premie
  - ● Indications
    - ❖ Surgical procedures that do not require prolonged postoperative monitoring
    - ❖ Minimal hemodynamic and fluid shifts
    - ❖ Minimal postoperative pain
    - ❖ Rapid resumption of daily activities
    - ❖ Suitable caretakers for recovery needs
  - ● Anesthetic considerations
    - ❖ Minimize the use of long-acting medications for rapid recovery
    - ❖ Use agents that minimize the risk of postoperative nausea and vomiting
    - ❖ Ensure adequate pain control
    - ❖ Choose techniques that do not require prolonged postoperative follow-up
    - ❖ If the child has apnea episodes, recommend transfer and admission to a hospital for at least 24 hours for monitoring
- ■ **Remote anesthesia**
  - ● Anesthesia services are increasingly necessary in locations out of the operating room
    - ❖ Interventional radiology, endoscopy, MRI, and radiation oncology
  - ● Setup
    - ❖ Although an anesthesia machine may not be present, monitoring capabilities should be equally rigorous
    - ❖ Supplemental oxygen and emergency equipment should be available
- ■ **Pediatric sedation**
  - ● Goals of sedation include patient safety, minimizing pain and anxiety, and minimizing patient movement for procedure
  - ● Incredibly difficult in pediatric populations due to rapid and difficult to predict swings from moderate sedation to general anesthesia
  - ● Requires hemodynamic monitoring and frequent assessments of consciousness level

Newborn assessment: APGAR

APGAR (0–2 points for each of the following)
Appearance (color)
Pulse
Grimace
Activity (muscle tone)
Respirations

APGAR 0 to 3: immediate resuscitation, suction, and bag mask with 100% O_2.

NEONATAL/PEDIATRIC CODES

- Pediatric advanced life support should be consulted for emergencies
  - Algorithms exist for arrest, tachycardia, and bradycardia
- Cardiac arrest
  - Ventricular fibrillation/tachycardia arrest
    - Initiate CPR with (pulse checks every 2 minutes)→ defibrillate at 2 J/kg → epinephrine at 0.01 mg/kg (repeat every 3 to 5 minutes) → consider amiodarone at 5 mg/kg
  - Pulseless electrical activity/asystole
    - Initiate CPR (pulse checks every 2 minutes) → epinephrine at 0.01 mg/kg (repeat every 3 to 5 minutes)
    - Investigate for reversible causes
- Effective resuscitation strategies
  - Chest compressions
    - In infants, done below intermammary line with 2 fingers to a depth of one-third of chest
    - Rate at 100 compressions per minute
    - Ratio of compressions to breaths
      - Children: 30:2
      - Infants: 3:1
  - Airway
    - If airway secured, deliver 8 to 10 breaths per minute
  - Shocks can be increased to 4 J/kg and up to 10 J/kg for refractory rhythms
- Newborn distress
  - Most cases of newborn distress are respiratory
    - 10% of newborns require tactile stimulation, suctioning, and supplemental O_2 after delivery
    - 1% require bag mask ventilation
      - Ventilate at 30 breaths per minute
    - 0.1% require CPR and epinephrine (0.01 mg/kg)
      - Done if HR <60
  - Vascular access
    - Umbilical vessels can be cannulated in emergency for vascular access
  - Normal umbilical blood gas values
    - Arterial: 7.25/50/20/22 (pH/$Paco_2$/Pao_2/)
      - Umbilical artery takes blood away from baby
    - Venous: 7.35/40/30/20 (pH/$Paco_2$/Pao_2/ HCO_3^-)
      - Fetal pH is more acidic than maternal, so drugs can be ionized and trapped in fetal circulation

QUESTIONS

1. Which of the following statements regarding the administration of spinal anesthesia in the infant compared with an adult is most correct?
   A. Infants need smaller dose (per kg) of spinal local anesthetic than adults
   B. Spinal anesthesia has shorter duration of action in infants than in adults
   C. Hypotension with spinal anesthesia is more profound in infants compared with adults
   D. Cerebrospinal fluid volume (per kg) is less in neonates compared with adults

2. An 11-month-old, 10-kg infant sustains a 12% scald burn injury from a coffee spill. An IV is placed and fluids are administered. What infusion rate will achieve the appropriate fluid goal for the first 12 hours post burn injury?

   A. 40 mL/hr
   B. 60 mL/hr
   C. 80 mL/hr
   D. 100 mL/hr

3. A male infant at 50 weeks postconceptual age is scheduled to undergo hernia repair. His Hb is 8.7 mg/dL. Which of the following management approaches is recommended to decrease the risk of postoperative apnea?

   A. Spinal anesthesia with sedation
   B. Transfusion to Hb >10
   C. Mild hypothermia
   D. Postpone surgery until anemia resolves

4. Administration of which of the following is associated with a decreased risk of propofol infusion syndrome?

   A. Corticosteroids
   B. Vasopressors
   C. Lactated ringers
   D. Carbohydrate intake

5. A 2-year-old girl with Tetralogy of Fallot has an acute episode of hypercyanosis immediately after anesthetic induction. Which of the following would be the most appropriate immediate treatment?

   A. Phenylephrine
   B. Propranolol
   C. Morphine
   D. Bicarbonate

PHYSIOLOGY OF LABOR

- **Central nervous system (CNS) changes**
  - Minimum alveolar concentration (MAC) is decreased by ~40%, which is likely a consequence of increased progesterone levels
  - The local anesthetic requirement for epidurals and spinals are decreased, as the epidural space is compressed and there is a theoretical decrease in cerebrospinal fluid.
- **Cardiovascular changes**
  - Blood pressure
    - Systolic blood pressure should remain within normal limits
      - Diastolic pressure may decrease
    - Hypotension can occur in the supine position secondary to aortocaval compression
      - Left uterine displacement will help relieve the aortocaval compression and associated hypotension
    - Hypertension should always be investigated (see below)
  - Cardiac output (CO)
    - Increases due to
      - Increased heart rate
      - Increased stroke volume
      - Increased blood volume → increased preload
      - Decreased systemic vascular resistance (SVR) → decreased afterload
    - Quantity of increase
      - First trimester: 30% to 40% increase
      - Second to third trimester: 30% to 60% increase
      - Delivery and autotransfusion: 75% to 80%
      - Postpartum: returns to nonpregnant levels in ~2 weeks
  - Murmurs and electrocardiogram (ECG)
    - Mechanical pressure from the fetus → heart is shifted upward during late pregnancy
    - ECG changes
      - Shortened PR
      - Left QRS axis shift
      - ST depression at precordial and limb leads
    - Physiologic murmurs are common due to increased blood flow
      - Systolic murmur from tricuspid valve regurgitation normal due to dilation of tricuspid annulus
      - S_3 flow murmur normal
      - S_4, severe systolic, or diastolic murmurs are pathologic
- Respiratory changes
  - **Lung volumes**
    - Increased
      - Tidal volume by 40% to 50%
      - Total lung capacity by 5%
    - Decreased
      - Functional residual capacity by 20%
      - Expiratory reserve volume by 20%
      - Residual volume by 20%

- ◆ Unchanged
  - ➤ Vital capacity
  - ➤ Forced expiratory volume 1 second
- • **Minute ventilation (MV)**
  - ◆ Progesterone stimulates respiratory drive
    - ➤ MV increases during first trimester → up to 50% by term
    - ➤ Driven by increased tidal volume, not respiratory rate
  - ◆ Causes a respiratory alkalosis
    - ➤ pH ~7.44
    - ➤ HCO_3 ~20
- • **Arterial blood gas (ABG)**
  - ◆ Pao_2 can increase by 10
  - ◆ Pco_2 can decrease by 10
- ■ Hematologic changes
  - • **Blood volume**
    - ◆ Begins to increase during first trimester → peaks at middle of third trimester
      - ➤ Aids perfusion of placenta and fetus
      - ➤ Preparation for blood loss at delivery
    - ◆ Oxygen consumption increases by 20%
    - ◆ **Plasma volume increases 50%**
      - ➤ Increased **volume of distribution** for drug effects
      - ➤ Plasma increases accommodated by decreased SVR
  - • Red blood cells (RBC)
    - ◆ Anemia of pregnancy is due to dilution, not absolute reduction
      - ➤ Anemia: Hb <11 g/dL
    - ◆ Erythropoietin levels increase 50% → RBC mass increases by 15% to 30% at term
    - ◆ 2,3-diphosphoglycerate decreases → right shift on oxyhemoglobin curve
    - ◆ Increased need for fetal hematopoiesis
      - ➤ Demand for iron, B_{12}, folic acid increases
  - • White blood cells (WBC)
    - ◆ Pregnancy associated with mild leukocytosis (9K to 15K cells/μL)
    - ◆ Leukocytosis can increase significantly with labor
  - • Platelets
    - ◆ Slightly decrease, but remains in normal range
    - ◆ Thrombocytopenia affects ~5% of pregnancies
  - • **Coagulation**
    - ◆ Procoagulation factors such as fibrinogen, II, XII, X and others increase
    - ◆ von Willebrand factor increases
    - ◆ Fibrinolytic inhibitors increase
    - ◆ Thrombin cleavage products increase
    - ◆ Resistance to protein C increases
    - ◆ Protein S decreases
    - ◆ Prothrombin time (PT)/partial thromboplastin time (PTT) should be normal
- ■ **Renal changes**
  - • Kidneys increase in size
  - • Increased risk of urinary stasis and pyelonephritis
  - • Urinary frequency and nocturia increase
  - • Creatinine and blood urea nitrogen (BUN) decrease
- ■ Gastrointestinal changes
  - • Increased **gastroesophageal reflux**
    - ◆ **Decreased lower esophageal sphincter pressure**
    - ◆ Enlarging uterus → increased intra-abdominal pressure → **mechanical pressure on stomach**
  - • **Gastric emptying affected by pregnancy**
  - • **Increased transit time in small and large intestine**
- ■ Hepatic changes
  - • Alkaline phosphatase, triglycerides increased

- **Albumin and total protein levels decrease**
- Liver function tests, bilirubin levels unchanged
- Gallbladder contractility decreases
- Increased risk of intrahepatic cholestasis of pregnancy
- Decreased pseudocholinesterase levels
  - The response to succinylcholine is NOT prolonged
- Decreased total protein levels
- Decreased albumin/globulin levels
- Uterine changes
  - **Uterine blood flow** (UBF) is 50 to 100 cc/min prior to pregnancy → 700 to 900 cc/min at term
  - UBF = (uterine arterial pressure – uterine venous pressure)/uterine vascular resistance
  - Blood supply to the uterus is NOT autoregulated
  - Oxygenated blood passes to the fetus via one uterine artery and one umbilical vein from the placenta
  - Deoxygenated blood returns to the placenta from the fetus via two umbilical arteries and to the mother via the uterine vein
  - Umbilical artery
    - PaO_2 20; $PaCO_2$ 50; pH 7.28; O_2 saturation 40%
  - Umbilical vein
    - PaO_2 30; $PaCO_2$ 40; pH 7.35; O_2 saturation 70%
  - Placental exchange from the mother to fetus occurs by diffusion
  - Fetal to mother CO_2 transfer enhances mother to fetus O_2 transfer
  - UBF must decrease by ~50% before fetal distress is noticeable
  - **Factors that decrease UBF**
    - Hypotension (uterus does not autoregulate)
    - **Aortocaval compression**
    - Uterine contraction
    - Sympathetic stimulation → vasoconstriction

FETAL WELL-BEING

- Monitoring
  - **Fetal heart rate (FHR) monitoring**
    - Technique
      - Commonly measured with a Doppler ultrasound on the maternal abdomen
      - Can also be measured invasively with a fetal scalp electrode
    - Normal FHR is 120 to 160 with variability
      - \>160: tachycardia
        - Fever, drugs, fetal distress
      - <120: bradycardia
        - Heart block, hypoxia
      - Should see beat to beat variability
        - Lack of variability can be secondary to
          - hypoxia
          - drugs: benzodiazepines, barbiturates, opioids, and volatile anesthetics can all ablate FHR beat to beat variability
          - atropine can as well, secondary to blocking parasympathetics in the fetus
        - Ephedrine can increase beat-to-beat variability
    - Decelerations are classified by their temporal relationship to contractions
      - Early: vagal response from uterine contractions
        - Fetal head compression
        - Not usually concerning
        - Supplemental O_2 does not help
      - Variable: transient cord compression
        - No relation to uterine contractions
        - Most common

- ❖ However: if they last >1 minute, can be indicative of severe fetal acidosis and imminent intrautero death
  - ➤ Late: uteroplacental insufficiency
    - ❖ Begin 10 to 30 seconds after beginning of uterine contraction and end 10 to 30 seconds after conclusion of contraction
    - ❖ Indicative of uteroplacental insufficiency
      - › Maternal hypotension
      - › Uterine hyperactivity
- Fetal scalp blood gases
  - ❖ Invasive test that detects for inadequate fetal oxygenation
- Fetal pulse oximetry
  - ❖ Sensor rests against fetal head/face and measures oxygen saturation
  - ❖ Value <30% is concerning for inadequate oxygenation
- Antepartum testing
  - **Maternal ultrasound**
    - ❖ Frequently done between weeks 18 and 20
    - ❖ Examination can detect cardiac, bone, brain, and other structural abnormalities
  - **Fetal nonstress test**
    - ❖ Noninvasive test performed during the third trimester
    - ❖ Measures fetal heart and contractions to determine FHR reactivity
    - ❖ Indications include reduced fetal movement, placental insufficiency, or postdate
  - **Contraction stress test**
    - ❖ A test to determine if the fetus will tolerate uterine contractions
    - ❖ Oxytocin is administrated intravenously to cause labor contractions
    - ❖ FHR is monitored for decelerations during contractions
  - **Biophysical profile**
    - ❖ Composed of a nonstress test plus ultrasonography
    - ❖ Measures five criteria (0 to 2 points/criteria)
      - ➤ Nonstress test
      - ➤ Fetal breathing movements
      - ➤ Fetal movement
      - ➤ Fetal tone
      - ➤ Amniotic fluid volume
- Amniotic fluid
  - Testing
    - ❖ **Amniocentesis** is an invasive procedure that samples amniotic fluid
    - ❖ Can diagnose genetic abnormalities
    - ❖ Ultrasound can diagnose fluid volume
  - **Oligohydramnios**
    - ❖ Insufficient amniotic fluid
    - ❖ Can be associated with fetal renal or urinary defects, placental insufficiency, leaking membranes, postdate pregnancy, or maternal comorbid disease
  - **Polyhydramnios**
    - ❖ Excessive amniotic fluid
    - ❖ Can be associated with maternal infection, fetal gastrointestinal abnormalities, renal disorders, and neurological abnormalities
- Postdelivery
  - APGAR neonatal score (see Table 16.1)
    - ❖ Measures five criteria (2 points/each) for up to 10 points
    - ❖ Developed to quickly assess health of newborn
      - ➤ Performed at 1 and 5 minutes
      - ➤ Low scores (<3) may necessitate immediate medical attention
        - ❖ Prolonged low scores associated with cerebral palsy
      - ➤ A score of 10 is rare due to cyanosis
  - Meconium
    - ❖ Meconium is composed of materials ingested by the fetus in utero

TABLE 16.1 APGAR

Criteria	0	1	2
Appearance (A) (color)	Blue	Blue extremities/pink body	Pink
Pulse (P)	Absent	<100	>100
Grimace/Irritability (G) (response to stimulation)	None	Feeble cry	Cry
Activity (A) (tone)	None	Flexion	Resists extension
Respiratory (R)	Absent	Weak	Strong

- ➤ Contents are sterile
- ➤ Normally retained in fetus's bowel until birth
- ◆ Meconium staining into the amniotic fluid occurs in ~10% of deliveries
  - ➤ No benefit to routine nasopharyngeal or oropharyngeal suction intrapartum
  - ➤ If baby is vigorous → suction with bulb syringe or catheter (do not intubate)
  - ➤ If baby is lethargic → intubate and suction
- ◆ Failure to pass meconium may indicate Hirschsprung disease or cystic fibrosis

LABOR

- ▪ Stages
  - ● First stage: onset of contractions to full cervical dilation
    - ◆ Latent phase: painful uterine contractions, cervical thinning and effacement
    - ◆ Active phase: rapid cervical dilation, typically from 3 to 4 cm to full
  - ● Second stage: delivery of infant
  - ● Third stage: delivery of placenta
  - ● Fourth stage: from delivery of placenta to 12 hours postpartum
- ▪ Drugs
  - ● **Labor stimulants**
    - ◆ Misoprostol (synthetic prostaglandin E_1)
      - ➤ Can be administered vaginally
      - ➤ Causes cervical ripening, uterine contractions
    - ◆ Oxytocin
      - ➤ Synthetic form can be administered IV/IM
      - ➤ Causes cervical dilation, uterine contractions
  - ● **Tocolysis (labor suppressants)**
    - ◆ β-adrenergic agonists: terbutaline
      - ➤ Mechanism
        - ❖ Bind β_2 receptors on myometrial cells → adenyl cyclase activation
        - ❖ Increase in cAMP decreases the intracellular concentration of calcium and interaction between actin and myosin → myometrial relaxation
      - ➤ Side effects
        - ❖ β_1 stimulation → tachycardia, anxiety, pulmonary edema
        - ❖ β_2 stimulation → smooth muscle dilation → hypotension
        - ❖ Increased glucagon secretion → hyperglycemia
        - ❖ Hypokalemia
        - ❖ Intraventricular hemorrhage
    - ◆ Magnesium
      - ➤ Mechanism
        - ❖ Depresses the excitability of the muscle fiber membrane
          - › Inhibits release of acetylcholine (ACh) at neuromuscular (NM) junction
          - › Decreases NM sensitivity junction to ACh

- ❖ Potentiates NM blocks (except succinylcholine)
- ❖ Competes with calcium and inhibits calcium-dependent processes
  - ➢ Effects
    - ❖ Improves uterine blood flow and decreases uterine vascular resistance
    - ❖ May provide fetal neuroprotection → decreases cerebral palsy risk associated with preterm labor
    - ❖ Neonate at risk for lethargy, hypotonia, respiratory depression
    - ❖ Ineffective for preventing preterm birth due to preterm labor
    - ❖ Sedative effect on parturient
  - ➢ Levels
    - ❖ 1.5 to 2 mEq/L: normal
    - ❖ 4 to 8 mEq/L: therapeutic
    - ❖ 5 to 10 mEq/L: ECG changes such as widened PR, QRS, QT intervals
    - ❖ 10 mEq/L: loss of deep tendon reflexes (DTR) (Test at biceps due to epidural)
    - ❖ 15 mEq/L: respiratory paralysis, heart block
    - ❖ 25 mEq/L: cardiovascular collapse
  - ➢ Treatment for overdose
    - ❖ Calcium
- ❖ Nonsteroidal anti-inflammatory drugs (NSAIDs)
  - ➢ Indomethacin has been shown to be a tocolytic, but serious risks prevent its common use
  - ➢ Risks
    - ❖ Reversible patent ductus arteriosus closure after 32 weeks
    - ❖ Decreased fetal renal function
    - ❖ Fetal intraventricular hemorrhage
    - ❖ Hyperbilirubinemia
    - ❖ Necrotizing enterocolitis
- ❖ Calcium-channel blockers
  - ➢ Nifedipine effective, but should be used cautiously in patients with cardiac and renal disease
- ● Treatment of uterine atony
  - ❖ Oxytocin
    - ➢ Produced and secreted from posterior pituitary gland → produces uterine contraction, smooth muscle constriction
    - ➢ Side effects
      - ❖ Relaxes vascular smooth muscle → hypotension
      - ❖ Increased nausea/vomiting
      - ❖ Structurally similar to vasopressin → rare causes of water intoxication
        - ⟩ Hyponatremia, confusion, seizures, coma
      - ❖ Tachycardia due to receptors at myocardium
      - ❖ Increases pulmonary artery pressures
  - ❖ Methylergometrine
    - ➢ Smooth muscle vasoconstrictor
    - ➢ Dose: 0.2 μg IM
    - ➢ Side effects and contraindication: hypertension
  - ❖ Carboprost tromethamine (Hemabate)
    - ➢ Induces uterine contractions
    - ➢ Dose: 250 μg IM
    - ➢ Side effects: bronchospasm, ventilation/perfusion mismatch due to shunting, hypoxemia, nausea, vomiting, fever, diarrhea
  - ❖ Misoprostol
  - ❖ Uterine artery embolization and hysterectomy if refractory

LABOR/C-SECTION ANESTHETIC: EPIDURAL AND SPINALS

- ■ Techniques
  - ● **A lumbar epidural** is the most common labor anesthetic and can be used for Cesarean section (C-section)

- ◆ Epidurals can increase uteroplacental blood flow and decrease catecholamines
  - ➤ High levels of catecholamines can decrease uteroplacental perfusion
- ◆ American Society of Anesthesiologists Practice Guidelines for Obstetric Anesthesia states that arbitrary cervical dilation is not needed for placement of epidural
- **A single shot spinal (SSS)** anesthetic is a common choice for C-section and it can also provide short-term analgesia for labor
- A **combined spinal-epidural (CSE)** utilizes both techniques and can be used effectively for both C-section and labor
- FHR monitoring is necessary pre and postneuraxial
  - ◆ Optimal during placement, but may not be possible
- ■ Dermatome levels
  - Pain during labor can cover a variety of spinal levels
    - ◆ First stage of labor: visceral pain via the T10-lumbar nerve roots
    - ◆ Second stage of labor: visceral pain via the sacral nerve roots
      - ➤ Descent of the fetus through the cervix and into the vagina → feeling of rectal pressure and pain via the pudendal nerve (S2-4)
  - During a C-section, coverage should reach as high as T4 to cover the peritoneum
  - Analgesic-sparing
    - ◆ Despite lumbar placement, labor epidurals can be sacral-sparing
    - ◆ L5-S2 nerve roots are especially large, making coverage difficult
- ■ Medication choices
  - **Drug selection and dosing**
    - ◆ Progesterone increases both local anesthetic and opioid sensitivity during labor → smaller doses needed
    - ◆ A local anesthetic and an opioid together offer synergism and superior analgesia for both epidurals and spinals
    - ◆ Drug selection should be based on timing, duration, and toxicity risks
    - ◆ Plasma protein concentration is decreased during pregnancy, so there is increased free fraction of local anesthetics systemically
  - Local anesthetics
    - ◆ Lidocaine
      - ➤ Intermediate onset, intermediate duration
      - ➤ Less risk of toxicity than bupivacaine
    - ◆ Bupivacaine
      - ➤ Slower onset, long duration
      - ➤ More potent than lidocaine
      - ➤ Greater risk of cardiac toxicity
    - ◆ 2-chloroprocaine
      - ➤ Rapid onset, shortest duration
        - ❖ Rapidity due to higher concentration (3%), not due to pKa or lipid solubility
      - ➤ Metabolized rapidly by pseudocholinesterase, so little risk of toxicity, even during intravascular injection
        - ❖ Half-life is ~20 seconds in maternal blood
        - ❖ Half-life is ~2 minutes in maternal blood for pseudocholinesterase deficient parturient
      - ➤ May antagonize epidural opioids
  - Opioids
    - ◆ Fentanyl
      - ➤ Lipid-soluble, commonly chosen for epidural infusions
      - ➤ Can enhance and speed the sensory, but not motor, block for spinal anesthetics
    - ◆ Morphine
      - ➤ Water-soluble, commonly chosen for long-acting analgesia after C-section
    - ◆ Meperidine
      - ➤ Opioid with local anesthetic properties, can cause patchy sympathectomy
- ■ **Temperature regulation**
  - Epidurals can alter thermoregulation and cause temperature elevation
    - ◆ Raises the threshold for sweating and prevents evaporative heat loss

TABLE 16.2 **Anticoagulants and neuraxials**	
Anticoagulant/antiplatelet drug	Time until neuraxial anesthesia placement from last dose
Heparin	No restrictions for subcutaneous prophylaxis If therapeutic anticoagulation, PTT needs to be less than 40
Enoxaparin	For prophylactic dosing, delay neuraxial until 12 hr For therapeutic dosing, delay neuraxial until 24 hr
Argatroban/bivalirudin/lepirudin	PTT <40
Clopidogrel	7 d
Dabigatran	3 d
Fondaparinux	48 hr/72 hr
Ticlopidine	14 d
Tirofiban/eptifibatide	8 hr
Abciximab	2 d

- Elevation typically <1°C, rarely reaches 38°C
- **Anticoagulation**
  - Risk of epidural hematoma and potential paralysis warrants careful attention to anticoagulation status
  - No need for checking platelets or coagulation factors prior to epidural placement in a parturient with no bleeding risk factors or history
  - Specific guidelines (see Table 16.2)
- **Risks**
  - Progress of labor
    - Misguided concern that epidurals may slow the progress of labor
    - Studies suffer from selection bias and loose starting points
      - Parturients with difficult labor may opt for early epidural
    - Epidurals may increase second stage of labor, but the overall effect is minimal
    - Epidurals associated with earlier intervention in third stage of labor when evacuation of placenta indicated
    - Meta-analysis shows epidurals do not increase the risk of C-section
  - Insufficient analgesia
    - May be due to epidural catheter position or dislodgement
    - Plica mediana dorsalis extends from dura mater to ligamentum flavum → can cause epidural catheter threading problems or a unilateral block
  - Postdural puncture headaches
    - Risks
      - 1% risk with small pencil point needle
        - Cutting needle leaves a hole equal to the diameter of the needle and dural fibers that have been cut
        - Pencil point leaves a tiny hole that spreads to the size of the needle
      - 80% risk when dura punctured with Tuohy
      - Ages 20 to 40 years at highest risk
      - Women have greater risk than men
    - Presentation
      - Develops within 5 days of dural puncture
      - Positional within 15 minutes of sitting up or 15 minutes of laying down
      - Accompanied by one of following symptoms
        - Nausea
        - Neck stiffness

- ❖ Hyperacusis
- ❖ Photophobia
- ❖ Nausea
- ➤ Onset within 1 hour → more likely pneumocephalus
  - ◆ Treatment
    - ➤ Resolves spontaneously at 1 week or within 48 hours after treatment of leak
    - ➤ Epidural blood patch
      - ❖ 70% to 80% success (return to normal function)
      - ❖ If no relief with first blood patch, second blood patch success is <50%
    - ➤ Caffeine
    - ➤ Sumatriptan
    - ➤ Methylergometrine
- ● Infection
  - ◆ Bacterial meningitis presents with fever, altered mental status, neck pain, and headache
  - ◆ Most cases develop 6 to 36 hours after dural puncture
  - ◆ Most common organism is strep viridians from oral bacteria of medical personnel (49%)
- ● Bleed
  - ◆ Symptoms: back pain, leg weakness, unexplained fever, delay in normal recovery
  - ◆ Treatment: deliver child rapidly, consult neurosurgeon
- ● **Horner syndrome**
  - ◆ Caused by local anesthetics covering the descending spinal sympathetic fibers
  - ◆ Benign and resolves spontaneously

C-SECTION: GENERAL ANESTHESIA

- ■ General anesthesia can be used for elective and nonelective C-sections
- ■ General anesthesia is used for C-sections when there is not sufficient time to use a neuraxial technique or it fails or there is too much hemodynamic instability in the mother
  - ● Fetal distress
  - ● Maternal hemorrhage (placental abruption or previa)
  - ● Cephalopelvic disproportion (CPD)
  - ● Uterine dystocia/atony
  - ● Breech presentation of the fetus
- ■ The most important factor determining fetal outcome after C-section is the time between uterine incision and delivery
- ■ Avoid maternal hyperventilation, as this can lead to hypoxemia and acidosis in the fetus via decreasing uterine and umbilical blood flow
  - ● PCO_2 should be 30 to 33
- ■ **Parturient airway**: eightfold increase in intubation failure (1/300)
  - ● Reduced functional residual capacity (FRC) and increased O_2 consumption → more rapid desaturation
  - ● Weight gain and breast size → difficulty inserting laryngoscope
  - ● Airway edema and increased Mallampati classification → inferior airway view
  - ● Capillary enlargement → increased risk of airway bleeding and need for smaller tube
  - ● Increased reflux and reduced lower esophageal sphincter tone → increased **aspiration** risk
  - ● Emergency situations → less optimal conditions during induction
- ■ **Induction drugs**
  - ● **All sedatives and hypnotics drugs pass to fetus**
    - ◆ **Opioids** can cause respiratory depression
      - ➤ Fetal metabolism of morphine can be limited due to immature organs
    - ◆ **Benzodiazepines** have limited fetal effects
    - ◆ **Propofol** is lipid soluble and crosses the placenta
    - ◆ **Ketamine** is lipid soluble and crosses the placenta
      - ➤ Oxytocic effects on uterine tone during second trimester, but not at term
  - ● All **inhalational agents** cross to the placenta
    - ◆ Small, non-ionized, and lipid soluble

- ◆ Little effects if the fetus is delivered rapidly and lower doses are used
- ◆ FRC is decreased, which leads to faster equilibration of the inhalational anesthetics and MAC is decreased in the pregnant woman
- **Local anesthetics**
  - ◆ **Placental transfer** determined by protein binding, pK_a, and maternal/fetal pH
  - ◆ Ionized local anesthetics can be trapped in fetal circulation
  - ◆ Specific drugs in fetal circulation
    - ➤ Lidocaine concentration most likely to be high
    - ➤ Bupivacaine less likely to be fetal circulation due to protein binding
    - ➤ Chloroprocaine is rapidly metabolized and is found at minimal concentration
- Muscle relaxants are ionized and do not transfer to the fetus
- Hemodynamic drugs
  - Commonly used pressors (phenylephrine and ephedrine) are passed to the fetus
  - Commonly used β-blockers, such as esmolol and labetalol, are passed to the fetus
    - ◆ Could be confused for decreased FHR and fetal distress
  - Adenosine, used to treat supraventricular tachycardia, does not cross the placenta
  - Atropine (tertiary ammonium) crosses the placenta, but glycopyrrolate (quaternary ammonium) does not
- Maintenance of anesthesia
  - Volatile anesthetics
    - ◆ Inhibit uterine contraction at >0.2 MAC
    - ◆ Inhibit oxytocin response at >0.5 MAC
  - Consider alternative options to volatiles in uterine atony such as nitrous or propofol

REGIONAL TECHNIQUES

- Can be used in emergency, as an alternative, or as an adjunct to techniques listed above for labor or C-section
- **Paracervical block**
  - Local anesthetic injected into vaginal fornices
  - Blocks visceral afferent fibers from uterus at the paracervical ganglion → effective for first stage of labor (T10-L1)
  - Side effects
    - ◆ Hypotension
    - ◆ Fetal bradycardia
- **Lumbar sympathetic block**
  - Local anesthetic injected at the anterolateral surface of the vertebral column just anterior to the medial attachment of the psoas muscle
  - Offers good analgesia for first stage of labor without motor block
  - Does not provide reliable anesthesia for the second stage of labor
  - Has almost entirely disappeared from practice and been replaced by epidurals
- **Pudendal block**
  - Local anesthetic injected into the pudendal canal allows relief to the perineum, vulva, and vagina
  - Effective for the second stage of labor (S2-S4)
  - Can be useful for episiotomy or laceration repair
- Skin infiltration for emergency C-section
  - Skin/muscle infiltration an option during emergency C-section without ability to do general or neuraxial anesthesia
  - 0.5% lidocaine or 3% chloroprocaine
    - ◆ Avoid bupivacaine due to local anesthetic toxicity at high doses
  - Supplementation with benzodiazepines and ketamine can maintain spontaneous respirations

LABOR/C-SECTION RISKS

- Hypotension
  - Etiology can include hemorrhage, hypovolemia, drugs, or aortocaval compression

- **Aortocaval compression** begins to occur at 20 weeks gestation
  - Relieved by left uterine displacement, pressor, and intravenous fluids
- Bezold–Jarish reflex
  - Bradycardia and hypotension typically following spinal or epidural anesthesia
- Medications
  - Phenylephrine
    - Direct α-mediated vasoconstriction
    - Increases blood pressure, but can be associated with reflex bradycardia
    - May decrease cardiac output
  - Ephedrine
    - Indirect α- and β-mediated vasoconstriction
    - Increases blood pressure through vasoconstriction of peripheral vessels
    - Increases risk of fetal acidosis compared to phenylephrine
- **Positioning injury**
  - Lumbosacral trunk at L4-5
    - Most common injury due to compression by fetal head or application of forceps
    - Risk increases with a large fetus and CPD
    - Presents with weakness of dorsiflexion and foot eversion as well as loss of sensation along lateral lower leg and dorsal surface of foot
  - Femoral nerve at L2-4
    - Caused by retractors during C-section and prolonged flexion and external hip rotation during pushing
  - Lateral femoral cutaneous at L2-3
    - Commonly injured at anterior superior iliac spine
    - Injured with excessive retraction of legs
  - Common peroneal nerve at L4-S3
    - Compression of fibular head while in stirrups
- **Aspiration**
  - Aspiration volumes of >0.4 cc/kg with pH < 2.5 → high risk of pneumonitis
    - Aspiration pneumonitis does not require antibiotics, but may require intubation and supportive care
      - Sodium citrate used prophylactically
    - 30 cc neutralizes 250 cc of gastric contents at a pH of 1.0
    - Works rapidly, effects last 1 hour
  - Guidelines advise against solid foods during labor, but clear liquids do not increase maternal complications
- Atony (see above)
- **Amniotic fluid embolism**
  - Immunologic process where vasoactive substances in the amniotic fluid reach circulation → pulmonary artery vasospasm → right ventricular failure → hypoxia and cardiovascular collapse
  - Presentation: dyspnea, hypoxemia, hemodynamic instability, unresponsiveness
  - Treatment: supportive care, extracorporeal membrane oxygenation (ECMO)
- Air embolism
  - Rare complication that can occur during C-sections when uterus is lifted above the level of the heart and veins are open to air
- **Disseminated intravascular coagulation (DIC)**
  - Associated with abruption, fetal demise, amniotic fluid embolism, sepsis, and severe hypertension
  - Manifests as excessive fibrin deposition and depletion of clotting factors
    - Decreased fibrinogen, decreased platelets, and prolonged coagulation times

COMPLICATED/HIGH-RISK PREGNANCIES

- Abnormal pregnancy/fetal loss
  - **Ectopic pregnancy**
    - Embryo does not implant in the uterine cavity and is not viable
    - Emergency that requires medical (methotrexate) or surgical treatment

- Spontaneous abortion
  - Often presents with bleeding
  - In an incomplete miscarriage, retained products will need evacuation through conservative management, misoprostol, or a dilation and evacuation (D&E)
- Molar pregnancy
  - Gestational trophoblastic disease where a nonviable egg implants into the uterus
  - Treatment requires evacuation of the mass through surgery
  - Diagnosed with an elevated hCG level and ultrasound showing honeycomb uterus, snowstorm uterus, or cluster of grapes.
  - Anesthetic implications
    - Hydatidiform mole could be associated with significant blood loss
    - Five percent of patients have associated hyperthyroidism where β-blockade is recommended
- Cervical incompetence
  - The cervix is thin or at risk for opening, increasing the risk of infection
  - Treatment requires a **cerclage** placed early in pregnancy and then removed after miscarriage risk has passed
- Hypertensive disorders
  - **Preeclampsia/eclampsia**
    - **Can occur not only DURING pregnancy, but AFTER delivery of the fetus as well**
    - Pathophysiology
      - Ineffective trophoblast migration into endometrium → trophoblast (and eventually placenta) is not properly seated in the endometrium
      - Spiral arteries are undilated, high resistance, and low flow
        - Lower vasodilating levels (NO, PGI_2)
        - Higher vasoconstricting levels (TxA_2, ET-1)
      - Endothelial dysfunction and vasoconstriction → platelet aggregation, platelet dysfunction, kidney proteinuria, hypertension, cerebral hemorrhage
    - Risk factors
      - Advanced maternal age
      - African racial background
      - Nulliparity
      - History of preeclampsia
      - Abruption
      - Fetal abnormalities
      - Obesity
      - Diabetes mellitus
      - History of renal or vascular disease
    - Diagnosis
      - Elevated blood pressure and one or more additional signs of organ dysfunction
      - Systolic blood pressure (SBP) >140 or diastolic blood pressure (DBP) >90
        - Must be on two separate readings taken at least 4 hours apart
        - Must be >20 weeks of gestation
          - Most commonly occurs after 24 weeks gestation
        - Must have normal baseline blood pressure
      - Organ dysfunction
        - Proteinuria ≥300 mg/24 hr
          - Proteinuria no longer mandatory to diagnose preeclampsia
        - Thrombocytopenia
        - Impaired liver function
        - Pulmonary edema
        - New onset headaches
        - Visual changes
      - Eclampsia is the development of **seizures** in a preeclamptic patient
    - Morbidity and mortality
      - No. 1 cause of death is intracerebral hemorrhage
        - Increased risk of ischemic or hemorrhagic strokes

- ➤ HELLP syndrome affects multiple organ systems
  - ❖ Hemolysis
  - ❖ Elevated liver enzymes
  - ❖ Low platelets
- ❖ Management and treatment
  - ➤ Blood pressure management
  - ➤ Prevent eclampsia with magnesium
  - ➤ Delivery is definitive treatment
- ❖ Anesthetic implications
  - ➤ Often volume-depleted with decreased central and pulmonary venous pressures on presentation
  - ➤ Epidurals can increase uterine blood flow during preeclampsia due to sympathectomy
  - ➤ Cautious management of blood pressure, especially during induction of general anesthesia, to avoid excessive hypertension
- ❖ Increased risk of reoccurrence with future pregnancies
- **Chronic hypertension (HTN)**
  - ❖ Persistent HTN before, during, and after pregnancy
  - ❖ Must be present before 20 weeks gestation
  - ❖ Aggressive treatment not recommended
    - ➤ Body may be accustomed to higher blood pressure
    - ➤ Tight blood pressure management associated with intrauterine growth retardation (IUGR)
  - ❖ Increased risk of superimposed preeclampsia, IUGR, abruption
- **Gestational HTN**
  - ❖ Newly diagnosed hypertension after 20 weeks gestation
  - ❖ Increase in BP without generalized edema or proteinuria
- Treatment of hypertension
  - ❖ Accepted drugs
    - ➤ Methyldopa
    - ➤ Labetolol
    - ➤ Nifedipine
    - ➤ Hydralazine
  - ❖ Contraindicated drugs
    - ➤ Thiazides
    - ➤ Angiotensin-converting enzyme inhibitors/Angiotensin receptor blockers
- Cardiac disorders
  - **Arrhythmias**
    - ❖ Pregnancy increases arrhythmias due to altered hormones, increased plasma volume, and states of increased sympathetic tone
    - ❖ Most arrhythmias of pregnancy are benign and do not require pharmacologic therapy
    - ❖ Common types of arrhythmias
      - ➤ Supraventricular tachycardias
        - ❖ Most common arrhythmia
        - ❖ Atrial fibrillation/flutter rare unless preexisting structural heart disease
        - ❖ Treatment: vagal maneuvers, adenosine, β-blockade, digoxin, conversion, catheter ablation
      - ➤ Ventricular tachycardias
        - ❖ Rare and often associated with preexisting structural heart disease
        - ❖ Treatment depends on underlying cause
          - ➢ Consider β-blockade, cardioversion, implantable cardioverter defibrillator (ICD) placement
  - **Congenital heart disease**
    - ❖ Due to advances in medical therapy and surgery, an increasing number of parturients have congenital or structural heart disease
    - ❖ Hemodynamic goals of delivery should be managed according to the goals of the underlying process (see cardiac section for specific diseases)
    - ❖ Anesthetic implications

- ➤ Consider additional hemodynamic monitors
- ➤ Epidurals allows minimal hemodynamic perturbations if medications are titrated slowly
- ➤ A denser epidural block can allow for a instrumented vaginal delivery, sparing the parturient the need to push
  - ❖ The valsalva act of pushing can have significant hemodynamic effects by decreasing preload
- ➤ While spinals and general anesthesia may be necessary in certain scenarios, there are increased risks for hemodynamic lability
- ● **Peripartum cardiomyopathy**
  - ❖ Dilated cardiomyopathy that presents in the last month of pregnancy up to the first month postpartum
  - ❖ No clear cause, but ejection fraction is less than 45%
  - ❖ Associated with congestive heart failure (CHF), arrhythmias, and even death
  - ❖ Treatment is supportive: diuretics, vasodilators, digoxin, potential anticoagulation, and even mechanical support
  - ❖ Mortality risk of 0.5% to 5.0%, with 50% having a complete recovery
- ■ **Obesity**
  - ● Morbid obesity carries multiple increased obstetrical risks
    - ❖ Increased hypertension and preeclampsia
    - ❖ Increased diabetes
    - ❖ Increased C-section rates
    - ❖ Increased maternal mortality
  - ● Anesthetic implications
    - ❖ Increased risk of aspiration from elevated gastric volumes
    - ❖ Increased obstructive sleep apnea and respiratory complications
    - ❖ More rapid desaturation
    - ❖ Worse supine hypotension
- ■ Endocrine disorders
  - ● **Gestational diabetes**
    - ❖ Parturient
      - ➤ Diagnosis by oral glucose tolerance test, screening glucose challenge test, or non-challenge blood glucose testing
      - ➤ Increases risk for preeclampsia, polyhydramnios, and C-section
      - ➤ In preexisting diabetes, insulin requirements decrease in early pregnancy, but increase during the second and third trimesters
        - ❖ Sharp decrease in insulin requirements postdelivery
      - ➤ Management can be with lifestyle and diet, oral agents, or insulin
        - ❖ Fasting glucose goal of 60 to 95 mg/dL
    - ❖ Fetus risks
      - ➤ Increased preterm delivery, fetal abnormalities, fetal macrosomia with increased birth trauma
      - ➤ Increased fetal insulin secretion → lack of glucose postdelivery → increased risk of hypoglycemia postdelivery
  - ● **Thyroid disorders**
    - ❖ The fetus depends on maternal thyroid hormone until the second trimester
      - ➤ Maternal hyperthyroidism or hypothyroidism during the first trimester may affect fetal organogenesis
    - ❖ Hypothyroidism
      - ➤ High TSH, low/normal T_4
      - ➤ Complications include anemia, miscarriages, preterm delivery, and placental disorders
    - ❖ Hyperthyroidism
      - ➤ Low TSH, high T_4
      - ➤ Complications include IUGR, preeclampsia
- ■ Autoimmune disorders
  - ● **Lupus**
    - ❖ Often flares during second and third trimester

- ◆ Renal disease worsens
- ◆ Associated with spontaneous abortion, intrauterine fetal demise (IUFD), and preterm delivery
- ◆ Fetal complications can include atrioventricular block
  - ➤ FHR monitoring may be inaccurate
  - ➤ Use other measures of fetal well-being
  - ➤ Fetal serial TTEs may be beneficial
- ◆ Treatment includes dexamethasone, plasmapheresis, and IVIG
- ● **Antiphospholipid disease**
  - ◆ Presents with increased risk of thrombosis and thromboembolism
  - ◆ Associated with spontaneous abortions and IUFD
  - ◆ Anesthetic implications
    - ➤ aPTT is prolonged, but this is a lab-testing artifact
    - ➤ Unless the patient is on anticoagulation, neuraxial is not contraindicated
- ● Marfan syndrome
  - ◆ Autosomal dominant connective tissue disorder
  - ◆ Obstetric complications include cervical incompetence, abnormal placentation, and postpartum hemorrhage
  - ◆ Cardiovascular risks are magnified during pregnancy
    - ➤ Cystic medial necrosis of aorta → aortic insufficiency and dissection
    - ➤ Hemodynamic changes of labor can increase risk of aortic rupture
      - ❖ Obstetricians may advise termination of pregnancy
    - ➤ If pregnancy continues
      - ❖ Serial echocardiograms and monitoring
      - ❖ Initiate β-blocker therapy
      - ❖ C-section or instrument-associated delivery advisable to avoid hemodynamic stresses of delivery
        - › Epidural catheter superior to spinal or general anesthesia
        - › Minimize inotrope usage
- ■ Neurologic disorders
  - ● **Myasthenia**
    - ◆ Autoimmune neuromuscular disease
    - ◆ Maternal consequences
      - ➤ Can flare, be stable, or remit during pregnancy
      - ➤ Concerns include respiratory failure and muscle fatigue during labor
    - ◆ Neonatal consequences
      - ➤ Maternal IgG antibodies can cross placenta → 10% to 20% of newborns affected
      - ➤ Anticholinesterase therapy may be required for the infant for 2 to 4 weeks until maternal antibodies are metabolized
  - ● **Spinal cord injury**
    - ◆ Despite spinal cord injury, uterus is capable of contraction
    - ◆ Injuries above T10 will not have uterine pain, but autonomic dysreflexia is a concern especially if the lesion is above T6
    - ◆ C-sections more frequently performed, but vaginal deliveries are also possible
  - ● **Multiple sclerosis**
    - ◆ Central nervous system disease that can present with muscle weakness, lack of coordination, spasticity, visual changes, lack of sensation, and other manifestations
      - ➤ May remit during pregnancy, but worsen postpartum
    - ◆ Pregnancy may be more difficult due to neuromuscular weakness and fatigue
    - ◆ Anesthetic implications
      - ➤ Spinals and epidurals have been used, but there is concern that spinals may worsen multiple sclerosis due to the effects of local anesthetics on the demyelinated cord
  - ● **Subarachnoid hemorrhage**
    - ◆ Occurs in pregnancy from many different causes, associated with 4% of pregnancy-related in-hospital deaths
    - ◆ More than half occur postpartum
- ■ Infectious disorders

- HIV
  - Highly active antiretroviral therapy (HAART) medications
    - Some may affect drug metabolism through modifying liver enzymes
    - Some may cause bone marrow suppression, including thrombocytopenia
  - Vertical transmission can occur in 15% to 40% of untreated mothers
    - HAART and C-section reduces risk to 2%
  - Neuraxial anesthesia and blood patches are safe
    - Spine is infected early in course of HIV

DELIVERY COMPLICATIONS

- Disorders of placental attachment
  - **Placental abruption**
    - Decreased maternal blood pressure and signs of fetal distress
    - Abnormal separation of placenta from the uterus
    - Presentation: painful vaginal bleeding
    - Anesthetic implications
      - Possible need for emergent C-section
      - Potential for significant blood loss
      - Increased risk of atony
      - High risk of fetal distress
  - **Placental previa**
    - Decreased maternal blood pressure and signs of fetal distress
    - Risk increases with increasing age and there is an increased risk of recurrence with future pregnancies
    - Placenta is partially or completely covering the lower uterine segment
    - Presentation: painless vaginal bleeding
    - Anesthetic implications
      - Possible need for emergent C-section
      - Potential for significant blood loss
  - Vasa previa
    - Fetal blood vessels run next to uterine orifice
    - Risks vessel rupture and fetal demise
    - Requires emergency C-section
  - Disorders of myometrial attachment
    - Types
      - Accreta: placenta adheres to myometrium
      - Increta: placenta invades myometrium
      - Percreta: placenta invades through myometrium into other structures
    - Risk increases with previous C-section and previa
      - Potential for rapid and substantial blood loss
- Uterine rupture
  - Severe abdominal pain and hypotension
  - Most common presenting sign is fetal bradycardia
    - Can be a complete loss of fetal heart tones
  - Risk increases with previous C-section(s)
    - Incidence is 0.8% to 1.6% after lower transverse C-section
    - Incidence is 0.01% without C-section history
  - Vaginal birth after C-section (VBAC)/trial of labor after C-section (TOLAC)
    - Advantages/disadvantages
      - Advantages: vaginal birth has decreased risk of deep vein thrombosis (DVT) and placental invasion
      - Disadvantages: vaginal birth has increased risk of uterine rupture and infection
    - Patient selection
      - Patient with one C-section should be offered TOLAC
      - Patient with two C-sections should be considered for TOLAC

> VBAC less likely to succeed during induction of labor
- Umbilical cord prolapse
  - Umbilical cord exits through the cervix, before fetus
  - Obstetric emergency due to cord compression
- Shoulder dystocia
  - After delivery of the fetal head, the shoulder cannot pass the pubic symphysis
  - Obstetric emergency because the umbilical cord is compressed at the birth canal
- Fetal malposition
  - Types
    - Breech: feet or buttocks first presentation
    - Transverse: sideways position
  - Version
    - Attempted at ~37 weeks to correct malposition
    - Anesthetic implications: prepare for stat general anesthetic due to possible abruption or umbilical cord compression during version
- Retained placenta
  - Part or all of placenta are unable to be delivered
  - Uterine bleeding continues until placenta is removed
- Chorioamnionitis
  - Bacterial infection of the fetal membranes
    - Bacteria from vagina tracts to uterus
    - Risk increases with more frequent vaginal exams
  - Presents with maternal fever and uterine tenderness
  - Treatment: antibiotics and delivery
- Preterm labor
  - Regular contractions of the uterus with cervical changes prior to 37 weeks gestation
  - Diagnosis: vaginal exam, transvaginal ultrasound, fetal fibronectin
  - Treatment
    - Corticosteroids (betamethasone) prior to 34 weeks for lung maturity
    - Tocolytics

NONOBSTETRIC SURGERY ON THE PARTURIENT

- Timing: second trimester ideal
  - First trimester key for organogenesis (2 to 8 weeks)
  - Third trimester risks stimulating preterm labor
    - FHR monitoring may be advisable during procedure
- **Techniques**
  - Maintain hemodynamics within normal limits
  - Target ETCO$_2$ of 32 to maintain normal maternal pH
  - Aspiration prevention if >13 weeks gestation
  - Avoid high intra-abdominal pressures if laparoscopic surgery
    - Target low insufflation pressures (12 to 15 mm Hg)
    - Open trocar technique

OBSTETRIC RESUSCITATION

- Trauma
  - Primary survey identifies life-threatening maternal injuries
    - FAST exam remains effective in parturients
  - Secondary survey includes fetal health
  - Hemorrhage risk
    - Fetomaternal hemorrhage
      > Kleihauer–Betke test: tests volume of fetal blood in maternal circulation
      > Risks Rh isoimmunization and hemolytic disease of newborn
    - Potential hemorrhage sites

➤ Uterine rupture
➤ Placental abruption
➤ Splenic laceration
➤ Hepatic injuries
- Preterm labor
    - Prostaglandin release with injury to myometrium → preterm labor
    - Most cases resolve spontaneously
- Advanced cardiovascular life support (ACLS) variations
    - 30° tilt (left uterine displacement) for chest compressions
    - Early intubation advised
    - C-section recommended within 4 minutes and fetus to be delivered within 5 minutes
        - Delivery improves ability to resuscitate mother due to decreased uteroplacental shunt, decreased oxygen consumption, and relief of cava
        - Neonate typically neurologically intact if delivered within 5 minutes, but rarely intact after 15 minutes
- Drug safety in pregnancy (see Table 16.3)

TABLE 16.3 **Drug safety in pregnancy**

Class	Safety
A	Safe
B	Safe in animals OR animal studies with risk, but safe in humans
C	No data in human and animal studies
D	Risk exists
X	Clear risk to fetus that outweigh benefit to mother

QUESTIONS

1. Which of the following is NOT consistent with a postdural puncture headache?
   A. Nausea
   B. Photophobia
   C. Worsening headache within 15 minutes of sitting up
   D. Onset within 1 hour of neuraxial procedure
   E. Hyperacusis

2. A 30-year-old G2P1 parturient at 39 weeks gestation with a history of severe mitral stenosis presents to the labor and delivery floor. She has never had cardiac surgical intervention. Upon questioning, she has mild shortness of breath and feels easily fatigued with very basic tasks. Which of the following anesthetics is most advisable for vaginal delivery?
   A. Spinal
   B. Epidural
   C. General
   D. Spinal or epidural
   E. Epidural or general

3. Which of the following changes is NOT consistent with a full-term pregnancy?
   A. Increased respiratory rate
   B. Reduced functional residual capacity
   C. Increased tidal volume
   D. Increased heart rate
   E. Increased systemic vascular resistance

4. A 28-year-old G1P0 patient with a history of asthma, gestational diabetes, and antiphospholipid syndrome presents for vaginal delivery. Her lab values are as follows: Hb 12.1, platelets 231, WBC 11K, PT 15, PTT 45. She requests an epidural. What should you do?
   A. Place epidural without further testing
   B. Tell patient she is not a neuraxial candidate due to the elevated PTT
   C. Recommend Vitamin K and then place epidural when PTT is within normal limits
   D. Transfuse FFP and then place epidural
   E. Order a TEG

5. Which of the following is an appropriate antihypertensive during pregnancy?
   A. Losartan
   B. Lisinopril
   C. Nifedipine
   D. Hydrochlorothiazide
   E. Clonidine

DEFINITIONS

- Pain terms
  - Allodynia: pain caused by stimulus; normally not painful
  - Hyperalgesia: increased response to normally painful stimulus
  - Hypoalgesia: decreased sensitivity to normally painful stimulus
  - Hyperpathia: painful syndrome where there is no response to repetitive stimulus until a threshold level is reached → explosive pain response
  - Anesthesia dolorosa: pain occurring in an insensate region
- Sensory terms
  - Hypoesthesia: decreased sensitivity to stimulation
  - Hyperesthesia: increased sensitivity to stimulation
  - Dysesthesia: unpleasant abnormal sensation
  - Paresthesia: abnormal, but not unpleasant, sensation
- Parestheticas
  - Meralgia paresthetica: entrapment of the lateral femoral cutaneous nerve → pain at the lateral thigh
  - Cheiralgia paresthetica: entrapment of radial nerve → pain at the back of the hand
  - Notalgia paresthetica (NP): compression of spinal nerves → pain between upper thoracic spine and scapula

TYPES OF PAIN

- Nociceptive pain: pain caused by simulation of nociceptors in visceral or somatic structures
  - Visceral pain
    - Pain due to nerve endings in the viscera
    - Responds to stretching more than cutting
  - Somatic pain
    - Pain due to nerves in the skin and musculoskeletal system
    - Complete relief through spinal anesthesia
- Neuropathic pain: pain caused by injury or dysfunction of the nervous system
- Psychogenic pain: pain inconsistent with an organic cause

PAIN FIBERS

- Types of pain fibers
  - A-α and A-γ fibers
    - Fibers that innervate muscle
  - A-β fibers
    - Fibers that carry sensory information
  - A-δ fibers
    - Fibers that respond to temperature, pressure, and pain
    - Thin and myelinated
  - B fibers
    - Fibers that communicate with the autonomic nervous system
    - Myelinated preganglionic fibers

- C fibers
  - Respond to pain
  - Unmyelinated → slow transmission
- Order of response
  - First pain: brief, well localized, sharp/pricking
    - A-δ fibers carry signal at 10 to 20 m/s
  - Second pain: longer, dull/burning, less well localized
    - C-fibers carry signal at 1 m/s

PAIN PATHWAYS

- **Pain transmission**
  - Painful stimuli at periphery → impulse transmitted through a first order neuron via the posterior nerve root → reaches cell body of first order neuron at the dorsal root ganglion
  - First-order neuron travels up or down up to three segments in Lissauer tract → synapses with second-order neuron (second-order neuron with cell body at the dorsal horn) → signal crosses to the contralateral cord → travels through the spinothalamic tract to the brain or synapses with wide dynamic range neurons to cause central sensitization of pain → central sensitization can disproportionately increase the firing rate to magnify transduction
  - Second-order neuron reaches the thalamus → synapses with third-order neurons at the thalamus → transmits signals to cerebral cortex
- **Sensitization**
  - Peripheral sensitization occurs through chemical mediators (bradykinin, prostaglandin, substance P), heat, and frequency of stimuli → decreased threshold for nociceptor stimulation
  - Central sensitization is due to windup and sensitization of second-order neurons and wide dynamic ranges through neurochemical mediators (calcitonin gene–related peptide, substance P), N-methyl-D-aspartate (NMDA) mechanisms, and expansion of receptive fields

WORLD HEALTH ORGANIZATION (WHO) ANALGESIC LADDER

- Recommended ladder for stepwise escalation of pain medications (Fig 17.1)
  - Initially created for cancer pain → now applied more broadly
  - Recommends widely available and inexpensive medications
  - Bottom level of ladder is for mild pain and the highest level of the ladder is for severe pain
- Levels
  - Bottom: nonopioids and adjuvants
    - Acetaminophen, nonsteroidal anti-inflammatory drugs (NSAIDs), antidepressants, antiepileptics
  - Middle level: weak opioids and adjuvants
    - Codeine, tramadol
    - The middle level is controversial due to concerns that the side effects of these medications may not justify their mild analgesic benefit
  - Top level: strong opioids and adjuvants
    - Morphine, hydromorphone, oxycodone, and fentanyl
- Recently, a new level has been proposed for invasive procedures
  - Invasive procedures would be the new top rung of the ladder
    - Nerve blocks, neurolysis, brain and nerve stimulators

OPIOIDS AND DELIVERY OPTIONS

- Oral and intravenous opioids
  - Parental opioids
    - As effective as intravenous opioids at appropriate doses, but without need for intravenous access
    - Recommended postoperatively as soon as oral medication is tolerated
  - Intravenous opioids

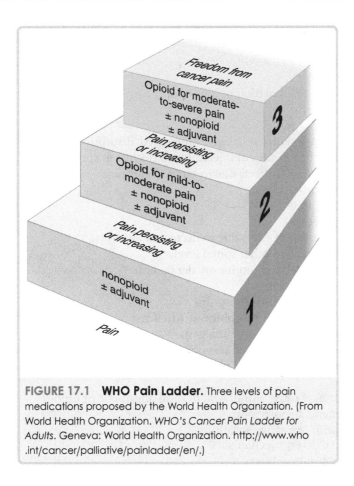

FIGURE 17.1   WHO Pain Ladder. Three levels of pain medications proposed by the World Health Organization. (From World Health Organization. *WHO's Cancer Pain Ladder for Adults.* Geneva: World Health Organization. http://www.who .int/cancer/palliative/painladder/en/.)

- ◆ Bolus delivery
  - ➤ Opioids are administered by nurses at periodic intervals based on patient demand
  - ➤ Benefits
    - ❖ Superior for patients unable to communicate pain or follow directions
    - ❖ Requires frequent checks and monitoring from nursing staff → increased awareness of patient pain
    - ❖ Avoids errors in pump programming and administration
- ◆ **Patient-controlled analgesia (PCA)**
  - ➤ Allows patient to self-administer opioids at small doses at the press of a button
  - ➤ PCA has option for basal rate and demand rate
    - ❖ Basal rates are associated with increased respiratory depression
    - ❖ Basal rates are not associated with improved pain or sleep
  - ➤ Benefits
    - ❖ Ease of use and rapid administration of analgesics
    - ❖ Ability to accommodate a wide range of patient pain thresholds based on programmability
    - ❖ Administration of small, titratable doses with more consistent steady state levels
    - ❖ Less risk of overdosing due to lack of demand by obtunded patients
- ■ Neuraxial analgesia for postoperative pain
  - ● Epidural vs. spinal
    - ◆ Epidurals are commonly used for postoperative pain due to the ability to thread off a catheter for long-term medication administration
      - ➤ Epidural opioids are 10× more potent than intravenous opioids
    - ◆ Spinals are rarely used for postoperative pain due to the short duration of analgesia
      - ➤ Intrathecal opioids are 100× more potent than intravenous opioids

- ➤ A single shot of spinal morphine can have up to 24 hours of analgesic effects
- Drug formulations
  - ➤ Neuraxial anesthesia for postoperative pain often combines a local anesthetic and opioid to maximize synergy
  - ◆ Opioid selection often based on opioid lipophilicity vs. hydrophilicity
    - ➤ Lipophilic opioids
      - ❖ Rapid onset
      - ❖ Shorter duration of action due to increased absorption
      - ❖ Better absorbed at sites of injection and decreased spread to other spinal levels
      - ❖ Increased systemic effects due to rapid absorption
      - ❖ Example: fentanyl
    - ➤ Hydrophilic opioids
      - ❖ Slower onset
      - ❖ Longer duration of effect due to decreased absorption
      - ❖ Increased spread to other spinal levels
      - ❖ May result in delayed respiratory depression
      - ❖ Example: morphine
  - ◆ Single-shot epidural or spinal morphine
    - ➤ A single shot of epidural morphine at 1 to 4 mg or intrathecal morphine at 0.1 to 0.4 mg can provide up to 24 hours of analgesia
    - ➤ Risks include pruritis, delayed respiratory depression, and urinary retention
    - ➤ Center must be capable of monitoring patients postoperatively to assess for respiratory depression
  - ◆ Side effects that may cause withdrawal of local anesthetic or opioid
    - ➤ Local anesthetic: hypotension
    - ➤ Opioid: pruritis, excessive sedation
- Epidural analgesia delivery mechanisms
  - ◆ Continuous epidural analgesia
    - ➤ Epidural is set at a constant infusion rate controlled by the medical team
  - ◆ **Patient-controlled epidural analgesia**
    - ➤ Epidural is set at a constant infusion rate controlled by the medical team
    - ➤ Patients are capable of self-bolusing supplemental doses of the epidural medication
- **Subarachnoid analgesia delivery mechanisms**
  - ◆ Long-term subarachnoid opioids are often indicated for chronic cancer pain requiring high doses of opioids with intolerable side effects
  - ◆ Delivered via implanted or external pump
  - ◆ Intrathecal granuloma is a complication of prolonged intrathecal catheters
    - ➤ Presents with paresthesias, neurological deficits, or loss of drug effect

NONOPIOID ANALGESICS AND ADJUVANTS

- ■ Acetaminophen
  - ● Mechanism
    - ◆ Central antinociceptive effect
      - ➤ Central cyclooxygenase (COX)-2 inhibitor → inhibits prostaglandin H_2 synthase
    - ◆ May block NMDA receptor activation and substance P at the spinal cord
    - ◆ Weak peripheral anti-inflammatory activity
  - ● Effectiveness
    - ◆ Synergistic with opioids
    - ◆ Has a ceiling effect
  - ● Metabolism
    - ◆ 90% conjugated with glucuronide → metabolite is excreted in bile
    - ◆ 5% to 15% oxidized via cytochrome P-450 to NAPQI → detoxified by glutathione
      - ➤ NAPQI is toxic to the liver
  - ● Liver failure
    - ◆ Excess acetaminophen ingestion → glutathione consumed → increased NAPQI → liver toxicity

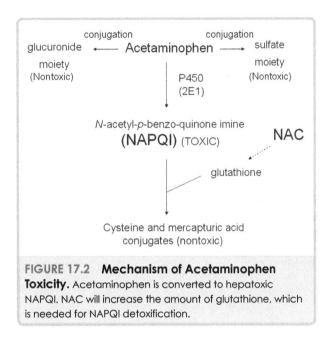

FIGURE 17.2 Mechanism of Acetaminophen Toxicity. Acetaminophen is converted to hepatoxic NAPQI. NAC will increase the amount of glutathione, which is needed for NAPQI detoxification.

- ➤ Approximately 10 g required for toxicity
- ➤ Alcohol lowers threshold for toxicity
- ✦ Acetaminophen toxicity is 51% of all hepatic failure (Fig. 17.2)
- ✦ Stages
  - ➤ Stage I: asymptomatic
  - ➤ Stage II: hepatitis-like findings (elevated transaminases)
  - ➤ Stage III: peak hepatotoxicity at 72 to 96 hours
  - ➤ Stage IV: hepatic recovery
- ✦ Treatment
  - ➤ N-acetylcysteine is a precursor for glutathione → increased glutathione decreases NAPQI
  - ➤ Loading dose of 140 mg/kg PO or 150 mg/kg IV
    - ❖ May require frequent re-dosing
- ■ NSAIDS
  - ● Mechanism
    - ✦ Peripheral nociceptive effect
    - ✦ Inhibits of cyclooxygenase (COX) → decreases prostaglandin synthesis
      - ➤ Prostaglandins sensitive peripheral nociceptors → hyperalgesia
    - ✦ COX-1 vs. COX-2
      - ➤ COX-1 is an enzyme that is produced under physiologic conditions
        - ❖ Associated with gastric protection
      - ➤ COX-2 is an enzyme produced under inflammatory conditions
        - ❖ Selective COX-2 inhibitors have less gastrointestinal side effects, but may have increased cardiovascular risk
  - ● Effectiveness
    - ✦ Synergistic with opioids
    - ✦ Ketorolac 30 mg IV has an effect of up to 10 mg of morphine
  - ● Side effects
    - ✦ Gastrointestinal ulcers and bleeding
      - ➤ Decreased prostaglandins → increased gastric acid secretion, decreased mucus production
    - ✦ Renal failure
      - ➤ Decreased prostaglandins → vasoconstriction and decreased kidney flow
      - ➤ NSAID-associated renal dysfunction worsened with increasing age, preexisting renal disease, and hypovolemia

- Decreased hemostasis
  - Increases platelet dysfunction
  - Inhibits procoagulant thromboxane
  - COX-2 inhibitors not associated with platelet dysfunction
- Gabapentin
  - Mechanism
    - Binds and inhibits $\alpha 2$-δ voltage-gated calcium channels at the central nervous system
    - $\alpha 2$-δ voltage-gated calcium channels are upregulated during nerve injury
  - Indications
    - Anticonvulsant
    - Analgesic activity
    - First-line agent for neuropathic pain
      - When administered preoperatively at a dose of 300 to 1,200 mg → decreases postoperative pain scores and short-term opioid consumption
      - Adjuvant that decreases opioid consumption postoperatively
  - Side effects
    - Excess sedation
    - Dizziness
- α_2 agonists
  - Clonidine
    - Mechanism
      - α_2 adrenergic agonist
      - Stimulates central adrenergic receptors → decreases sympathetic response
    - Indications
      - Reduces anesthetic and opioid requirements
      - Decreases postoperative shivering
      - Supplementation for neuraxial anesthesia
        - Adds to quality and duration of neuraxial block
          - Reduce area of increased sensitivity to pain (hyperalgesia) at site around the wound
          - Lower rates of postoperative pain
        - Increase sedation
      - Hemodynamic changes are typically minimal, but bradycardia and hypotension can occur
  - Dexmedetomidine (see Chapter 3)
- Antispasmodics
  - Baclofen
    - Agonist at $GABA_B$ channels
    - May have analgesic properties
    - Commonly used for spasticity associated with neuromuscular disorders such as multiple sclerosis, cerebral palsy, spinal cord injury, or amyotrophic lateral sclerosis
    - Can be administered orally or intrathecally
    - Side effects include drowsiness, fatigue, and orthostatic hypotension
  - Cyclobenzaprine
    - Antispasmodic agent that relieves painful muscle spasms
    - Side effects include sedation, dry mouth, and syncope
  - Tizanidine
    - α_2 agonist that reduces spinal motor neuron activity
    - Decreases sympathetically medicated pain
    - Side effects include sedation, weakness, and dizziness
- Antidepressants
  - Tricyclic antidepressants (TCA)
    - Mechanism for analgesia
      - Inhibit reuptake of norepinephrine and serotonin
      - Used for depression and chronic pain
    - Side effects
      - Anticholinergic effects (dry mouth, blurred vision, urinary retention)
      - Sedation and drowsiness

- TCA overdose
  - Presentation
    - Anticholinergic effects
    - Hypertension and tachycardia
    - ECG changes: prolonged QRS, QT
  - Treatment: sodium bicarbonate
    - Increases gradient of sodium across neuronal membranes to overcome the blockade of sodium channels by TCA
    - pH elevation keeps TCA in neutral form
- Serotonin and norepinephrine reuptake inhibitors
  - Mechanism for analgesia
    - Inhibit reuptake of norepinephrine and serotonin
    - Used for depression and chronic pain
  - Side effects
    - Loss of appetite
    - Sedation
    - Sexual dysfunction
- Topical agents
  - Lidocaine
    - Mechanism
      - Block voltage-gated sodium channels at neuronal cell membrane → inhibit neuron depolarization
    - Formulations
      - Patches can be used at topical areas of painful skin
      - Gels and ointments can be used at mucus membranes
    - Minimal systemic side effects
      - Doses should be monitored for systemic toxicity
  - Capsaicin
    - Mechanism
      - Capsaicin is a temperature-sensitive transient release potential voltage-gated channel (TRPV1) agonist → activation of sensory neurons → longer refractory state with desensitization of channel
      - TPRV1 channel targeted for analgesic development
    - Formulation
      - Capsaicin patch (8%) approved for postherpetic neuralgia
    - Side effects
      - Degenerates epidermal nerve fibers
      - Side effect is mostly on skin
- Ziconotide
  - N-type voltage-sensitive calcium channel blocker with potent analgesic activity
    - Ziconotide is an amino acid found in the venom of deep-sea snail *Conus magus*
    - No reliance on opioids
    - No tolerance, withdrawal, or addiction
  - Routes
    - IV: profound hypotension (contraindicated)
    - Intrathecal: approved for use for refractory pain to analgesics and intrathecal opioids

BACK PAIN

- **Evaluating back pain**
  - Assessing severity
    - 90% of acute back pain resolves within 4 to 6 weeks with conservative therapy
    - Risk factors warranting further or urgent evaluation
      - Neurological deficits (numbness, motor deficits, loss of bowel, or bladder control)
      - Unintentional weight loss
      - Fevers

- ➤ History of cancer
- Assessing location
  - ◆ Axial pain is along the spine
    - ➤ Due to disc degeneration, facet arthropathy, or myofascial cause
  - ◆ Radicular pain extends to extremities
    - ➤ Due to nerve root involvement
- **Types of pain**
  - Facet joint pain
    - ◆ Pain along the axial spine worsened by extension and lateral bending
    - ◆ Caused by stress on facet joint due to degenerative disc disease or loss of vertebral height
  - Sacroiliac joint pain
    - ◆ Pain along the upper buttock and lower thigh with tenderness at the sacroiliac joint
    - ◆ Cause is not clear and onset is gradual
  - Discogenic pain
    - ◆ Presents with midline axial pain that does not extend to the distal extremities
    - ◆ Caused by degenerative disc disease
  - Myofascial pain
    - ◆ Presents with aching muscle pain that worsens with activity
    - ◆ Caused by trauma or motion injury
  - Cauda equina
    - ◆ Presents with severe back pain, saddle anesthesia, and bowel and bladder dysfunction
    - ◆ Trauma or compression to the cauda equina containing the lumbar and sacral nerve roots
  - Spinal stenosis
    - ◆ Pain in the extremities caused by calcification of the central canal
      - ➤ Worsened by activities that extend the spine (e.g., walking downhill)
      - ➤ Improved by activities that flex the spine (e.g., walking uphill)
  - Failed back surgery syndrome
    - ◆ Pain that is not relieved or continues after back surgery
- **Procedures for back pain**
  - Steroid injections
    - ◆ Mechanism
      - ➤ Anti-inflammatory through decreased prostaglandins, thromboxanes, and leukotrienes
    - ◆ Types
      - ➤ **Epidural steroid injection**
        - ◆ Indicated for radicular pain due to root irritation and spinal stenosis
          - ⟩ Injection into radicular or vertebral arteries can cause spinal cord injury or neurological damage
          - ⟩ Recent evidence has questioned the efficacy of cervical steroid injections
      - ➤ **Facet medial branch blocks:** indicated for degenerative arthropathy of facet
      - ➤ **Sacroiliac joint block:** indicated for sacral and low back pain
  - **Radiofrequency ablation**
    - ◆ Mechanism
      - ➤ Uses elevated temperatures to denervate peripheral nerves that cause pain
    - ◆ Indicated for facet pain
      - ➤ Associated with brief increase in pain before clinical improvement
  - Electrical stimulation
    - ◆ **Transcutaneous electrical nerve stimulation**
      - ➤ Transcutaneous electrical nerve stimulation is a low intensity electrical stimuli at 2 to 100 Hz that produces tingling/vibratory sensation
      - ➤ Produces analgesia by releasing endogenous endorphins → inhibitory effect at spinal cord
    - ◆ **Spinal cord stimulator**
      - ➤ Procedure
        - ◆ Large bore needle is placed in the epidural space via a paramedian approach
        - ◆ Stimulation electrode is passed through the needle and threaded to appropriate vertebral level causing discomfort

- ❖ Electrodes are connected to an implantable pulse generator controlled via the programmer
- ❖ Stimulation is initiated to cause a paresthesia → further stimulation and pain is ignored by patient
  - ➤ Mechanism
    - ❖ Stimulation of spinal cord results in inhibition of vasoconstricting mediators
    - ❖ Inhibits spino-cortico transmission of nociceptive signals
  - ➤ Indications
    - ❖ Failed back surgery syndrome
      - › Radicular pain responds best (over mechanical or nociceptive pain)
    - ❖ Lower extremity peripheral vascular disease

PAIN SYNDROMES AND CONDITIONS

- ■ Complex regional pain syndrome (CRPS)
  - ● Types
    - ❖ Type I: reflex sympathetic dystrophy
      - ➤ Most common type of CRPS
      - ➤ No evidence of nerve lesions
    - ❖ Type II: causalgia
      - ➤ Follows injury to large nerves
  - ● Symptoms
    - ❖ Pain, edema, spasms, and sympathetic dysfunction
      - ➤ Small subset with skin changes (smooth, shiny, edematous, or scaly skin)
      - ➤ Nail bed changes and hair loss can occur
      - ➤ Pain may shift to other locations or jump to the other extremity
      - ➤ 50% with tremor and 82% with poor coordination
    - ❖ Most resolve with time
  - ● Diagnosis
    - ❖ Budapest criteria
      - ➤ Continuing pain that is disproportionate to the inciting event
      - ➤ Symptoms in three of four categories: sensory, vasomotor, edema, or motor
        - ❖ Symptoms are problems that patients report
      - ➤ Signs in two of four categories: sensory, vasomotor, edema, or motor
        - ❖ Signs are visually observed or felt
      - ➤ No other diagnosis better explains symptoms
  - ● Treatment
    - ❖ Physical therapy to diminish secondary injury
    - ❖ Sympathetic block
      - ➤ Examples: stellate ganglion block, cervical sympathetic block, or lumbar sympathetic block
    - ❖ Spinal cord stimulation
    - ❖ Regional nerve block
- ■ **Peripheral neuropathy**
  - ● Mechanism
    - ❖ Damage to peripheral nerves causing pain and loss of sensation
    - ❖ Common causes include long-term diabetes, autoimmune diseases, genetic conditions, and medication side effects
  - ● Presentation
    - ❖ Numbness, tingling, pain, pins and needles sensation
    - ❖ Motor weakness and loss of coordination
  - ● Treatment
    - ❖ Treat the underlying case (e.g., improved glucose control, remove offending medications)
    - ❖ Neuropathic pain medications including gabapentin, TCA, serotonin and norepinephrine reuptake inhibitors, and capsaicin

- **Herpes zoster**
  - Mechanism
    - Reactivation of varicella zoster virus (shingles) that presents with a painful skin rash
    - Varicella zoster virus remains dormant at the dorsal root ganglion
      - Reactivation by stress, surgery, UV light, trauma, malignancy, systemic steroids, HIV, and immune suppression
  - Presentation
    - Rash that follows a dermatomal pattern → typically heals within a month
      - Thoracic dermatome is the most common distribution
      - Ophthalmic distribution of the trigeminal is second most common distribution
    - Postherpetic neuralgia
      - Residual pain >3 months after onset of rash
      - Pain may be present years after resolution of herpes zoster rash
      - Often with sympathetic component
        - Sympathectomy can treat pain
          - Epidural can prevent recurrence
          - Other drugs treat pain, not prevent
      - Antivirals decrease duration, but not effective at prevention
  - Treatment
    - Zoster vaccine for prevention
    - Antiviral drugs
    - Analgesics
      - TCAs, anticonvulsants, topical local anesthetics, topical capsaicin, transcutaneous electrical nerve stimulation
- **Trigeminal neuralgia**
  - Mechanism
    - Compression of the trigeminal nerve → hyperactive nerve functioning
    - Chronic entrapment may cause demyelination in the **Gasserian ganglion**
  - Presentation
    - Sudden, unilateral, severe, brief, stabbing, recurrent pain at a branch of the fifth CN
      - Maxillary division most commonly affected
      - Exacerbated by mechanical pressure
    - More likely unilateral
    - Women > men
    - Age >50 years
  - Treatment
    - Carbamazepine (tegretol)
      - Sodium and calcium channel blocker → suppresses glutamate release and action of NMDA, potentiates GABA
        - NNT: 8
      - Side effect
        - Sedation, rash
        - Serious effects include leukopenia and Stevens Johnsons syndrome
    - **Trigeminal rhizotomy**
      - Prior to rhizotomy, a local anesthetic block should be performed to test if the trigeminal nerve is the source of nociception
      - If the local anesthetic block is successful at relieving pain → radiofrequency trigeminal rhizotomy, **glycerol rhizotomy**, or balloon compression should be effective
      - Side effects
        - 90% with facial numbness
        - 10% with dysesthesias
        - 2% with anesthesia dolorosa
    - Posterior fossa microvascular decompression
- **Phantom limb pain (PLP)**
  - Mechanism
    - Painful sensation following limb amputation that missing limb is still present

- Etiology remains unclear
  - Theorized to be due to cortical reorganization or defects in signaling from the peripheral nervous system
- Presentation
  - Patients may present with phantom sensations, PLP, or stump pain
  - Incidence is 60% to 85% in first week of limb loss, but pain can occur years later
    - Pain typically fades with time, but rarely disappears
    - Sensations include stabbing, pricking, squeezing, and shooting pain
  - Incidence same for traumatic/nontraumatic amputees
  - Incidence increases with more proximal amputation
  - PLP can be reactivated by epidural/spinal anesthetics
- Treatment
  - Nerve blocks
  - Antiepileptics
  - Antidepressants
  - NMDA antagonists
  - Clonidine
  - Opioids
- Fibromyalgia
  - Mechanism
    - Disseminated musculoskeletal pain with generalized tenderness due to a central cause
    - Patients commonly with low serotonin, elevated substance P at cerebrospinal fluid, and low androgen levels
  - Presentation
    - Commonly associated with sleep disturbances, depression, anxiety, fatigue, and other debilitating conditions
    - Demographics
      - More common in women than men
      - Incidence increases up to 80 years of age, then decreases
    - American College of Rheumatology diagnostic requirements
      - Must affect all four quadrants of the body
      - >3 months duration
      - Presence of tender points (18 designated)
        - Pain at $\geq$11/18 sites via 4 kg/cm^2 pressure
  - Treatment
    - Antidepressants
    - Neuropathic pain medications
    - NSAIDS are not effective
    - Opioids only if severe
- **Myofascial pain syndrome**
  - Mechanism
    - Unknown
  - Presentation
    - Deep aching that is poorly circumscribed
    - Deep muscle pain caused by trigger points and fascial constrictions
    - Can see associated erythema and stiffness
    - Trigger points exacerbated by vascular or muscular spasm
  - Treatment
    - Acetaminophen or NSAIDs
    - Antidepressants
    - Neuropathic pain medications
    - Antispasmodics
    - Ultrasound therapy
    - Trigger point injections
    - Acupuncture

HEADACHES

- Migraines
  - Presentation
    - Migraine headaches are typically unilateral, pulsating, aggravated by physical activity, associated with photophobia and phonophobia, and cause nausea and vomiting
    - A migraine with aura is defined as the addition of abnormal visual or sensory symptoms
  - Treatment
    - Avoid triggers that exacerbate migraines
    - NSAIDs, acetaminophen, and caffeine may be sufficient for mild migraines
    - Triptans may reduce pain, but may increase cardiovascular risk
- Tension
  - Presentation
    - Tension headaches are nonpulsatile and not aggravated by physical activity
    - Most common type of headache
  - Treatment
    - NSAIDs, acetaminophen generally effective
    - TCAs may be considered as second-line agents
- Cluster
  - Presentation
    - Cluster headaches are severe, unilateral orbital or supraorbital, and often accompanied by conjunctival injection, nasal congestion, or rhinorrhea
    - Frequent attacks are termed "clusters"
    - More common in men than women
  - Treatment
    - Oxygen therapy may yield rapid improvement
    - Triptans

ALTERNATIVE MEDICINE

- **Acupuncture**
  - Anxiolysis
    - Preoperative acupuncture at auricular points → anxiolysis
  - Anesthesia and analgesia
    - Acupuncture does not reduce minimum alveolar concentration requirements
    - Acute pain
      - Increases endogenous opioid release and activates structures in the descending antinociceptive pathway → decreases inflammation and postoperative pain
    - Chronic pain
      - May be effective for headaches, low back pain, rheumatoid conditions, and facial pain
  - Postoperative nausea and vomiting (PONV)
    - Stimulation of P6 pressure point decreases PONV
- **Hypnosis**
  - Studies have shown hypnosis can reduce postoperative pain requirements and decrease PONV
  - Hypnosis may alter the processing of pain and influence pain perception

QUESTIONS

1. A 50-year-old man complains of localized pruritis and diffuse mild burning of the left shoulder. These symptoms are most consistent with a diagnosis of:
   A. Meralgia paresthetica
   B. Cheiralgia paresthetica
   C. Notalgia paresthetica
   D. Analgia paresthetica

2. An epidural nerve block falls into which step of the World Health Organization's (WHO) analgesic ladder?
   A. Step 1
   B. Step 2
   C. Step 3
   D. Step 4
   E. Does not apply

3. Which of the following is most consistent with the mechanism of action of gabapentin's analgesic activity?
   A. Blockade of NMDA receptors
   B. Inhibition of $\alpha 2-\delta$ voltage-gated calcium channels
   C. Inhibition of reuptake of norepinephrine and serotonin
   D. Activation (agonist) of $GABA_B$ channels
   E. Blockage of voltage-gated sodium channels

4. Which of the following statements regarding PLP is most correct?
   A. Commonly disappears after the first year
   B. The time of onset is greatest after the first week of limb loss
   C. Incidence is increased with traumatic (compared with nontraumatic) amputations
   D. Can be reactivated by spinal anesthetics

5. Which of the following is most consistent with the diagnosis of CRPS?
   A. Dermatomal distribution of pain
   B. Pain that is proportional to the inciting event
   C. Absence of allodynia
   D. Presence of tremor

LOCAL ANESTHETICS

- ■ Classification
  - ● Local anesthetics contain a substituted amine through an ester or amide linkage
  - ● Amino esters
    - ◆ Name contains one "i"
      - ➤ Examples: procaine, chloroprocaine
    - ◆ **Metabolized by cholinesterase** → forms para-aminobenzoic acid
    - ◆ Short half-life in circulation
  - ● Amino amides
    - ◆ Name contains two or more "i's"
      - ➤ Examples: lidocaine, bupivacaine, ropivacaine, mepivacaine
    - ◆ **Metabolized by the liver** through dealkylation
    - ◆ Longer half-life in circulation
- ■ **Mechanism** (Fig. 18.1)
  - ● Local anesthetics must diffuse into the nerve cell membrane uncharged → protonated to take on positive charge once inside the cell membrane → inhibit the α-subunit of voltage-gated sodium channels → inhibit sodium ion influx → inhibit nerve conduction
  - ● Different nerves are inhibited at different concentrations of local anesthetics
    - ◆ Susceptibility to local anesthetic is determined by the size of the nerve and myelination
    - ◆ Myelin enhances ability to block nerves

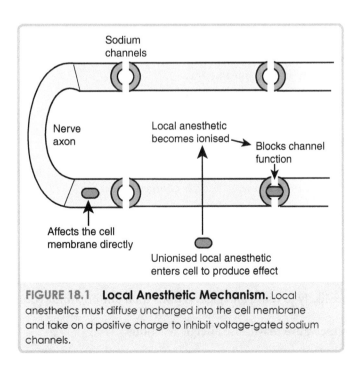

FIGURE 18.1 **Local Anesthetic Mechanism.** Local anesthetics must diffuse uncharged into the cell membrane and take on a positive charge to inhibit voltage-gated sodium channels.

- Block order
  - First: small unmyelinated sympathetic fibers
  - Second: unmyelinated C fibers
  - Third: myelinated fibers for proprioception, touch, and pressure
  - Fourth: large myelinated motor fibers
- Application
  - Block order can be used to assess the onset of a regional and neuraxial anesthesia and predict whether the block will be effective

■ **Qualities of local anesthetics**
- **Potency**
  - Increased lipophilicity → increased diffusion through cell membrane → increased potency
- **pK$_a$**
  - Lower pK$_a$ → more molecules are uncharged at physiologic pH → increased diffusion through cell membrane → increased speed of onset
  - With rare exceptions, most local anesthetics are weak bases
- **Protein binding**
  - Increased protein binding → increased duration of action

■ **Systemic absorption**
- Local anesthetic classification
  - Amino esters are rapidly cleared once they reach circulation → unlikely to cause systemic toxicity
  - Amino amides require liver metabolism → potential for elevated serum levels
- Site of injection
  - Absorption of local anesthetic depends on the vascularity of the site of injection
  - Rank of highest to lowest plasma concentration based on site of injection
    - Intravenous
    - Tracheal
    - Intercostal
    - Caudal
    - Paracervical
    - Epidural
    - Brachial plexus
    - Peripheral nerve
    - Subcutaneous tissue

■ Additives to local anesthetics
- **Epinephrine**
  - Benefits of epinephrine
    - Aids detection of intravascular injections
    - Prolongs duration of local anesthetics
    - Minimizes systemic toxicity of local anesthetics
  - Disadvantages of adding epinephrine
    - Decrease in local blood flow → ischemia if injection site is poorly vascularized
    - Systemic absorption → hypertension, tachycardia
  - Onset time
    - Local anesthetics premade with epinephrine are formulated at a lower pH to stabilize epinephrine → more local anesthetic is charged → decreased absorption into tissue → slower onset time
    - Adding epinephrine to a local anesthetic immediately before injection → local anesthetic retains natural pK$_a$ → does not affect onset time
- Sodium bicarbonate
  - Increases pH → increased uncharged local anesthetic → increases speed of onset

■ Allergic reactions
- Amino esters more likely to cause allergic reactions than amino amides due to para-aminobenzoic acid metabolite
- Methylparaben preservative may cause allergic reactions

■ Systemic toxicity

- Causes of toxic intravascular levels
  - ◆ Direct intravascular injection
  - ◆ Rapid absorption from tissue
  - ◆ High doses of administered local anesthetics
  - ◆ Impaired metabolism of local anesthetics
- **Central nervous system**
  - ◆ Symptoms can include metallic taste, dizziness, visual changes, tinnitus, loss of consciousness, and seizures
  - ◆ Treatment
    - ➤ Supportive care
    - ➤ Supplemental oxygen
    - ➤ Mild hyperventilation (may require intubation)
      - ✦ Hyperventilation → decreases cerebral blood flow, increases alkalosis → increases seizure threshold
    - ➤ Benzodiazepines for seizure activity
    - ➤ Lipid emulsion
- **Cardiovascular system**
  - ◆ Presents with arrhythmias, hypotension, and cardiovascular collapse
  - ◆ Molecular metabolisms of systemic cardiovascular toxicity
    - ➤ Block potassium channels → lengthen cardiac action potential
    - ➤ Block calcium channels → depress contractility
    - ➤ Block β-receptors → decreases inotropy and impairs resuscitation
    - ➤ Block sodium channels → decrease depolarization rate
  - ◆ Risk increased with bupivacaine
    - ➤ Highly lipophilic → enters neuron rapidly and diffuses out of neuron more slowly
    - ➤ High protein binding → longer duration
    - ➤ Ropivacaine may be less cardiotoxic than bupivacaine
  - ◆ Treatment
    - ➤ Supportive care
    - ➤ Supplemental oxygen
    - ➤ Mild hyperventilation (may require intubation)
      - ✦ Hyperventilation → corrects acidosis and hypercarbia that promote local anesthetic ion trapping
    - ➤ Cardioversion or antiarrhythmic
    - ➤ Lipid emulsion
- Lipid emulsion
  - ◆ Twenty percent intralipid used for cardiotoxicity associated with local anesthetics
  - ◆ May increase local anesthetic clearance from cardiac tissues by acting as a "lipid sink"
  - ◆ Bolus at 1.5 cc/kg (about 100 cc) with infusion at 0.25 cc/kg/min × 10 minutes
    - ➤ Additional boluses may be necessary

REGIONAL ANESTHESIA PRINCIPLES

- Injection selection
  - Single shot
    - ◆ Duration and quality of regional block depends on local anesthetic used, volume of injection, and proximity to target nerve
  - Catheters
    - ◆ Used to provide prolonged postoperative analgesia
    - ◆ Increased risk of infections
      - ➤ 20% to 40% of catheters with colonization of bacteria
      - ➤ Axillary and femoral sites are the highest risk for infection
      - ➤ Catheter use >48 hours increases risk
      - ➤ Tunneling may decrease risk
      - ➤ Risk of serious infection is low, but case reports of abscesses have been published
- Localization

- Nerve stimulator
  - ◆ Deliver a current to illicit nerve stimulation → motor response
  - ◆ $Q = I \times T$ (Charge = intensity × duration)
  - ◆ Twitches of the appropriate muscle at a current ≤0.5 mA indicate desired location
- Ultrasound
  - ◆ Needle insertion and nerve localization are done under visual guidance
  - ◆ Diminished risk of direct nerve or vascular injury

HEAD AND NECK BLOCKS

- **Stellate ganglion**
  - **Technique**
    - ◆ Local anesthetic injection toward the C6 transverse process to cause sympathetic inhibition
  - Indications
    - ◆ Treats pain with a sympathetic component
    - ◆ Complex regional pain syndrome, acute herpes zoster, and postherpetic neuralgia
  - Side effects/complications
    - ◆ Intravascular injection into the vertebral artery → central nervous system toxicity
    - ◆ Block recurrent laryngeal nerves → hoarseness
    - ◆ Epidural or subarachnoid injection → high spinal or epidural anesthesia
- **Trigeminal nerve block**
  - Technique
    - ◆ Individual blocks are required for each division of the trigeminal nerve
      - ➤ Ophthalmic nerve blocked at the supraorbital notch
      - ➤ Maxillary nerve blocked at the pterygopalatine fossa
      - ➤ Mandibular nerve blocked just posterior to the pterygoid plate
  - Indication
    - ◆ Blocks are commonly used to diagnose trigeminal neuralgia (see Chapter 8)
    - ◆ Can be used for minor facial or eye procedures

CERVICAL PLEXUS BLOCKS AND LANDMARKS

- Anatomy
  - Cervical plexus formed by C1-4
  - Location of plexus
    - ◆ Deep to sternocleidomastoid
    - ◆ Anterior to middle scalene
  - Innervates the back of the head, lateral neck, and anterior and lateral shoulder
- Block types
  - Superficial cervical plexus
    - ◆ Injection of local anesthetic along posterior border of the sternocleidomastoid → covers cutaneous tissue
  - Deep cervical plexus
    - ◆ Injection of local anesthetic in the cervical paravertebral space around C2-C4 → covers deeper tissue
- Side effects/complications
  - Injection into nearby structures
    - ◆ Vertebral arteries → central nervous system toxicity
    - ◆ Subarachnoid space → high spinal
    - ◆ Epidural space → cervical anesthesia
  - Blocking nearby nerves
    - ◆ Unilateral phrenic nerve → respiratory distress in those with low pulmonary reserve
    - ◆ Recurrent laryngeal nerve → hoarseness
    - ◆ Sympathetic block → unilateral Horner syndrome (miosis, ptosis, anhidrosis)

UPPER EXTREMITY BLOCKS AND LANDMARKS

- Anatomy
  - Brachial plexus formed by C5-T1 (Fig. 18.2)
  - **Location of plexus**
    - Roots are between the anterior and middle scalene muscles
    - Trunks pass over the first rib near the subclavian artery
    - Cords pass to the axilla near the axillary artery
- Block types
  - Interscalene
    - Technique
      - Injection of local anesthetic at the three roots between the anterior and the middle scalene muscles
    - Coverage
      - Blocks both the cervical and brachial plexus → effective for shoulder surgery
      - Spares the inferior trunk at C8-T1 (ulnar nerve)
      - If anterior shoulder is spared, perform a superficial cervical plexus block
    - Side effects/complications
      - Intravascular injection → central nervous system toxicity
      - Phrenic nerve is blocked ~100% of the time → respiratory distress in those with low pulmonary reserve
      - Recurrent laryngeal nerve → hoarseness
      - Sympathetic block → unilateral Horner syndrome (miosis, ptosis, anhidrosis)
  - Supraclavicular
    - Technique
      - Injection of local anesthetic at the trunks lateral to the subclavian artery at the supraclavicular fossa

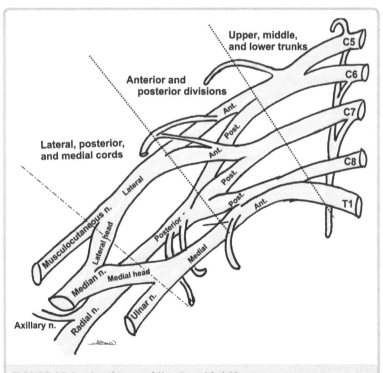

FIGURE 18.2   Anatomy of the Brachial Plexus. Ant., Anterior; Post., Posterior; n., nerve. (Reproduced from Tsui BCH, Rosenquist RW. Peripheral nerve blockade. In: Barash PG, Cullen BF, Stoelting RK, et al., eds. *Clinical Anesthesia.* 7th ed. Philadelphia, PA: Wolters Kluwer; 2013:949.)

- ◆ Coverage
  - ➤ Blocks the brachial plexus at the trunks → effective for surgery at the elbow, forearm, and hand
- ◆ Side effects/complications
  - ➤ Injection is close to the pleura by the first rib → pneumothorax
  - ➤ Phrenic nerve is blocked in 40% to 60% of patients → respiratory distress in those with low pulmonary reserve
- ● Infraclavicular
  - ◆ Technique
    - ➤ Injection of local anesthesia at the cords inferior to the mid-clavicle
  - ◆ Coverage
    - ➤ Blocks the brachial plexus at the cords → effective for surgery of the forearm or hand
  - ◆ Side effects/complications
    - ➤ Intravascular injection → central nervous system toxicity
    - ➤ Inserting the needle too medially → increases risk of pneumothorax
    - ➤ Inserting the needle too laterally → risks missing the musculocutaneous nerve as it branches off the brachial plexus
- ● Axillary
  - ◆ Technique
    - ➤ Injection of local anesthetic at the terminal nerves of the brachial plexus
    - ➤ Radial, ulnar, and median nerve are oriented around the axillary artery
      - ❖ Radial nerve is posterior
      - ❖ Ulnar nerve is inferior
      - ❖ Median nerve is superior
    - ➤ Musculocutaneous nerve lies in the coracobrachialis muscle
      - ❖ Blocked at two possible locations
        - ⟩ Blocked at axilla just superior to the axillary artery
        - ⟩ Blocked at arm at the intercondylar line deep to the lateral margin of the biceps tendon
    - ➤ Intercostobrachial nerve lies in the intercostalis externus and serratus anterior
      - ❖ Blocked at the axillary fossa
  - ◆ Coverage
    - ➤ Blocks terminal nerves → effective for surgery of forearm and hand
    - ➤ May require supplementation of the musculocutaneous nerve
      - ❖ Covers radial forearm
    - ➤ May require supplementation of the intercostobrachial nerve
      - ❖ Covers posteromedial arm
  - ◆ Side effects/complications
    - ➤ Intravascular injection → central nerve system toxicity
    - ➤ Direct nerve injury
- ● Bier block
  - ◆ Technique
    - ➤ Place an IV in the operative hand as distally as possible
    - ➤ Elevate the arm for exsanguination
    - ➤ Inflate a proximal blood pressure cuff greater than the arterial blood pressure
    - ➤ Inject local anesthetic → onset ~5 minutes
    - ➤ If patient complains of tourniquet pain
      - ❖ Inflate distal tourniquet
      - ❖ Release proximal tourniquet
    - ➤ After 30 minutes, release tourniquet
  - ◆ Local anesthetic selection
    - ➤ Used local anesthetics
      - ❖ Lidocaine at 1.5 to 3 mg/kg
      - ❖ Prilocaine at 3 to 4 mg/kg
      - ❖ Ropivacaine at 1.2 to 1.4 mg/kg
    - ➤ Avoided local anesthetics

- ❖ Bupivacaine → increased cardiac toxicity
- ❖ Chloroprocaine → increased thrombophlebitis
- ◆ Coverage
  - ➤ Provides analgesia to area distal to the cuff
  - ➤ Can also be used for treatment of complex regional pain syndrome with local anesthetic or other agents (guanethidine, reserpine, bretylium, phentolamine)
- ◆ Side effects/complications
  - ➤ Tourniquet pain
  - ➤ Direct nerve injury from tourniquet compression
  - ➤ Local anesthetic toxicity during cuff deflation

LOWER EXTREMITY BLOCKS AND LANDMARKS

- ▪ Anatomy
  - ● Nerves
    - ◆ Lumbar plexus is formed by T12-L4 (Fig. 18.3)
    - ◆ Sacral plexus is formed by L4-S3
  - ● Location
    - ◆ Lumbar plexus passes between the psoas major and quadratus lumborum muscles
      - ➤ Lumbar plexus gives rise to the femoral nerve → becomes the saphenous nerve distally
    - ◆ Sacral plexus passes through the greater sciatic foramen
      - ➤ Sciatic nerve forms from the sacral plexus and a branch of the lumbar plexus
- ▪ Lumbar plexus blocks
  - ● Psoas block
    - ◆ Technique
      - ➤ Local anesthetic injected between psoas major and quadratus lumborum muscles from a posterior approach
    - ◆ Coverage
      - ➤ Covers the hip and the anterolateral thigh
    - ◆ Side effects/complications
      - ➤ Injection into other spaces

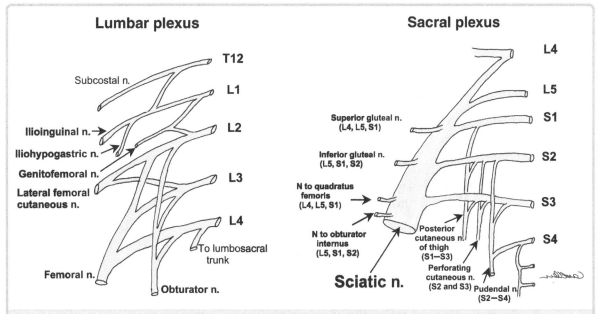

FIGURE 18.3 Anatomy of the Lumbar Plexus and Sacral Plexus. n., nerve. (Reproduced from Tsui BCH, Rosenquist RW. Peripheral nerve blockade. In: Barash PG, Cullen BF, Stoelting RK, et al., eds. *Clinical Anesthesia.* 7th ed. Philadelphia, PA: Wolters Kluwer; 2013:952.)

- ❖ Subarachnoid
- ❖ Epidural
- ❖ Intravascular
  - ➤ Retroperitoneal hematoma
- Femoral
  - ❖ Technique
    - ➤ Local anesthetic injected lateral to the femoral artery
    - ➤ Two fascial layers traversed are the fascia lata and fascia iliaca
  - ❖ Coverage
    - ➤ Anterior thigh and knee
    - ➤ Indicated for knee arthroplasty or repair of femoral shaft fractures
  - ❖ Side effects/complications
    - ➤ Intravascular injection
    - ➤ Nerve injury
- Obturator
  - ❖ Technique
    - ➤ Local anesthetic injected into obturator canal through an insertion near the pubic tubercle
  - ❖ Coverage
    - ➤ Medial thigh
    - ➤ Rarely blocked for regional anesthesia
  - ❖ Side effects/complications
    - ➤ High failure rate due to depth of obturator canal
- Lateral femoral cutaneous
  - ❖ Technique
    - ➤ Local anesthetic injected at the anterior superior iliac space after passage through the fascia lata
  - ❖ Coverage
    - ➤ Lateral thigh
  - ❖ Side effects/complications
    - ➤ Nerve injury
- ■ Sacral plexus blocks
  - Sciatic nerve block
    - ❖ Technique
      - ➤ Local anesthetic injected as the sciatic nerve passes through the sacrosciatic foramen at the lower border of the gluteus maximus
    - ❖ Coverage
      - ➤ Blocks the posterior tibial and common peroneal nerve
      - ➤ Used for any procedure below the knee when supplemented with a saphenous nerve block
    - ❖ Side effects/complications
      - ➤ Nerve injury
      - ➤ Vascular injury
  - Popliteal block
    - ❖ Technique
      - ➤ Local anesthetic injected into the popliteal fossa between the biceps tendon laterally and semimembranosus tendon medially
        - ❖ Target the sciatic nerve as it bifurcates into the posterior tibial and common peroneal nerve
      - ➤ Posterior tibial nerve is medial and larger
        - ❖ Responsible for plantarflexion and foot inversion
      - ➤ Common personal nerve is lateral and smaller
        - ❖ Responsible for dorsiflexion and foot eversion
    - ❖ Coverage
      - ➤ Covers the foot and ankle when supplemented with a saphenous block
    - ❖ Side effects/complications
      - ➤ Nerve injury
      - ➤ Intravascular injection

- Ankle block
  - Technique
    - Local anesthetic injected near five nerves of the ankle
      - Often done in a ring technique to cover the entire ankle
    - Nerves are the saphenous, superficial peroneal, deep peroneal, sural, and posterior tibial nerve
  - Coverage
    - Saphenous: branch of the femoral nerve that innervates the medial ankle and foot
      - Blocked anterior to the medial malleolus
    - Posterior tibial: branch of the common peroneal that innervates the sole of the foot
      - Blocked posterior to the medial malleolus
    - Sural: branch of the common peroneal nerve that innervates the lateral malleolus and lateral foot
      - Blocked posterior to the lateral malleolus
    - Superficial peroneal: branch of the common peroneal nerve that innervates the dorsum of the foot
      - Blocked anterior to the lateral malleolus
    - Deep peroneal: branch of the common peroneal that innervates the web space between the first and second toe
      - Blocked between the tendons of the anterior tibial and extensor digitorum longus muscles
  - Side effects/complications
    - Nerve injury

THORACIC, ABDOMINAL, AND PELVIC BLOCKS

- Thoracic blocks
  - Paravertebral block (Fig. 18.4)
    - Technique
      - Local anesthetic injected or catheter placed as the spinal nerves emerge from the vertebral foramina
      - Insert needle 2 cm deeper than the posterior surface of the transverse process in a caudal direction until loss of resistance or localization of the paravertebral space with ultrasound
    - Coverage
      - Although commonly performed at the thoracic level, a paravertebral block can be done along the entire lumbar and thoracic spine
      - Unilateral coverage for thoracic, breast, or abdominal procedures
        - Will cover several dermatomes above and below the entry site assuming sufficient volume is injected
        - Tendency is for spread to be more caudad than cephalad
    - Side effects/complications
      - Injection near pleural → pneumothorax
      - Injection too medial → risks epidural or intrathecal injection
      - Injection too lateral → risks becoming an intercostal block without sufficient coverage
  - Intercostal block
    - Technique
      - Local anesthetic injected at the inferior border of the rib
        - Vein is superior, artery is in the middle, and nerve is inferior along the lower border of the rib
    - Coverage
      - Blocks intercostal nerves at injected levels
    - Side effects/complications
      - Intravascular injection
      - Increased vascular absorption and systemic levels → increased risk of toxicity
- Abdominal blocks
  - Neurolytic blocks

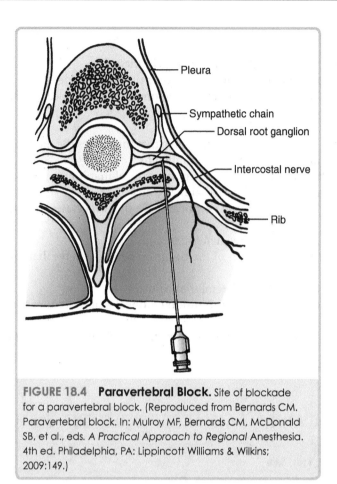

FIGURE 18.4 **Paravertebral Block.** Site of blockade for a paravertebral block. (Reproduced from Bernards CM. Paravertebral block. In: Mulroy MF, Bernards CM, McDonald SB, et al., eds. *A Practical Approach to Regional Anesthesia.* 4th ed. Philadelphia, PA: Lippincott Williams & Wilkins; 2009:149.)

- ◆ Indicated for chronic pain through use of neurolytic agent on nerves
  - ➤ Alcohol or phenol commonly used for neurolysis
- ◆ Diagnostic block with local anesthetic recommended prior to neurolytic block to demonstrate that the target nerve is the source of pain
- ● Celiac plexus block
  - ◆ Celiac plexus supplies the abdominal organs
    - ➤ Ascending colon, gallbladder, and pancreas
  - ◆ Indications
    - ➤ Commonly used for pancreatic cancer pain
  - ◆ Side effects/complications
    - ➤ Hypotension following sympathectomy
    - ➤ Subarachnoid injection
    - ➤ Aortic injury
    - ➤ Direct organ injury
    - ➤ Diarrhea
- ● Hypogastric plexus block
  - ◆ Hypogastric plexus supplies the pelvic organs
    - ➤ Uterus, bladder, rectum, vaginal fundus, prostate, testes, and ovaries
  - ◆ Indications
    - ➤ Chronic pelvic pain of various etiologies
  - ◆ Side effects/complications
    - ➤ Impotence
    - ➤ Direct organ injury
- ■ Pelvic blocks
  - ● Ilioinguinal

- ◆ Local anesthetic injected between the internal oblique and transversus muscle at the level of the iliac crest
  - ➤ Covers pain from the abdominal wall around the levels of injection
- ◆ Indicated for lower abdominal surgery, particularly inguinal surgery
- ● Genitofemoral
  - ◆ Local anesthetic injected at genital branch of the genitofemoral nerve at the inguinal canal
  - ◆ Indicated for pain along the groin and upper medial thigh
- ● Pudendal
  - ◆ Local anesthetic injected into the ischiorectal fossa
    - ➤ Covers external genital organs, perineum, distal two-third of vagina, and anus
  - ◆ Indicated for surgery on the pelvic floor or vaginal delivery

COMMON NERVE INJURIES

- ■ Brachial plexus
  - ● Injured via stretch (head of the humerus) or compression (between the clavicle and first rib)
- ■ Radial nerve
  - ● Wrist drop and weakness of thumb abduction
- ■ Median nerve
  - ● Inability to oppose thumb and pinky finger
  - ● Decreased sensation of palmer surface of thumb, pointer, middle, and half of ring finger
- ■ Ulnar nerve
  - ● Injured via compression against the posterior aspect of the medial epicondyle of the humerus
  - ● Inability to abduct pinky finger
  - ● Decreased sensation to dorsal and palmer surfaces of pinky and half of ring finger
- ■ Sciatic nerve
  - ● Injured via stretching
    - ◆ Lithotomy position
  - ● Weakness below the knee
  - ● Decreased sensation over the majority of the foot with the exception of the inner arch (that is innervated by the saphenous)
- ■ Common peroneal nerve
  - ● Branch of the sciatic nerve
  - ● Most commonly injured nerve of the lower extremity
    - ◆ Injured in lithotomy position when the nerve is compressed against the fibular head
    - ◆ Results in foot drop, loss of dorsiflexion, and the inability to evert the foot
- ■ Anterior tibial nerve
  - ● Injured if the foot is flexed for a prolonged period of time
  - ● Results in foot drop
- ■ Femoral nerve
  - ● Injuries occur at the level of the pelvic brim
  - ● Result in loss of hip flexion and knee extension
  - ● Decreased sensation over the superior aspect of the thigh
- ■ Obturator nerve
  - ● Injured during forceps delivery of a baby or with excessive flexion of the thigh
  - ● Results in the inability to adduct leg
  - ● Decreased sensation over the medial aspect of the thigh

QUESTIONS

1. A 42-year-old male presents for a left rotator cuff repair under general anesthesia with an interscalene catheter for postoperative analgesia. The catheter is placed successfully and uneventfully under ultrasound guidance. Prior to his expected discharge home, you are called to the recovery area as the patient is complaining that his eyelid is drooping. On examination, he also has miosis of the right pupil. Which of the following is the correct diagnosis?
   A. Atypical anxiety reaction
   B. Intravascular placement of the nerve catheter
   C. Horner syndrome
   D. Phrenic nerve block

2. An otherwise healthy 18-year-old male presents after fracturing his elbow while skiing. You decide to perform an axillary nerve block for pain relief. Which of the following is the correct orientation of the median, radial, and ulnar nerves in relation to the axillary artery?

   A. Posterior, inferior, superior
   B. Superior, posterior, inferior
   C. Inferior, posterior, superior
   D. Superior, inferior, posterior

3. After performing a popliteal nerve block, you realized you dosed the patient by pounds instead of kilograms and administered over 9 mg/kg of lidocaine without epinephrine.

Which of the following symptoms are some of the earliest signs of local anesthetic toxicity?
   A. Vomiting and diarrhea
   B. Dizziness and tinnitus
   C. Circumoral numbness and nystagmus
   D. Lightheadedness and seizures

4. A 55-year-old female has recently been diagnosed with metastatic pancreatic cancer. Due to the extent of her disease she is not a surgical candidate. She reports that she has been taking increasing doses of narcotics with little-to-no effect on her abdominal pain. She now presents for a celiac plexus block. Which of the following is the one of the most common complications?

   A. Pneumothorax
   B. Aortic puncture
   C. Orthostatic hypotension
   D. Local anesthetic toxicity

5. A 68-year-old male with a long-standing history of diabetes presents for amputation of the left fourth and fifth metatarsal. Which of the following nerves must be blocked to achieve adequate anesthesia for the procedure?

   A. Superficial peroneal, tibial, sural
   B. Superficial peroneal, deep peroneal, tibial
   C. Deep peroneal, sural, saphenous
   D. Saphenous, sural, tibial

CHAPTER 19 Intensive Care Medicine

SHOCK STATES

- **Sepsis**
  - **Definitions**
    - Systemic inflammatory response syndrome (SIRS; 2 or more)
      - Temperature >38.3°C or <36°C
      - Heart rate (HR) >90
      - Respiratory rate >20
      - White blood cells >12K or <4K
    - Sepsis (SIRS + suspected source of infection)
      - Infectious sources can be pneumonia, urinary tract infection, bacteremia, and many others
    - Severe sepsis (sepsis + organ dysfunction)
      - Organ dysfunction can be marked by hypotension, hypoperfusion, oliguria, creatinine increase, lung injury, coagulopathy, or hyperbilirubinemia
    - Septic shock (severe sepsis + hypotension despite fluid resuscitation)
  - **Pathophysiology**
    - Derangements during sepsis are caused by the interaction between the infectious organism and the host's inflammatory response
    - Cellular mechanism
      - Proinflammatory mediators
        - Cytokines include IL-1, IL-6, and TNF-α
        - Activation of neutrophils and lymphocytes
        - Complement system
      - Endothelial dysfunction
        - Increase in nitric oxide (NO) → vasodilation
          - Inducible NO synthase is stimulated by IL-6 and TNF-α, which leads to the increase in NO
        - Capillary leakage → tissue edema
        - Endothelial surfaces normally have anticoagulant properties
          - Disturbed in sepsis by procoagulant inducers (C-reactive protein)
          - Leads to intravascular thrombosis
    - **Organ system dysfunction**
      - Cardiac
        - Decreased myocardial contractility
        - Impaired oxygen delivery
      - Pulmonary
        - Increased work of breathing
        - Capillary leak in lungs impairs oxygenation
          - Risk of acute respiratory distress syndrome (ARDS)
      - Renal
        - Hypoperfusion and hypotension can lead to acute renal failure
          - Acute tubular necrosis
      - Hepatic
        - Hypoperfusion and hypotension can lead to "shock" liver
          - Possible increased bilirubin, transaminases, and international normalized ratio (INR)
      - Endocrine

- ❖ Adrenal insufficiency
  - ⟩ Impaired stress response as there is an inadequate increase in serum cortisol levels
- ❖ Insulin deficiency
  - ⟩ Impaired function of pancreatic beta cells
  - ⟩ Ensuing hyperglycemia leads to increased risk of infection, delay in wound healing, and reduced granulocyte function
- ❖ Vasopressin deficiency
- ● **Treatment**
  - ❖ **Hemodynamic support**
    - ➤ Support blood pressure (BP) with intravenous fluids
    - ➤ If fluid resuscitation insufficient → initiate vasopressors to maintain mean arterial pressure >65 mm Hg
      - ❖ Norepinephrine and vasopressin are the most commonly selected vasopressors
      - ❖ Dobutamine or epinephrine may be added if cardiac support is needed
      - ❖ Dopamine should be avoided in septic shock
    - ➤ Consider central line placement for vasopressors administration, central venous pressure monitoring, and measurement of central venous saturation
      - ❖ Early goal-directed therapy trial included using a central line to monitor resuscitation, but more recent studies have challenged this need
  - ❖ Respiratory support
    - ➤ Sepsis and fluid resuscitation may lead to need for respiratory support, including intubation and mechanical ventilation
    - ➤ Avoid etomidate for intubation → increased mortality in septic shock
    - ➤ Initiate lung-protective ventilation to minimize risk or effect of ARDS
  - ❖ **Antimicrobial coverage**
    - ➤ Obtain blood, urine, sputum, and other cultures prior to antibiotic initiation (if possible)
    - ➤ Target source control (treating infection, surgery, or drainage)
    - ➤ Initiate broad-spectrum antibiotics within the first hour
- ■ **Hypovolemic**
  - ● Defined by decreased intravascular volume causing inadequate tissue perfusion
    - ❖ Common causes are hemorrhage and severe dehydration
  - ● Stages of hypovolemic shock
    - ❖ Stage I: blood loss <15%
      - ➤ Compensated shock due to ability to physiologically adjust
      - ➤ Associated with minimal hemodynamic changes
    - ❖ Stage II: blood loss 15% to 30%
      - ➤ Mild shock
      - ➤ Associated with increased HR, slight decrease in urine output
    - ❖ Stage III: blood loss 30% to 40%
      - ➤ Decompensated shock
      - ➤ Associated with systolic BP <100, decrease in urine output, and reduced capillary refill
    - ❖ Stage IV: blood loss >40%
      - ➤ Severe shock
      - ➤ Associated with HR >140, systolic BP <100, respiratory failure, minimal urine output, and cold mottled skin
  - ● Triad of death
    - ❖ Triad: hypothermia, acidosis, and coagulopathy
    - ❖ Combination of the three makes resuscitation incredibly difficult and survival unlikely
  - ● Treatment
    - ❖ Large-bore vascular access
      - ➤ Consider transfusing an equal ratio of blood:FFP:platelets
      - ➤ Minimize nonblood products during acute bleeding
    - ❖ Rapid control of hemorrhage if bleeding
    - ❖ Rapid fluid resuscitation
- ■ **Cardiogenic**
  - ● Defined by hypoperfusion due to cardiac failure

- ◆ Acute coronary syndrome
- ◆ Right or left ventricular failure
- ◆ Cardiomyopathy
- ◆ Cardiac tamponade
- ◆ Pulmonary embolism
- ● Markers of circulatory failure
  - ◆ Hypotension
  - ◆ Low cardiac index (<1.8 L/min/m^2)
  - ◆ Left ventricular end-diastolic pressure >18 mm Hg
  - ◆ Right ventricular end-diastolic pressure >10 mm Hg
- ● Treatment
  - ◆ Treat underlying cause (e.g., reperfusion if acute coronary syndrome)
  - ◆ Vasopressors and inotropes to maintain perfusion
  - ◆ Mechanical support (e.g., ventricular assist device or balloon pump)

INFECTION CONTROL

- ■ **Antibiotic classification**
  - ● **Antibacterial agents**
    - ◆ Primary gram-positive antimicrobials
      - ➤ β-lactams
      - ➤ First- and second-generation cephalosporins
      - ➤ Vancomycin
      - ➤ Linezolid
      - ➤ Daptomycin
    - ◆ Primary gram-negative antimicrobials
      - ➤ Third- and fourth-generation cephalosporins
      - ➤ Piperacillin/tazobactam
      - ➤ Aminoglycosides
      - ➤ Fluoroquinolones
      - ➤ Carbapenems
      - ➤ Aztreonam
  - ● Anaerobes
    - ◆ Metronidazole
    - ◆ Clindamycin
  - ● **Antifungal agents**
    - ◆ Azoles
    - ◆ Echinocandins
    - ◆ Amphotericin B
  - ● **Antivirals**
    - ◆ Oseltamivir
    - ◆ Acyclovir
  - ● **Antiparasitics**
    - ◆ Mebendazole
    - ◆ Albendazole
- ■ **Antimicrobial resistance**
  - ● Antimicrobial resistance is increasing
    - ◆ 50% of all nosocomial infections have antimicrobial strains
  - ● Risk factors for multidrug-resistant organisms
    - ◆ Prolonged hospitalization
    - ◆ Previous antibiotic exposure
    - ◆ Prolonged ventilation
    - ◆ Prolonged urinary catheter
    - ◆ Immunosuppression
    - ◆ Malnutrition
  - ● Examples of antibiotic resistance organisms

- Vancomycin resistant enterococci
- Extended-spectrum β-lactamases
- Klebsiella pneumonia carbapenemase
- Multidrug-resistant pseudomonas
- Strategies to reduce antibiotic resistance
  - Consider and treat other causes of presentation besides infection
  - Obtain cultures prior to initiating antibiotics
  - Target antibiotics toward likely organisms
  - Start antibiotics broadly in the intensive care population → narrow when culture data available
  - Avoid treating colonized organisms
  - Reduce ventilator time, remove Foley catheters when not needed, and daily assessment of the need for invasive vascular access
  - Perioperative antibiotics should be limited to 24 hours
- **Central line infections**
  - Central line–associated bloodstream infections are a significant source of morbidity and mortality
    - Increase length of stay up to 21 days
    - One of the leading causes of deaths (mortality as high as 25%)
  - Risk factors
    - Patient immunosuppression
    - Patient malnutrition
    - Prolonged hospital stay
    - Multiport catheter
    - Catheter duration >7 days
    - Catheter location
      - Increased infection rate with femoral lines, least with subclavian
      - Some studies have suggested that femoral line infection risk is not greater if done aseptically
  - Prevention
    - Aseptic technique during placement
    - Use of central line checklist
    - Appropriate catheter-site care
    - Daily reassessment of need for central line
    - Chlorhexidine-impregnated sponges
    - Consider antibiotic impregnated catheters if risk is high
- Infection control
  - **Universal precautions**
    - Method of preventing employee exposure to infectious pathogens
    - Should apply to all patients
      - Assumes all bodily fluids and blood should be considered potentially hazardous
      - Includes gloves, masks, and gowns as necessary when there is potential for contact with bodily fluids
      - Limit exposure to infectious agents as much as possible
  - Special precautions
    - Contact precautions
      - Applies to patients with antibiotic-resistant bacteria (methicillin-resistant *Staphylococcus aureus*, vancomycin-resistant enterococci)
      - Organisms are transmitted by direct contact
      - Includes gloves and gown
    - Airborne precautions
      - Applies to patients with diseases that can be transmitted through droplets or the air (*Mycobacterium tuberculosis*, multiple viruses)
      - Organisms are smaller than droplets, remain in the air longer
      - Include N95 respirator and negative pressure room
    - Droplet precautions
      - Applies to patients with respiratory viruses (influenza, parainfluenza, adenovirus, respiratory syncytial virus)
      - Organisms are larger than airborne particles, rarely transmit >3 ft
      - Includes surgical mask

TRAUMA SURVEYS

- Purpose
  - Primary and secondary surveys are done in a systematic manner to assess, prioritize, and treat life-threatening injuries
  - Primary survey consists of ABCDEs (see below) and should be done first
  - Secondary survey is a complete examination of all body parts, necessary x-rays, and a collection of patient history
    - Secondary survey should be done only after the primary survey is completed
    - The primary survey will require frequent reassessment during the secondary survey
- Primary survey
  - Airway
    - Establish a definitive airway if airway integrity is questionable
      - Definitive airway is via an endotracheal tube or tracheostomy
    - Jaw thrust, chin lift, oral airways are temporizing measures until a definitive airway can be secured
  - Breathing
    - Assess ventilation, oxygenation, and need for mechanical assistance
    - Chest tube placement for suspected pneumothorax
  - Circulation
    - Intravenous access for volume resuscitation
    - Control hemorrhage
    - Monitor for arrhythmias
  - Disability
    - Neurologic examination for level of consciousness, pupil reaction, lateralizing signs, and spinal injury
    - Assess Glasgow Coma Score (GCS)
  - Exposure
    - Patient should be undressed for thorough examination
- Secondary survey
  - History
    - Collect patient allergies, medications, past medical history, last meal, and details of the trauma
  - Physical
    - Head
      - Evaluation of scalp and head for laceration and contusions
      - Assessment for ocular injuries
      - Palpate bony structures of face
    - Neck
      - Presume cervical neck injury and take necessary precautions until injury is definitely excluded
      - Inspect and palpate neck
    - Chest
      - Assess bones of chest wall
      - Reassess breathing and auscultate lungs
    - Abdomen
      - Assess for abdominal injuries
    - Perineum
      - Assess for hematoma or bleeding
      - Rectal examination
    - Musculoskeletal
      - Assess for pelvic fracture
      - Assess extremities for orthopedic injuries
      - Tourniquet can be used to stop hemorrhage from extremities
- Radiological evaluation
  - Focused assessment with sonography for trauma (FAST) (Fig. 19.1)
    - Four ultrasound views to assess for fluid in the abdomen and pericardium
      - Allows rapid assessment at the beside in 2 to 3 minutes

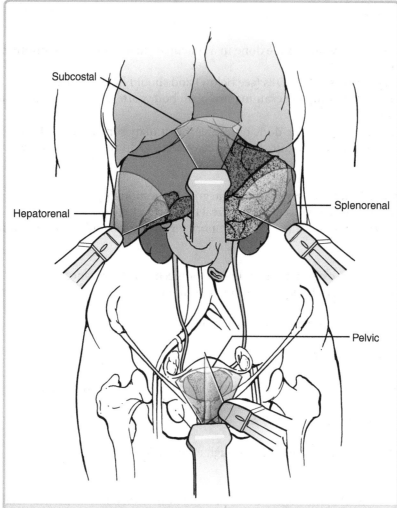

FIGURE 19.1 FAST Exam Locations. Four sites of focused assessment of sonography for trauma (FAST) examination: subcostal, hepatorenal, splenorenal, and pelvic.

- ➤ High sensitivity and specificity
- ◆ Views
  - ➤ Subcostal
    - ❖ Probe at the subxiphoid and angled cephalad
    - ❖ Assess for fluid in the pericardium
  - ➤ Hepatorenal
    - ❖ Probe at the right midaxillary line around the 10th rib
    - ❖ Assess for fluid in Morrison pouch
  - ➤ Splenorenal
    - ❖ Probe at left mix-axillary line around the ninth rib
    - ❖ Assess for fluid in the splenorenal space
  - ➤ Pelvic views
    - ❖ Probe at pubic symphysis–directed caudad
    - ❖ Assess for fluid in the pouch of Douglas and rectovesical pouch
- ● C-spine
  - ◆ CT (computed tomography) is test of choice for acute diagnosis of C-spine injuries
    - ➤ Patients with negative CT and positive signs on examination → MRI
  - ◆ **C-spine x-rays** are not sufficiently sensitive or specific for C-spine injuries

- **CT scan**
  - ◆ If patients are hemodynamically stable, a CT scan of injured areas can yield valuable information on degree of injury, presence of active bleeding, and need for surgical intervention

TRAUMA-SPECIFIC INJURIES

- Traumatic brain injury
  - Physical examination should consist of comprehensive neurological examination and Glasgow Coma Scale (GCS)
    - ◆ CT scan essential to diagnose injuries and determine if surgical intervention is needed
      - ➤ Focal injuries include epidural, subdural, or intracerebral hematomas
    - ◆ Goal is to prevent secondary injury
      - ➤ Prevent hypotension, hypovolemia, hypoxia, and intracranial pressure (ICP) elevation
      - ➤ See traumatic brain injury in Chapter 8
- C-spine injuries
  - Types of injuries
    - ◆ Atlanto-occipital dislocation
      - ➤ Commonly due to severe traumatic flexion
      - ➤ Most die at the scene
    - ◆ C1 fracture
      - ➤ Commonly due to axial loading
      - ➤ Unstable injury, but rarely with spinal cord injury
    - ◆ C2 fracture
      - ➤ Largest cervical vertebra and susceptible to various injuries
      - ➤ Most involve odontoid process
    - ◆ C3 and C4 fractures
      - ➤ Rarely injured due to curvature of C-spine
    - ◆ C5, C6, and C7 fractures
      - ➤ C5 is the most commonly fractured cervical vertebrae
  - Management
    - ◆ Immobilization
      - ➤ Airway management should include in-line stabilization
        - ❖ Assistant's arms on upper chest and clavicles, hands/wrists on neck and head
        - ❖ Assistant stands across from the intubator and uses heels of hands to immobilize the occiput
      - ➤ Collar can be removed for intubation if in-line stabilization is done
        - ❖ Collars inhibit mouth opening and do not reduce neck movement during laryngoscopy
    - ◆ Imaging
      - ➤ CT is immediate imaging modality of choice for C-spine injury
      - ➤ MRI may be obtained if CT is negative and collar cannot be cleared
      - ➤ C-spine x-rays are not sensitive or specific
        - ❖ 3-view C-spine misses 15% of C-spine injuries
    - ◆ Consult surgeon for further assessment and need for collar, halo, or surgical intervention
- Thoracic injuries
  - Tension pneumothorax
    - ◆ Develops when air enters the pleural space without the ability to exit → collapses the affected lung and displaces the mediastinum → decreases venous return → circulatory collapse
      - ➤ Works by a flap-valve mechanism permitting only one-way flow
    - ◆ Presents with chest pain, respiratory distress, deviated trachea, and absent breath sounds
    - ◆ Treatment
      - ➤ Immediate needle decompression with large caliber needle (14 or 16 G) at midclavicular line, second intercostal space → converts tension pneumothorax to simple pneumothorax
      - ➤ Chest tube is definitive treatment
  - Hemothorax
    - ◆ Develops with accumulation of blood in the chest cavity → impairs ventilation
      - ➤ Massive hemothorax is defined as > one-third patient's blood volume in the chest

- ◆ Presents with respiratory distress and hypovolemic shock
- ◆ Treatment
  - ➤ Chest tube
  - ➤ Massive resuscitation
  - ➤ Potential for surgical thoracotomy
- ● Flail chest
  - ◆ Develops with multiple rib fractures that are fractured at ≥ 2 places
  - ◆ Presents with paradoxical motion of chest wall, pain, and respiratory distress
  - ◆ Treatment
    - ➤ Analgesia
      - ◈ Consider epidural anesthesia for effective long-term analgesia that does not impair ventilation
    - ➤ Potential need for intubation if in respiratory distress
    - ➤ Potential rib fixation
- ● Pulmonary contusion
  - ◆ Develops after injury to lung parenchyma
    - ➤ Most due to motor vehicle collisions
    - ➤ Majority of patients have overlying rib fracture
  - ◆ Presents with respiratory distress, hypoxia, and impaired ventilation
    - ➤ Causes alveolar edema, hemorrhage, decreased compliance, and impaired diffusion
  - ◆ Treatment
    - ➤ Supportive care with mechanical ventilation and chest physical therapy
- ■ Abdominal and pelvic trauma
  - ● Penetrating vs. blunt injury
    - ◆ Blunt injury can involve shearing and deceleration injuries → organ lacerations
      - ➤ Common organs injured are the spleen and liver
    - ◆ Penetrating injury involves direct injury
      - ➤ Common organs injured are the liver and bowel
  - ● Pelvic instability
    - ◆ Source of major blood loss in trauma due to fracture or ligament disruption
    - ◆ May require pelvic binder, embolization, or surgical fixation
- ■ Burns
  - ● Burns can be from a thermal, electrical, or chemical source
  - ● Thermal burns
    - ◆ Fire or excessive heat can cause injury at the skin and underlying structures
    - ◆ Extreme capillary leak
      - ➤ Decreased cardiac output secondary to decreased preload from hypovolemia
    - ◆ Secure airway in cases of inhalational injury
      - ➤ Urgent intubation should be highly considered in the presence of singed nasal hairs or nasal/oral mucosa
      - ➤ Assess for carbon monoxide poisoning
        - ◈ Carboxyhemoglobin levels can reach 100% in fire victims
      - ➤ High risk for ARDS
    - ◆ Aggressively fluid resuscitate by Parkland formula or institutional protocol
      - ➤ 4 mL/kg/hr for 0 to 10 kg, plus 2 mL/kg/hr for 10 to 20 kg, plus 1 mL/kg/hr for each kg more than 20 kg
    - ◆ Wound care, surgical debridement, and grafting
  - ● Electrical burns
    - ◆ High-voltage injuries (>1,000 V) can damage underlying muscle, nerves, and other tissues → damage often more significant than appearance on skin
    - ◆ High risk of cardiovascular conduction abnormalities
    - ◆ Require more volume resuscitation than thermal burns
      - ➤ Myoglobinuria: frequent cause of renal failure
    - ◆ Muscle edema can rapidly progress to compartment syndrome
      - ➤ May require escharotomy or fasciotomy
  - ● Chemical burns

- ◆ Caused by cleaners or industrial products
  - ➤ Alkali products: ammonia, bleach, lye, cement, sodium and potassium hydroxide
    - ❖ Results in liquefactive necrosis and saponification of fat
  - ➤ Acidic products: sulfuric acid, hydrochloric acid, hydrofluoric acid
    - ❖ Results in coagulation necrosis and formation of an eschar
      - › Prevents further tissue penetration of the chemical/acid
      - › Acid burns tend to be more superficial as compared to alkali burns
    - ❖ Absorption of hydrofluoric acid leads to hypocalcemia and cardiac arrhythmias
  - ◆ Tissue damage results from protein denaturation
  - ◆ Treatment involves copious irrigation and removal of chemicals
    - ➤ Avoid neutralizing chemical on skin → causes thermal reaction
  - ◆ May require debridement and wound care
- ■ Drowning
  - ● Pathophysiology
    - ◆ Submersion in fluid → voluntary breath hold → fluid entrained in larynx → laryngospasm → hypoxia, hypercapnia → loss of consciousness → entrainment of fluid in lungs → cardiac arrest
  - ● Morbidity and mortality
    - ◆ At 3 minutes → PaO_2 falls below 30 mm Hg → anoxic brain injury
  - ● Treatment
    - ◆ Support airway first
      - ➤ Hemodynamics often improve with improved ventilation and oxygenation
    - ◆ Address cardiovascular system after airway management

ACUTE RESPIRATORY DISTRESS SYNDROME

- ■ Characteristics
  - ● Acute onset
  - ● Bilateral patchy infiltrates on chest x-ray
  - ● No evidence of left atrial hypertension
  - ● Reduced PaO_2/FIO_2 (P:F) ratio
    - ◆ Historical definition
      - ➤ P:F ≤ 300 → acute lung injury
      - ➤ P:F ≤ 200 → ARDS
    - ◆ Berlin definition of ARDS
      - ➤ 200 < P:F ≤ 300: mild ARDS
      - ➤ 100 < P:F ≤ 200: moderate ARDS
      - ➤ P:F ≤ 100: severe ARDS
  - ● Pathophysiology
    - ◆ Characterized by inflammatory injury at lung
      - ➤ Common causes include pneumonia, aspiration, pancreatitis, and sepsis
    - ◆ Phases of ARDS
      - ➤ Alveolar injury: initial phase of injury characterized by diffuse damage to alveoli
      - ➤ Exudative phase: second phase of injury characterized by injury to epithelium and increased alveolar permeability → interstitial and alveolar edema
      - ➤ Proliferative phase: type II pneumocytes proliferate → pulmonary edema resolves, but lungs poorly compliant
      - ➤ Fibrotic phase: chronic phase of injury characterized by collagen deposition and destruction of airspaces
    - ◆ Disability
      - ➤ Of survivors, two-thirds do not return to normal lifestyle
      - ➤ Cause of death is typically multiorgan failure
  - ● Treatment
    - ◆ Lung protective ventilation → reduces barotraumas → improves mortality
      - ➤ Small tidal volumes at ≤6 cc/kg if possible
      - ➤ Minimize peak and plateau pressures
      - ➤ Permissive hypercapnia

- ◆ Conservative fluid management
- ◆ Neuromuscular blockade
  - ➤ Cisatracurium for 48 hours may reduce mortality
- ◆ Prone positioning
  - ➤ Controversial, but may offer mortality benefit in experienced centers
- ◆ Recruitment maneuvers, NO, high frequency oscillation, inverse ratio ventilation, and extracorporeal membrane oxygenation (ECMO) may be considered in cases refractory to other modes of treatment, but evidence of mortality benefit is limited

NUTRITION

- Caloric needs
  - Patients in the intensive care unit frequently do not receive their daily caloric needs
    - ◆ NPO status for surgery or procedures
    - ◆ Bowel rest after surgery
    - ◆ Gastrointestinal complications that prevent feeding
    - ◆ Aspiration risk
    - ◆ Impaired mental status
  - Nutritional requirements
    - ◆ Basal requirements
      - ➤ Calculated through conventional equations
      - ➤ Calculating through assessing the patient's energy expenditure through carbon dioxide production
    - ◆ Sources of calories
      - ➤ Carbohydrates: 4 kcal/g
      - ➤ Protein: 4 kcal/g
      - ➤ Fat: 9 kcal/g
  - Malnourishment
    - ◆ Many patients may be malnourished prior to admission due to their underlying illness, malignancy, or poor nutritional status
      - ➤ Poor nutritional status correlated with increased complications and mortality
      - ➤ Obese patients are malnourished
    - ◆ Albumin levels can be a marker of nutritional status
  - Conditions that require increased nutritional support
    - ◆ Inflammatory diseases, burns (up to 200% increase in metabolic rate!), and pancreatitis have increased metabolic demands → require increased nutritional support
- Methods of nutritional support
  - **Enteral**
    - ◆ Preferred mode of feeding
      - ➤ Prevents gut atrophy
      - ➤ Minimal infectious risks
      - ➤ Ability to deliver a high number of calories
      - ➤ Formulations can be tailored to specific needs (renal failure, fluid status, etc.)
    - ◆ Patients can eat, have an orogastric/nasogastric tube, or a gastric/jejunal tube to assist feeding
  - **Parenteral**
    - ◆ Highly concentrated and hypertonic solution infused through a central vein
    - ◆ Utilized in situations when the gut cannot be used for an extended duration
    - ◆ Associated with increases risks
      - ➤ Increased infectious risks (fungal)
      - ➤ Requires central access
      - ➤ Increased gut atrophy and fatty liver disease
        - ❖ Cholestasis
        - ❖ Bacterial translocation secondary to intestinal mucosal atrophy
      - ➤ Acetate in solution may cause metabolic alkalosis
      - ➤ Calories may be limited based on volume of solution
      - ➤ Insulin addition to TPN may cause hyperglycemia or hypoglycemia upon termination

- Early parenteral nutrition completing enteral nutrition in adult critically ill patients (EPaNIC) study found late initiation of parenteral nutrition was associated with fewer infections, reduced costs, and unchanged mortality
- Re-feeding syndrome
  - A chronically malnourished patient is deficient in electrolytes and minerals, especially phosphate
  - Rapid re-feeding → increased insulin secretion → consumption of electrolytes and minerals → phosphate depletion → inability to form sufficient ATP → inadequate oxygen delivery to vital organs
    - Consequences include neuromuscular weakness, respiratory failure, arrhythmias, heart failure, rhabdomyolysis, hemolytic anemia, and death
  - Treatment
    - Phosphate, magnesium, and electrolyte repletion
    - Caloric intake should start slowly with continued escalation after prolonged fasting

GLUCOSE CONTROL

- Hyperglycemia is a common finding in the intensive care unit
  - Preexisting diabetes
  - Inflammatory response to injury
  - Increased insulin resistance
  - Nutritional supplementation
- Hyperglycemia is associated with mitochondrial injury, neutrophil dysfunction, endothelial dysfunction, oxidant injury, and complement inhibition
- Management
  - NICE-SUGAR (Normoglycemia in the Intensive Care-Evaluation) trial recommended glucose target of 140 to 180
  - Further reductions in glucose increased risk of hypoglycemia

CRITICAL CARE MYOPATHY

- Presentation
  - Presents with muscle weakness and neuropathy following prolonged ICU hospitalization
  - Risk factors
    - Steroids, sepsis, immobility, hyperglycemia, and neuromuscular blockers
- Diagnosis
  - EMG (electromyogram) testing
    - Specific, but not very sensitive (<50%)
    - Findings included prolonged latency and spontaneous motor discharges
  - Increased creatine phosphokinase
    - Increased muscle necrosis
- Complications
  - Increased duration of mechanical ventilation
  - Increased ICU complications
    - Deep vein thrombosis, pulmonary embolism, pneumonia
  - Impaired rehabilitation

QUESTIONS

1. A 22-year-old man is brought to the emergency department after sustaining a stab wound during a fight. His examination is notable for tachypnea and tachycardia, decreased systolic BP, oliguria, and confusion. On the basis of these findings, his estimated blood loss is at least:

   A. 10%
   B. 20%
   C. 30%
   D. 50%

2. A 65-year-old man is admitted to the ICU with respiratory failure due to community acquired *Haemophilus influenza* pneumonia. The minimum level of infection-prevention precautions appropriate for care of this patient is?

   A. Standard precautions
   B. Droplet precautions
   C. Airborne precautions
   D. Contact precautions

3. Which of the following criteria correctly corresponds to the Berlin definition of ARDS?

   A. Acute lung injury is defined as $Pao_2/Fio_2 < 200$
   B. Heart failure must be excluded
   C. Pao_2/Fio_2 is based on zero positive end-expiratory pressure
   D. Lung injury within 1 week of an apparent clinical insult

4. A 55-year-old man with history of colon cancer develops a small bowel obstruction requiring exploratory laparotomy and small bowel resection. Postoperatively he develops an ileus, which prevents enteral feeding for 1 week. When enteral feeding is initiated which of the following electrolyte abnormalities would be most suggestive of re-feeding syndrome?

   A. Hypercalcemia
   B. Hypophosphatemia
   C. Hyperkalemia
   D. Hypomagnesemia

5. A 65-year-old woman undergoes right upper lobe wedge resection for asymptomatic nodule identified on routine chest x-ray. Her past medical history is notable for hypertension. On arrival in the PACU she has a temperature of 100.2, HR of 105, respirations of 24, and systolic BP of 85. Her white blood cell count is 16. Which of the following diagnoses is most appropriate for this patient?

   A. Systemic inflammatory response syndrome (SIRS)
   B. Sepsis
   C. Severe sepsis
   D. Septic shock

CHAPTER 20

Toxins and Drugs of Abuse

SUBSTANCE ABUSE

- Definitions
  - **Tolerance:** diminishing effect of a substance at a given dose
  - Dependence: **withdrawal** symptoms during cessation of substance
  - **Addiction:** compulsive behavior despite adverse consequences to using the substance
- **Mechanisms for tolerance, dependence, and addiction**
  - Increased metabolism of substances
    - Induction of liver enzymes
  - Drug receptor changes
    - Nerve receptor desensitization after prolonged exposure
    - Increased or decreased receptor quantity based on the substance abused
  - Alteration in neurotransmitter levels
- Perioperative assessment
  - Preoperative history and physical examination
    - Collect history of substance(s) abused and dosages used
      - Depressants
        - Alcohol
        - Benzodiazepines
        - Opioids
      - Stimulants
        - Cocaine
        - Amphetamines
      - Psychotropic substances
        - Cannabis
    - Consider and address patient concerns regarding surgery
      - Physician judgment
      - Inadequate dosing of analgesics
      - Risk of relapse
    - Assess need for further preoperative testing based on whether the substances used have affected other organ systems (e.g., endocarditis, cardiomyopathy)
  - **Preoperative planning**
    - Consider postponing elective surgery in cases of acute intoxication or high risk of withdrawal
    - Consider preoperative detoxification or maintenance programs for patients actively abusing substances
    - Consider halting medications that may inhibit the ability to titrate anesthetics and opioids
      - Examples: buprenorphine, naltrexone
  - **Anesthetic planning**
    - Consider opioid and anesthetic-sparing modalities
      - Local, regional, and neuraxial anesthesia
    - Consider anesthetic requirements
      - Acute intoxication with depressants reduces anesthetic requirements
      - Chronic intoxication with depressants increases anesthetic requirements
      - Intoxication with stimulants increases anesthetic requirements

- ◆ Consider hemodynamic fluctuations
  - ➤ Intoxication with stimulants may require intraoperative management for tachycardia and hypertension
- ■ **Specific agents of abuse**
  - ● Alcohol
    - ◆ Alcohol abusers are at increased risk of liver disease, cardiomyopathy, dementia, Wernicke–Korsakoff syndrome, and anemia
    - ◆ Increased risk of delirium tremens (DT) postoperatively
      - ➤ DT is caused by downregulation of $GABA_A$ receptors and upregulation of glutamate
      - ➤ Presentation
        - ◆ Fever, visual changes, hallucinations, feeling of impending doom, autonomic hyperactivity
      - ➤ Timeframe: typically presents 2 to 4 days after alcohol cessation
      - ➤ Associated with significant mortality increase
    - ◆ DT can be treated or prevented with benzodiazepines, chlordiazepoxide, barbiturates
      - ➤ Propofol useful as a $GABA_A$ agonist for those intubated in the ICU
  - ● Cocaine
    - ◆ Intoxication presents with euphoria, agitation, dilated pupils, sweating, tachycardia, hypertension, and seizures
    - ◆ Cocaine prevents reuptake of catecholamines → increased risk of intraoperative hypertension and tachycardia
      - ➤ Chronic cocaine use may deplete catecholamine stores
    - ◆ Increased risk of coronary vasoconstriction and arrhythmias
      - ➤ Treatment is with benzodiazepines and nitroglycerin
      - ➤ Do not β-block cocaine intoxication before α-blockade → risks unregulated α-agonism and severe hypertension
  - ● Cannabis
    - ◆ Acute intoxication acts as a central nervous system (CNS) depressant and decreases anesthetic requirements
    - ◆ Cardiovascular effects include tachycardia, hypotension, and arrhythmias → increased risk of myocardial ischemia
    - ◆ Cannabis smokers are at increased risk of airway irritation, have increased carbon monoxide levels, and may have decreased forced expiratory volume in 1 (FEV_1) values → increased risk of adverse respiratory events

SUBSTANCE ABUSE IN THE ANESTHESIOLOGIST

- ■ Rates of abuse
  - ● Drug abuse among anesthesiology residents and attending anesthesiologists range from 1% to 2%
    - ◆ Residents are more likely to abuse substances than attending anesthesiologists
  - ● Anesthesiologists are 4% of the physician population, but account for 12% of physicians in treatment programs
- ■ Risk factors for substance abuse
  - ● Age <35 years
  - ● Family history of addictive disease
  - ● Comorbid depression and alcohol use
- ■ Causes of increased abuse
  - ● Increased drug availability
    - ◆ Increased drug accounting measures have not reduced drug abuse
  - ● Highly addictive profile of drugs abused
    - ◆ Fentanyl is the most commonly abused drug
  - ● Occupational stress
- ■ Signs of abuse
  - ● Withdrawal from activities
  - ● Changes in behavior

- Increased agitation
- Impaired job performance is often the last sign
- Treatment
  - Consists of long-term therapy and rehabilitation
  - Involvement in peer groups
  - Recovery rates are higher for health-care professionals than the general population
- Reentry into the workforce
  - Reentry may be restricted based on the policies of the state or hospital
  - Reentry often requires a substantial amount of time away from the job
  - 14% death rate due to substance abuse in residents reentering anesthesiology after abuse

POISONS AND WEAPONS

- Biological agents
  - Smallpox
    - Caused by viral agent (variola)
      - Transmitted through droplets, bodily fluids, or contact with contaminated items
      - Highly contagious
    - Presentation
      - After a 1- to 2-week incubation period, presents with rash, headaches, fevers, nausea, vomiting, and malaise
      - Maculopapular rash with lesions at the same stage → develops into fluid-filled blisters → ruptured blisters can transmit the virus
    - Treatment
      - Smallpox was eradicated in 1979 through global vaccination efforts
      - If exposed, patients should be vaccinated within 4 days to lessen symptoms
      - Cidofovir is an antiviral with activity against smallpox
  - Anthrax
    - Caused by *Bacillus anthrasis*
      - Transmitted by spores
        - Spores are highly resilient and can survive in extreme conditions
    - Presentation
      - Presentation depends on site of infection
        - Pulmonary: flu-like symptoms, pneumonia, and respiratory failure
        - Inhalational: hematemesis, diarrhea
        - Gastrointestinal: bloody diarrhea, difficulty swallowing
        - Cutaneous: painless, necrotic skin lesions
      - Pulmonary and inhalational anthrax are associated with high mortality rates than cutaneous anthrax
      - Spores infecting a human can reach the lymph nodes and bloodstream → systemic illness
    - Treatment
      - Ciprofloxacin for treatment
      - Consider ciprofloxacin prophylaxis if exposure suspected
      - Vaccine is available
        - Frequent side effects limit routine use
      - Decontaminate infected material
  - Plague
    - Caused by *Yersinia pestis*
      - Transmitted by droplets, physical contact, contaminated surfaces, or bodily fluids
    - Presentation
      - Bubonic plague causes lymph node swelling, cyanosis, and gangrene (black death)
      - Septicemic plague causes fever, bleeding, and shock
      - Pneumonic plague causes coughing, hemoptysis, and generalized weakness
        - Mortality is near 100%
    - Treatment

- Antibiotics include streptomycin, gentamicin, tetracycline, doxycycline, and chloramphenicol
- Botulism
  - Caused by *Clostridium botulinum*
    - Transmitted through spores in oil, water, or contaminated food
    - Spores release neurotoxin → inhibit acetylcholine release at the neuromuscular junction
  - Presentation
    - Presents with diffuse weakness, vision changes, respiratory collapse, ileus, urinary retention, and autonomic dysfunction
    - May affect infants <6 months due to weakened immune system
      - Honey is frequently implicated in infants
  - Treatment
    - Trivalent botulinum antitoxin
    - Effective against circulating toxin, not toxin that has entered the nerve
    - High risk of allergy since it is from horses
      - Do not give prophylactically without symptoms
- Tetanus
  - Caused by *Clostridium tetani*
    - Transmitted through wounds or cuts
  - Presentation
    - After incubation period, presents with muscle spasm
    - Tetany is a prolonged and painful contraction of a collection of muscles
    - Tetanus can cause sympathetic hyperactivity
  - Treatment
    - Tetanus immunoglobulin
    - Supportive care to prevent spasms and manage labile hemodynamics
    - Mechanical ventilation may be needed
- Ebola
  - Caused by Ebola virus
    - Transmitted by bodily fluids or contaminated surface
  - Presentation
    - After incubation period, presents with fever, sore throat, headaches, vomiting, and bleeding
  - Treatment
    - Supportive care through fluid resuscitation, transfusions, and hemodynamic monitoring
    - No vaccine or treatment is available
- Chemical agents
  - Organophosphates (e.g., sarin nerve gas)
    - Causes symptoms through inhibition of cholinesterase
    - Presents with symptoms consistent with excess acetylcholine at the muscarinic and nicotinic junctions
      - Altered mental status, bradycardia, miosis, drooling, seizures, fasciculations, wheezing, diarrhea, and paralysis
    - Treatment
      - Atropine antagonizes acetylcholine
        - Repeated administration at escalating doses often needed
        - Start at 2 mg → up to 20 mg total may be needed
      - Pralidoxime frees acetylcholinesterase from the organophosphate compound
  - Cyanide
    - Causes symptoms through binding of iron in cytochrome oxidase enzymes → inhibits the electron transport chain → lactic acidosis
    - Presents with hyperventilation, loss of consciousness, convulsions
      - Severe cases cause respiratory arrest
    - Treatment
      - Sodium thiosulfate detoxifies cyanide to thiocyanate

- ➤ Sodium nitrate increases methemoglobin to scavenge cyanide
- ➤ Supportive care
- Phosgene
  - ◆ Causes symptoms through inhalation into the alveoli → carbonyl chloride gas is an extreme airway irritant
    - ➤ Previously used for chemical warfare
    - ➤ Now used in industry to make plastics and pesticides
  - ◆ Presents with airway irritability including coughing, retching, and choking
    - ➤ Severe immediate bronchospasm and laryngospasm → hypoxia and death
    - ➤ Gradual pulmonary edema → cardiac and respiratory arrest
  - ◆ Treatment is supportive
- ■ Radiation
  - Dose
    - ◆ Sieverts (Sv) is the unit used to quantify routine medical radiation (e.g., interventional radiology, chest x-ray)
    - ◆ Gray (Gy) is the unit used to quantify radiation absorption during a mass casualty event
      - ➤ >0.1 Gy can cause radiation sickness
      - ➤ >0.25 Gy can cause more severe symptoms
      - ➤ >2 Gy with increased mortality risk
  - Symptoms
    - ◆ Low dose
      - ➤ Nonspecific symptoms including headache, nausea, and vomiting
    - ◆ High dose
      - ➤ Thermal burn injuries
      - ➤ Dizziness and altered mental status
      - ➤ Bone marrow suppression → aplastic anemia → infections and bleeding
  - Prevention
    - ◆ Minimize time around radiation
    - ◆ Increase distance from radiation source
    - ◆ Appropriate shields
  - Treatment
    - ◆ Supportive care

QUESTIONS

1. A 25-year-old man is scheduled for hand surgery from a fracture sustained during a fight. He has a history of daily alcohol, cocaine, and marijuana use. He previously lost his job and was incarcerated in relation to his polysubstance abuse. His compulsive drug use despite the harmful consequences is best described as:

   A. Addiction
   B. Withdrawal
   C. Tolerance
   D. Dependence

2. The most consistent early sign of a substance abuse problem among anesthesiologists is:

   A. Failure to show up for work
   B. Weight loss
   C. Social isolation
   D. Impaired clinical performance

3. A 55-year-old man underwent open reduction and internal fixation (ORIF) of a tibial fracture sustained in a fall. He has a history of heavy daily alcohol use. Which of the following signs is most consistent with the diagnosis of DT?

   A. Visual hallucinations
   B. Whole body tremor
   C. Withdrawal seizures
   D. Global confusion

4. Acute cocaine overdose is most likely to prolong the duration of action of which of the following commonly used drugs:

   A. Succinylcholine
   B. Propofol
   C. Midazolam
   D. Rocuronium

5. A 55-year-old microbiologist is admitted to the ICU with acute respiratory failure and shock. Four days prior to admission he developed nonspecific flu-like symptoms. Chest x-ray reveals a widened mediastinum, and gram-positive bacilli can be seen on blood culture after 2 to 3 days. Which of the following is the most likely causative agent?

   A. Anthrax
   B. Botulism
   C. Plague
   D. Smallpox

CHAPTER 21 Statistics and Data

BINARY STATISTICAL ANALYSIS

- **Sensitivity and specificity**
  - Sensitivity
    - Proportion of positives that are correctly identified
    - Sensitivity = true positives/(true positives + false negatives)
  - Specificity
    - Proportion of negatives that are correctly identified
    - Specificity = true negative/(true negatives + false positives)
  - Application
    - Used to assess the strength and accuracy of diagnostic tests
    - Not influenced by prevalence of the condition
- Predictive value
  - Positive predictive value (PPV)
    - Proportion of individuals with a positive test who are truly positive
    - PPV = true positives/(true positives + false positives)
  - Negative predictive value (NPV)
    - Proportion of individuals with a negatives test who are truly negative
    - NPV = true negatives/(true negatives + false negatives)
  - Application
    - A high NPV is desired for screening tests
      - Does not necessarily rule in, but does rule out, the condition
    - A high PPV test is good for confirming the disease
      - Does not necessarily rule out, but does rule in, the condition
  - Predictive value tests are influenced by the prevalence of the condition
- Likelihood ratio
  - Positive likelihood ratio
    - Odds of having the disease with a positive test
    - Sensitivity/(1 – specificity)
  - Negative likelihood ratio
    - Odds of having the disease with a negative test
    - (1 – sensitivity)/specificity

STUDY DESIGN

- Types of studies
  - Case-control studies: compare patients who already have a condition to patients without the condition
    - Seeks to identify factors that may be associated with the condition
    - Generates odds ratios
  - Cross-sectional studies: evaluates the relationship between a condition and its factors at a point in time
    - Used to measure prevalence of a disease and associated factors
  - Cohort studies: identify individuals with a condition and follow them over time to assess the impact of specific interventions
    - Can be prospective or retrospective
    - Generates relative risk

- Randomized control trial: planned study where an intervention is introduced in one arm and compared to another arm
  - Best method to determine causality
  - Randomization done to prevent confounding variables
- Meta-analysis: a collection of trials are pooled together for analysis
  - Beneficial if a series of small studies trended toward, but did not reach, statistical significance
- Types of variables
  - Continuous
    - Variables that can fall along an entire spectrum of ranges
    - Example: height of patients undergoing surgery
  - Interval
    - Categorical variables that are regularly ordered
    - Example: pain on a scale of 1 to 10
  - Nominal
    - Two or more categories without a distinct order
    - Example: specialties in medicine such as anesthesiology, surgery, and internal medicine
  - Ordinal
    - Two or more categories with a distinct order
    - Example: small, medium, large
  - Dichotomous
    - Only two categories of variables
    - Example: yes or no
- Null hypothesis
  - Hypothesis of no association
    - Refers to a default position that no difference exists between arms of a trial
    - Experimental trials seek to have sufficient evidence to reject the null hypothesis
  - Type I error: null is rejected, but true
  - Type II error: null is accepted, but false

STATISTICAL RESULTS

- Statistical tests
  - Continuous variables
    - **The *t* test**
      - Used to determine if two sets of data are statistically different
        - Requires a normal distribution
      - Unpaired test
        - Compare two sets of samples
        - Example
          - 100 people are enrolled in a study
            - 50 receive an intervention and 50 do not receive an intervention
          - Unpaired *t* test compares the outcome of the intervention vs. the outcome with no intervention
      - Paired test
        - Compare matched pairs of samples where each patient acts as his/her own control
        - Example
          - 100 people enrolled in a study
            - Data is recorded before the intervention and data is recorded after the intervention
          - Paired *t* test compares the results of the intervention using each patient as their own control
    - **Analysis of variance (ANOVA)**
      - Statistical test for comparing whether multiple means are equal
      - Used for three or more variables (two variables would be a *t* test)
    - Linear regression
      - Statistical test comparing multiple normally distributed numbers

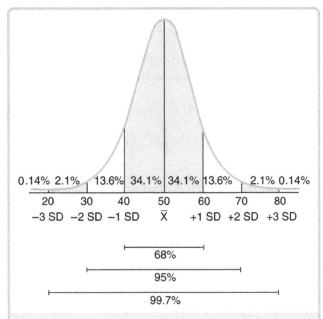

FIGURE 21.1 Standard Deviation. A standard deviation (SD) created from a normal distribution. (Reproduced from Polit DF, Beck CT. *Nursing Research.* 9th ed. Philadelphia, PA: Wolters Kluwer; 2011.)

- Categorical variables
    - **Chi-square**
        - Statistical test used to determine if there is a significant association between two or more categorical variables
    - McNemar test
        - Statistical test used to compare paired nominal data using a 2 × 2 table with matched pairs
- Interpreting data
    - **Standard deviation** (Fig. 21.1)
        - Standard deviation (SD) represents amount of variation from the mean, assuming data is normally distributed
            - Increased scatter of data → increased SD
            - Decreased scatter of data → decreased SD
        - Interpreting SD
            - 1 SD of a normal sample includes 68% of the population
            - 2 SDs of a normal sample includes 95% of the population
        - **Standard error of the mean** (SEM)
            - SEM = SD/$\sqrt{\text{sample size}}$
            - SEM decreases with an increased sample size
            - Mean is more likely accurate with an increased sample size to draw from
    - Risk assessment
        - **Relative risk**
            - Risk of disease in exposed group divided by risk of disease in unexposed group
            - (Disease in exposed/total exposed)/(disease in unexposed/total unexposed)
        - **Hazard ratio**
            - Risk of event in exposed group divided by risk of event in unexposed group with respect to time
                - Calculation requires plotting risk of event against time

- ➤ Hazard ratio is an assessment of risk across a studied time interval
  - ❖ Relative risk is an assessment of risk at one point in time
  - ❖ **Odds ratio**
    - ➤ Odds of disease in exposed group divided by odds of disease in unexposed group
    - ➤ (Disease in exposed/no disease in exposed)/(disease in unexposed/no disease in unexposed)
  - ❖ Application
    - ➤ Relative risk and odds ratio are used to compare the effect of an environment or intervention on a disease
    - ➤ Hazard ratios are used to compare the rate of events occurring over a time interval
- ● Risk reduction
  - ❖ Risk difference
    - ➤ Difference in absolute risk between the exposed and unexposed group
    - ➤ Risk difference = (Disease in exposed/total exposed) – (disease in unexposed/total unexposed)
  - ❖ Number needed to treat/harm
    - ➤ Measure of the number of patients who need to be exposed to an intervention to prevent or cause an outcome
    - ➤ Number needed to treat = 1/risk difference
- ● Statistical significance
  - ❖ Determined by hypothesis testing
  - ❖ Statistical significance
    - ➤ Term used to indicate whether the results of the study are meaningful and not merely due to chance
    - ➤ Determined by p value
      - ❖ p value is the probability of obtaining such a result if the null hypothesis is true
      - ❖ p values are arbitrarily set at 5% (or $p = 0.05$) as the cutoff for statistical significance
    - ➤ Decreased p values → decreased Type I error (false positive)
  - ❖ **Confidence intervals** are often used to indicate significance
    - ➤ Reflects 95% confidence that the true value lies within the calculated intervals
  - ❖ Receiver operating characteristic (ROC) curves
    - ➤ Graphs binary systems
      - ❖ Plots sensitivity and (1 – specificity) on each axis
      - ❖ Used to create predictive models for association
    - ➤ Area under the curve is reflected as a value between 0 and 1
      - ❖ ROC ≥0.8 indicates strong association
- ● **Power analysis**
  - ❖ Statistical power is the probability that a test will reject a false null hypothesis
    - ➤ An adequately powered study will detect a difference between two groups if one exists
    - ➤ Increased power → decreased Type II error (false negative)
  - ❖ Power analysis is done prior to starting a trial to determine the sample size required
    - ➤ Estimate is done based on the expected difference of the intervention
    - ➤ If the intervention causes a significant difference → smaller sample needed for adequate power
    - ➤ If the intervention causes a small difference → larger sample needed for adequate power
  - ❖ When individual studies have been inadequately powered, a **meta-analysis** can be used to improve power and increase the likelihood of detecting statistical significance
- ■ Validity
  - ● Internal validity
    - ❖ Interval validity is an assessment for how well a study was done
      - ➤ Weakened by confounding variables and study bias
    - ❖ Interval validity is high when no other causes for the trial outcome other than the intervention seem reasonable
  - ● External validity
    - ❖ External validity represents the likelihood a study result can be extrapolated to other populations than the group studied

QUESTIONS

1. A researcher is interested in determining whether viewing a preoperative video by patients improves knowledge about their postoperative care. Patients are given a knowledge test before watching a video and then the test is repeated after viewing the video. The change in test scores (pre vs. post) is calculated for each patient. Which of the following statistical tests is most appropriate for analyzing this data?

    A. Regression analysis
    B. Two-sample t test
    C. ANOVA
    D. Paired t test

2. In a sample of post anesthesia care unit (PACU) discharge times for 100 patients the mean is 63 minutes and SD is 100 minutes. What is the estimated standard error for the distribution of mean discharge times?

    A. 63 minutes
    B. 0.63 minutes
    C. 1 minute
    D. 10 minutes

3. A new screening test is designed to detect undiagnosed obstructive sleep apnea among patients scheduled to undergo general anesthesia. The probability that a patient has obstructive sleep apnea given a positive test result is referred to as the test's?

    A. Sensitivity
    B. Specificity
    C. Positive predictive value
    D. Negative predictive value

4. A researcher is interested in determining whether the anesthetic type (regional vs. general) is associated with patient satisfaction (satisfied vs. not satisfied). Thirty patients are randomly assigned to each group. Data for the study are provided in the table below. Which statistical test is most appropriate to analyze the data?

	Satisfied	Not satisfied
Regional	18	12
General	25	5

    A. Chi-square
    B. Log rank test
    C. t test
    D. ANOVA

5. A randomized controlled trial is designed to compare a new drug for post operative nausea and vomiting (PONV) prophylaxis to ondansetron. It is determined that 100 patients will be needed in each group to detect a 15% difference in PONV with 90% power and $\alpha = 0.01$. Which of the following changes would require an increase in sample size?

    A. Detect a difference of 10%
    B. Detect a difference of 20%
    C. Use an alpha (α) of 0.05
    D. Use a power of 80%

CHAPTER 22 · Ethics and Practice Management

PROFESSIONALISM AND LICENSURE

- **Certification** for anesthesiologists
  - Certification is through the American Board of Anesthesiology (ABA)
    - Training requirements
      - Satisfactory completion of an accredited residency program by the Accreditation Council for Graduate Medical Education (ACGME)
      - Completion of Part I and Part II of the board exam certification process
    - Qualities of certified anesthesiologists
      - Possesses the knowledge, judgment, adaptability, skills, and personal characteristics necessary for an anesthesiologist
      - Can effectively communicate with colleagues and patients
      - Can lead an anesthesiology care team
  - **Primary certification**
    - Available to anesthesiologists who have completed the residency training requirements, but have not been certified by the ABA
    - Composed of Part I written and Part II oral examination
  - **Maintenance of Certification of Anesthesiology (MOCA)**
    - Test required every 10 years after primary certification for recertification
    - Offered between years 7 and 10 following last certification
- **ACGME core competencies**
  - **Patient care**
  - **Medical knowledge**
  - **Professionalism**
  - **Practice-based learning and improvement**
  - **Systems-based practice**
  - **Interpersonal skills and communication**

LEGAL ISSUES AND MALPRACTICE

- **Medical malpractice**
  - Causes of malpractice lawsuits
    - Negligence: breach of standard of care causing harm
    - Lack of informed consent: providing inadequate information for a reasonable person
    - Vicarious liability: obligation to provide reasonable supervision for those working for the anesthesiologists
    - Battery/assault: touching or attempting to touch another person without expressed or implied consent
  - Negligence is most common malpractice lawsuit for physicians
    - **Requirements of negligence**
      - A standard of care exists
      - A breach of that care took place
      - That breach was the direct cause of patient injury
    - Negligence can be prosecuted as criminal medical negligence if severe and unethical violations have taken place

- **Trial timeframe**
  - ◆ Plaintiff files complaint
  - ◆ Defendant must answer
  - ◆ Motions can occur
  - ◆ Discovery with expert testimony and depositions
  - ◆ Settlements with alternative dispute resolution
  - ◆ Pretrial conference
  - ◆ Trial
- Anesthesia Closed Claims Project
  - Funded by the Anesthesia Quality Institute and located at the University of Washington
  - Database and registry created to identify and address safety concerns in anesthesia
    - ◆ Created through case summaries collected by anesthesiologists from malpractice insurance claim files
    - ◆ Information consists of surgical procedure, injury sustained, events leading to injury, outcome of lawsuit, and efforts at prevention
  - Database is used extensively for research and to target safety efforts
- **National Practitioner Data Bank**
  - Data bank of physicians and their professional credentials
  - Contains clinical privileges, malpractice information, and adverse actions taken against physician
- **Professional liability insurance**
  - Insurance policy options and coverage vary by state, hospital, and practice
    - ◆ Several states cap malpractice lawsuits → less coverage needed
    - ◆ Several states prone to increased malpractice lawsuits → supplemental coverage needed
  - Policies often specify a policy limit per occurrence and policy limit for the year (e.g., $1 million/ $3 million)

OPERATING ROOM MANAGEMENT

- Operating room interests
  - Surgeons: desire convenient operating room access, ability to use state-of-the-art equipment
  - Anesthesiologists: desire high utilization during business hours, case intensity to match staffing ability, efficient turnover
  - Nursing: desire predictable staffing, standardization of equipment
- **Operating room scheduling**
  - Open-block systems
    - ◆ First-come, first-serve system
    - ◆ Suitable at hospitals where there is little demand for operating rooms
    - ◆ Creates scheduling unpredictability in high-demand environments
  - Surgeon or service-specific block systems
    - ◆ A surgeon or service is granted a block of operating room time
    - ◆ System used at most hospitals
    - ◆ Improved ability for surgeons to schedule procedures ahead of time
    - ◆ Improves predictability for anesthesiologist staffing needs
    - ◆ Staggering block times for surgeons who use the same equipment improves resource utilization
  - Adjustments to schedule
    - ◆ Block scheduling requires adaptations to the schedule as the day of surgery approaches
      - ➤ Unused time is released
      - ➤ Urgent and waitlist cases are added
      - ➤ Certain operating rooms may be opened or closed based on equipment needed
    - ◆ Block time may be adjusted regularly based on surgeon utilization
    - ◆ Open rooms should be made available to handle emergent cases
  - Time management
    - ◆ On-time starts and turnover efficacy depend on collaboration between surgeons, anesthesiologists, nurses, and patients
      - ➤ Parallel processing can significantly minimize delays
    - ◆ Studies have shown that surgeons are most responsible for first case delays

- **Operating room costs**
  - Operating room utilization
    - A target of 70% to 85% operating room utilization is ideal to maximize profits and minimize stress on employees and patients
      - Increased utilization beyond 85% increases case delays and overtime expenses
      - Decreased utilization below 75% decreases revenue
  - Types of costs
    - **Fixed costs**
      - Overhead, administrative support, salaried employees, operating room maintenance
        - Most operating room costs are fixed
      - Adjusting the scheduling and improving operating room flow have little effect on fixed costs
    - **Variable costs**
      - Surgical and disposable supplies, overtime labor
      - Improved scheduling, decreased case cancellations, better utilization can have a significant effect on variable costs
  - **Strategies to improve operating room profits**
    - Increase case volume (most profitable strategy)
      - Decreased surgical case time
      - Decrease turnover time
    - Improve operating room utilization
    - Reduce costs of supplies

ETHICAL ISSUES

- Ethical tenets
  - Autonomy: right to make own decisions
  - Beneficence: obligation to provide good care or prevent harm
  - Justice: fair distribution of resources that provides the greatest benefit
  - Nonmaleficence: not inflicting harm
- **Informed consent**
  - Based on principle of autonomy
  - Requirements
    - Patient capacity
      - Ability to understand information, interpret consequences and benefits, and formulate and communicate a decision
    - Disclosure of procedure, risks, and benefits
      - Reasonable person standard
        - Physician is required to disclose what a reasonable person would want to know
      - Subjective standard
        - Physician is required to disclose additional information that the patient would want to know based on their medical history, needs, or beliefs
  - Informed consent does not protect against liability when adverse events occur
    - Settlements are larger when an adverse event occurs and informed consent was not done properly
- **Informed refusal**
  - Patients may refuse specific forms of treatment based on religious or personal beliefs
    - Example: do not resuscitate/do not intubate (DNR/DNI) orders, Jehovah Witnesses and blood transfusions
  - Patients are allowed to refuse care under the same principle as informed consent
    - Patients must have capacity
    - Physicians must explain the risks of refusal
  - Physicians are under no obligation to provide care to a patient whose demands would be considered negligent care
- **Advanced directives**
  - Document created by patients to guide their wishes in the event they are not capable of making decisions for themselves

- A surrogate decision maker may be specified, or family members may be asked to make decisions on behalf of patients
  - Decision-making hierarchy: power of attorney > spouse > children > parents > siblings
  - Surrogate decision makers are asked to make decisions based on what the patient would have wanted, not their own preferences
- Advanced directives, including do not resuscitate orders, apply to the operating room unless otherwise reversed
  - DNR/DNI orders are frequently reversed in the operating room due to the ability to reverse most cases requiring immediate resuscitation in the operating room
- Organ donation
  - Donation after brain death
    - Brain death is an irreversible loss of function of the entire brain and brainstem
    - Due to potential conflict of interest, organ donation should not be discussed by the physician caring for the patient
  - Donation after cardiac death
    - Cardiac death should be imminent following the withdrawal of life-sustaining treatment
    - Amnestic and analgesic care for the patient supersedes organ transplantation
- Privacy
  - The **Health Insurance Portability and Accountability Act (HIPPA)** provides rules for protecting identifiable health information and prevents loss of health insurance when changing jobs

PATIENT SAFETY

- Definitions
  - **Error:** a mistake in patient care
    - An error does not require harm be done to the patient
    - Most errors do not result in harm, but would likely result in harm if multiple errors occurred
      - "Swiss-cheese" model of errors
  - **Adverse event:** action that causes harm or potential harm to a patient
    - Adverse events are not necessarily caused by an error
    - A known consequence or side effect of treatment can be considered an adverse event
  - **Sentinel event:** unexpected event causing significant harm or death
    - Warrants immediate investigation into cause
- **Systems-based** approach to patient safety
  - Patient injury is primarily caused by poorly designed systems
  - Human errors play a role and are inevitable, but a well-designed system can mitigate and prevent many errors
- **Reporting systems**
  - Reporting systems for patient safety have greatly improved safety and reduced errors
    - Goal of a reporting system should be correcting errors, not placing blame
  - Features of a successful reporting system
    - Access for all employees
    - De-identification
    - Review by people who are not direct supervisors of those involved in the report
    - No punishment for reporters or people involved
    - Legal protection
    - Timely feedback and implementation

QUESTIONS

1. Which of the following is NOT part of the ACGME core competencies?

   A. Medical knowledge
   B. Practice-based learning and improvement
   C. Systems-based knowledge
   D. None of the above

2. A 76-year-old female was recently diagnosed with metastatic ovarian cancer. She has recovered well from her first procedure; however, she now requires a second operative procedure. Her projected outcome remains grim. She refuses surgery and expresses to her medical care team that she would like to go home and spend time with her family. What is your next step?

   A. Speak to her family and explain to them that she is refusing further medical care and you do not agree
   B. Suggest a family meeting with the patient and her health-care providers to help determine the best plan of action
   C. Explain to her that she is refusing medical care and you cannot support this decision
   D. Try to convince her to have the second procedure and then she can decide if she still would like to go home

3. A 54-year-old female is involved in a motor vehicle crash. Her injuries include a pelvic fracture, liver laceration, and splenic rupture. She is scheduled for an emergent exploratory laparotomy. Before you anesthetize her she states that she is a Jehovah Witness and refuses any blood products, even if they are needed to save her life. During the procedure her Hb is 5.4 and she continues to hemorrhage. You have already given her over 6 L of IVF. What is your next step?

   A. Call her husband and tell him she is continuing to bleed and ask him if you can give her blood
   B. Start giving blood products, as she is going to die without them
   C. Do nothing; continue with IVF resuscitation
   D. Give her albumin and have the perfusionist set up cell saver

4. Which of the following comprise the three fundamental findings for declaring a patient "brain dead?"

   A. Coma, absence of brainstem reflexes, and apnea
   B. Coma, core temperature of 36°C, apnea
   C. Absence of brainstem reflexes, core temperature of 36°C, and apnea
   D. Coma, absence of brainstem reflexes, and core temperature of 36°C

5. Which of the following is the most common cause for medical malpractice claims filed against physicians?

   A. Negligence
   B. Lack of informed consent
   C. Vicarious liability
   D. Battery/assault

CHAPTER 1

1. *Answer: C*
Sensitivity refers to the pacemaker's ability to detect electrical activity generated by the patient's own heart to prevent any competition between the hearts intrinsic activity. The lower the setting, the more sensitive the pacemaker is to intracardiac signals. The general range of sensitivity for a normal pacemaker box is 0.4 to 10 mV for the atria, and 0.8 to 20 mV for the ventricles.

The sensitivity threshold can be determined by dialing up the sensitivity to find the minimum R-wave amplitude needed to be detected by the pulse generator. However, use of maximal sensitivity settings could cause the pacemaker to mistake various random fluctuations of electrical activity for cardiac activity. This could lead to either it not firing at all (convinced the myocardium is depolarizing normally) or firing constantly, mistaking the electrical interference for atrial activity and placing the patient at risk for "R on T." Thus, the sensitivity needs to be set intelligently.

2. *Answer: B*
A quench occurs when an MRI magnet turns resistive and catastrophically releases all of the stored energy as heat, boiling off the stored cryogens as gas. The most common cause of quench is an intentional shutdown of the magnet for a life-threatening emergency. Quench may also be the consequence of an unintentional shutdown. If not properly vented, a quench can result in the complete dissipation of oxygen in zone IV, risking hypoxia to the patient and MRI personnel. When a quench occurs, team members should perform their institution's protocol in reaction to this occurrence. If possible, the patient should immediately be removed from zone IV and oxygen administered to the patient. Powerful static magnetic fields may persist after a quench, and therefore the usual precautions apply when entering zone IV. Emergency response personnel should be restricted from entering zone IV during any environmental emergency because of the persistent magnetic field.

3. *Answer: C*
Radiographic examinations represent the largest source of radiation exposure to the U.S. population. The risk for adverse health effects from cancer is proportional to the amount of radiation dose absorbed, and the amount of dose depends on the type of radiographic examination. Standard radiographic examinations have effective doses (and potential detriment) that vary widely by over a factor of 1,000 (0.01 to 10 mSv). A chest radiograph has an effective dose of 0.05 to 0.25 mSv, while CT examinations tend to be in a more narrow dose range but have relatively high effective doses (approximately 2 to 20 mSv), and doses for interventional procedures usually range from 5 to 70 mSv. For comparison the mean effective dose in atomic bomb survivors was 40 mSv, a dose similar to that incurred from five to six routine chest CT scans.

4. *Answer: B*
CO_2 absorbers contain strong bases (sodium hydroxide and potassium hydroxide) that can extract labile protons from anesthetic molecules, resulting in the production of CO. Desiccated CO_2 absorbers such as soda lime and Baralyme can degrade inhaled anesthetics and produce carboxyhemoglobin concentrations in excess of 30%. CO production varies with the volatile anesthetic administered: (desflurane > enflurane > isoflurane) >> (halothane = sevoflurane). CO production is also increased with Baralyme as compared to soda lime and also with higher temperatures. The reactions that produce CO do not occur while the anesthesia machine is idle; rather, they occur only when agent vapor flows through the absorber. Therefore, flushing the breathing circuit with fresh gas before use (such as during a pre-use check) will not prevent or relieve the problem.

CO exposure is unlikely to be detected intraoperatively; thus, it is important to ensure that the conditions under which CO can be produced during inhalation anesthesia do not occur. Specifically, it is important to discontinue the flow of medical gas whenever an anesthesia machine will not be promptly used on another patient, change absorbent regularly, and use low flows (which will tend to keep granules moist).

5. *Answer: D*
Mapleson breathing systems are used for delivering oxygen and anesthetic agents and to eliminate CO_2. They consist of different components: Fresh

gas flow, reservoir bag, breathing tubes, expiratory valve, and patient connection. There are five basic types of Mapleson system: A, B, C, D, and E, depending upon the different arrangements of these components. Mapleson F was added later. For adults, Mapleson A is the circuit of choice for spontaneous respiration because dead space gas is reused at the next inspiration, and exhaled alveolar gas passes out through the expiratory valve. Mapleson D (Option B) is the best circuit for controlled ventilation.

CHAPTER 2

1. *Answer: B*

There are two main types of Doppler echocardiographic systems in common use—continuous wave and pulsed wave. Each has important advantages and disadvantages.

Continuous wave (CW) Doppler involves continuous generation of ultrasound waves coupled with continuous ultrasound reception. A two-crystal transducer accomplishes this dual function, with one crystal devoted to each function. The main advantage of CW Doppler is its ability to measure high blood velocities accurately. The continuous production of sound energy allows one to measure very high Doppler shifts and thus obtain information on higher velocities. The main disadvantage of CW Doppler is its lack of selectivity or depth discrimination. Since CW Doppler is constantly transmitting and receiving from two different transducer heads (crystals), there is no ability to locate the tissue reflecting the energy is lost; instead, an average of the velocities along the path of the ultrasound beam is acquired.

Pulsed wave Doppler uses one crystal for both the emission and the reception of the ultrasound energy. The crystal emits ultrasound for a specified period of time and then waits for the reflected energy to return. The advantage is that the location of the tissue with the velocity being measured is known. Because the crystal will not emit another sound until the reflected sound energy returns, the velocities it can measure using this technique are necessarily slow. The main disadvantage of PW Doppler is its inability to accurately measure high blood flow velocities, such as may be encountered in certain types of valvular and congenital heart disease. This limitation is technically known as "aliasing" and results in an inability of PW Doppler to faithfully record velocities above 1.5 to 2 m/sec when the sample volume is located at standard ranges in the heart.

Doppler color flow imaging is based upon the principles of PW Doppler echocardiography. With color flow imaging, velocities are displayed using a color scale, with flow toward the transducer typically displayed in orange/red and flow away from the transducer displayed as blue. Color flow imaging is typically used in the screening and assessment of regurgitant flows, in the assessment of intracardiac shunts, and to assist in continuous wave Doppler alignment for determination of regurgitation velocities.

2. *Answer: B*

Mixed venous oxygen saturation ($S\bar{v}_{O_2}$) is the percentage of oxygen bound to hemoglobin in blood returning to the right side of the heart. $S\bar{v}_{O_2}$ is a global representation of total body oxygen supply and demand (i.e., it reflects the amount of oxygen "left over" after the tissues remove what they need). Mixed venous oxygen saturation is measured from blood drawn from the tip of the pulmonary artery catheter. It measures the "mixture" of the venous blood returning from the head and arms (via superior vena cava), the gut and lower extremities (via the inferior vena cava), and the coronary veins (via the coronary sinus). It reflects the average amount of oxygen remaining after all tissues in the body have removed oxygen from the hemoglobin and before it is reoxygenated in the pulmonary capillaries. Normal $S\bar{v}_{O_2}$ is approximately 40 mm Hg with a saturation of 75%. A reduction in $S\bar{v}_{O_2}$ may be attributed to a reduction in O_2 delivery (secondary to a reduction in O_2 content per deciliter or a reduction in cardiac output), or an increase in O_2 consumption (secondary to an increased metabolic state).

3. *Answer: C*

Pulmonary capillary wedge pressure (PCWP) provides an indirect estimate of left atrial pressure (LAP). In the absence of mitral stenosis, this pressure reflects left ventricular diastolic pressure (the filling pressure of the left ventricle). Measurement of pulmonary artery wedge pressure may be useful for differentiating between cardiogenic and noncardiogenic causes of pulmonary edema. Normal occlusive pressure is about 8 to 12 mm Hg. An occlusive pressure more than 20 mm Hg can cause the onset of fluid movement into alveoli and a pressure more than 30 mm Hg indicates frank pulmonary edema.

4. *Answer: C*

The CVP waveform consists of three positive waves referred to as *a*, *c*, and *v* and two negative slopes called the *x* and *y* descents. The *a* wave represents the right atrial pressure increase during the phase of atrial contraction. The *c* wave is caused by the bulging of the closed tricuspid valve into the right atrium during the beginning of ventricular systole. Following the *c* wave is the first major descent in the CVP waveform, the *x* descent. The *x* descent is a drop in atrial pressure during ventricular systole caused by atrial relaxation. At the trough of the *x* descent, there is an increase in atrial pressure as the atrium begins to fill during late systole. This is called the *v* wave. The final aspect of the CVP waveform is the *y* descent, which is due to an atrial pressure drop as blood enters the ventricle during diastole.

CVP WAVEFORM

a = atrial contraction
c = closing and bulging of the tricuspid valve
x = atrial relaxation
v = passive filling of atrium
y = opening of the tricuspid valve

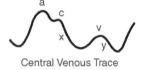
Central Venous Trace

5. *Answer: C*
The placement site of the arterial catheter determines the shape of the systemic blood pressure waveform. As the pressure wave is measured at sequentially farther distances from the heart, the high-frequency components such as the dicrotic notch begin to disappear. There is more resonance such that the systolic peak is higher and the diastolic trough is lower as the blood pressure wave travels away from the heart. The mean arterial pressure remains approximately the same at all measurement sites. Compared with the radial artery, the dorsalis pedis artery shows a delay in pulse transmission, sharper initial upstroke (therefore, a higher systolic pressure), and loss of the dicrotic notch.

CHAPTER 3

1. *Answer: A*
Etomidate is a unique intravenous anesthetic agent possessing a carboxylated imidazole structure. Etomidate preserves hemodynamic stability and therefore is a popular induction agent for patients with limited cardiopulmonary reserve.

Etomidate inhibits the action of 11β-hydroxylase in the adrenal cortex, causing a reduction in cortisol and aldosterone synthesis and an elevation of adrenocorticotrophic hormone (ACTH). This effect is apparent even after a single induction dose, but is more pronounced with continuous infusion. As

a result of the 11β-hydroxylase inhibition by etomidate, levels of the steroid precursors 11-deoxycorticosterone, 11-deoxycortisol, progesterone, and 17-hydroxyprogesterone become elevated.

Etomidate does not cause release of histamine.

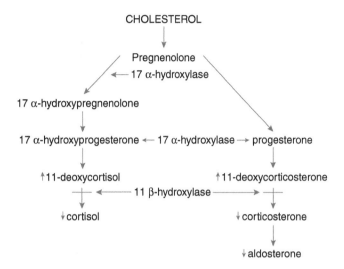

2. *Answer: A*
The context-sensitive half-time (CSHT) is the time required for blood or plasma concentrations of a drug to decrease by 50% after drug administration is discontinued. It is a useful measure because it describes the clinical duration of action of a drug in the "context" of the duration of infusion. The CSHToften cannot be predicted by the elimination half-life (the time needed for actual drug metabolism or elimination) because it also depends on drug redistribution. For drugs such as fentanyl, in which redistribution is the primary mechanism responsible for the decline in plasma concentration after a brief infusion or bolus, the CSHT will initially be short. As the duration of infusion continues, redistribution becomes progressively less important and the CSHT increases, until ultimately it equals the elimination half-life. For a drug with a small volume of distribution, such as remifentanil, redistribution is very limited and the CSHT changes little even with prolonged infusion.

3. *Answer: D*
Pseudocholinesterase (PChE) deficiency is a genetic or acquired alteration in the metabolism of choline esters such as succinylcholine and ester-linked local anesthetics. The most common clinical manifestation of PChE deficiency is prolonged paralysis after administration of succinylcholine. If a patient shows no response to TOF stimulation 15 minutes after receiving succinylcholine, PChE deficiency should be suspected.

A dibucaine number is useful to decipher whether the PChE deficiency is genetic in origin, and can imply hetero- or homozygosity. Dibucaine is a local anesthetic that inhibits PChE activity when mixed with a blood sample. The percentage of PChE inhibited will yield a dibucaine number: 80 to 100 indicates normal PChE function, 40 to 70 indicates heterozygous, and less than 30 indicates homozygous for atypical genotype. A patient that is homozygous for atypical genotype can have prolonged paralysis after receiving succinylcholine for more than 4 hours.

Activity of the PChE can be also be impaired by kidney or liver disease, malnutrition, major burns, cancer, or certain drugs. In this situation the PChE enzyme functions normally but the levels are decreased. The patient in the question has prolonged paralysis despite a normal dibucaine number suggesting that her PChE levels are low.

4. *Answer: C*
Sugammadex is a modified gamma cyclodextrin designed to selectively reverse the effects of the neuromuscular blockers rocuronium and vecuronium. It works by forming a complex with these drugs, reducing their availability to bind to nicotinic receptors in the neuromuscular junction. Sugammadex does not reverse the benzylisoquinoline neuromuscular blocking agents such as atracurium and cisatracurium.

5. *Answer: C*
Tramadol is an analgesic used for treatment of mild to moderate pain. Its postulated mechanisms of action include augmentation serotonergic and noradrenergic neurotransmission and direct action of its major metabolite, O-desmethyltramadol, which is an opioid. A number of studies suggest the presence of a drug interaction between tramadol and ondansetron in the postoperative period that potentially decreases the effectiveness of tramadol.

CHAPTER 4

1. *Answer: B*
A number of potentially adverse effects have been attributed to nitrous oxide exposure including megaloblastic anemia, neurologic toxicity, immunodeficiency, impaired wound healing, and possible increased risk of teratogenicity. The postulated mechanism for these adverse effects is the irreversible inhibition of vitamin B_{12}, which in turn inhibits methionine synthase, folate metabolism, and deoxyribonucleic acid synthesis. In addition, inactivation of methionine synthase is associated with increased plasma homocysteine concentrations,

http://anesthesiology.pubs.asahq.org/article.aspx?articleid=1931781, which may increase the risk of postoperative cardiovascular complications. In addition, inactivation of methionine synthase is associated with increased plasma homocysteine concentrations. Long-term elevation of plasma homocysteine concentration is a risk factor for cardiovascular disease, and an acute increase in plasma homocysteine has been associated with endothelial dysfunction and hypercoagulability. Methemoblobin is a known toxicity of inhaled nitric oxide therapy not nitrous oxide.

2. *Answer: D*
Metabolic degradation products of volatile anesthetics can injure tissues. The type of injury depends on the extent of metabolism and the nature of the metabolites. Desflurane, halothane, and isoflurane all are metabolized to trifluoroacetate, which can cause hepatotoxicity through an immunologic mechanism involving trifluoroacetyl hapten formation and a resulting autoimmune response. The incidence of hepatic injury depends on the extent of metabolism, with the highest rates associated with halothane and much lower rates with isoflurane and desflurane. Unlike other halogenated anesthetics, sevoflurane is not metabolized to hepatotoxic trifluoroacetylated proteins; hence, hepatotoxic potential of sevoflurane is considered to be low.

3. *Answer: C*
The rapid uptake of high concentrations of nitrous oxide at induction of inhalational anesthesia produces an increase in alveolar concentrations of oxygen and the accompanying volatile anesthetic agent. This process is known as the second gas effect. The effect is caused by the concentrating effect of nitrous oxide uptake on the partial pressures of the other gases in the alveolar mixture. During emergence, nitrous oxide enters the alveoli far more rapidly than nitrogen leaves, causing dilution of oxygen within the alveoli of patients breathing air and may cause "diffusion hypoxia." Patients that have undergone anesthesia with nitrous oxide should receive supplemental oxygen in the PACU to allow resolution of the effects of diffusion hypoxia. Hypoventilation is common in the postoperative period and can contribute to hypoxemia. However, the minute ventilation for this patient remained constant suggesting that hypoventilation was not contributing to the patient's hypoxemia.

4. *Answer: A*
The MAC of an inhaled anesthetic is the alveolar concentration that will produce immobility to a

standardized surgical incision in 50% of patients. The standard deviation of MAC is ~10%, thus 95% of patients will not respond to 1.2 MAC, and 99% will not respond to 1.3 MAC. For desflurane: 1.3 MAC = 1.3 × 6 ≅ 8 vol%.

5. *Answer: C*
A time constant (τ) is defined as volume divided by flow. Complete equilibration with any tissue takes approximately 3 time constants. The time constant for isoflurane is 3 to 4 minutes while for sevoflurane, desflurane, or nitrous oxide it is approximately 2 minutes. Therefore, the amount of time required for complete equilibration with the brain is closest to 2 minutes × 3 = 6 minutes.

CHAPTER 5

1. *Answer: B*
The Revised Cardiac Risk Index (RCRI) is a tool used to estimate a patient's risk of perioperative cardiac complications. The RCRI consists of a six-point index score, which includes the following variables and risks:

- High-risk surgery (intrathoracic, intra-abdominal, or suprainguinal vascular)
- Ischemic heart disease (defined as a history of MI, pathologic Q waves on ECG, use of nitrates, abnormal stress test, or chest pain secondary to ischemic causes)
- Congestive heart failure
- History of cerebrovascular disease
- Diabetes requiring insulin therapy
- Preoperative serum creatinine level higher than 2 mg/dL

Each of the six risk factors was assigned one point. Patients with none, one, or two risk factor(s) are assigned to RCRI classes I, II, and III, respectively, and patients with three or more risk factors were considered class IV. The risk associated with each class was 0.4%, 1%, 7%, and 11% for patients in classes I, II, III, and IV, respectively. The patient in the stem question would receive points for high-risk surgery and ischemic heart disease (2 points total).

2. *Answer: C*
Poor functional capacity is associated with increased cardiac complications in noncardiac surgery. A patient's functional capacity can be expressed in METs. (1 MET is defined as 3.5 mL O_2 uptake/kg per min, which is the resting oxygen uptake in a sitting position—the oxygen consumption of a 70-kg, 40-year-old man in a resting state.) Greater than 7 METs of activity tolerance is considered excellent, whereas less than 4 METs is considered poor activity

tolerance. The Duke Activity Status Index suggests questions that correlate with MET levels; for example, walking on level ground at about 4 miles per hour or carrying a bag of groceries up a flight of stairs expends approximately 4 METs of activity. Patients limited in their activity from noncardiac causes, such as severe osteoarthritis or general debility, are categorized as having poor functional capacity, because one cannot discern if significant cardiac conditions exist without the benefit of a functional study (noninvasive testing).

3. *Answer: C*
Careful management is important to increase rates of successful transplantation. Lungs may get injured in the hours before and after brain death resulting from direct trauma, resuscitation maneuvers, neurogenic edema, aspiration of blood or gastric content, or ventilator-associated trauma, and pneumonia. Early donor guidelines recommended tidal volumes of 10 to 15 mL/kg body weight. However, the introduction of "lung protective ventilation" to active donor management (using tidal volumes of 6 to 8 mL/kg, PEEP, and measures to prevent derecruitment) has been associated with increased numbers of transplantable lungs. Avoiding high inspired oxygen concentrations may limit bronchiolitis obliterans syndrome in lung recipients. http://bja.oxfordjournals.org/content/108/suppl_1/i96–i107. Recruitment maneuvers are an important component of donor optimization, especially when the oxygenation is subnormal and pulmonary abnormalities are visible on chest x-ray. Re-recruitment is particularly important after tracheal suction or after apnea testing. Extravascular lung water can be minimized by the early use of methylprednisolone and avoiding a positive fluid balance.

4. *Answer: C*
Postoperative cognitive dysfunction (POCD) is a new cognitive impairment arising after a surgical procedure. Its manifestations may be subtle depending on the particular cognitive domains that are affected. The most commonly seen problems are memory impairment and impaired performance on intellectual tasks. POCD can affect patients of any age but is more common in the elderly. Factors that elevate the risk of POCD include old age, preexisting cerebral, cardiac, and vascular disease, alcohol abuse, low educational level, and intra- and postoperative complications. The method of anesthesia, that is, general vs. regional does not play a causal role for the development of POCD.

5. *Answer: A*
Neurokinin-1 receptor antagonists are a promising new class of antiemetics that were originally

developed and approved for chemotherapy-induced nausea and vomiting. Neurokinin-1 antagonists compete with substance P, an endogenous ligand with a high density of receptors in the area postrema and the nucleus tractus solitarii, believed to be involved in terminal emetic pathways. Administrated orally before surgery, aprepitant, the first neurokinin-1 antagonist approved by the U.S. Food and Drug Administration, has similar efficacy against nausea and greater efficacy against vomiting compared with other commonly used antiemetics. Aprepitant is not associated with QTc prolongation or sedative effects, but its high cost limits its use to high-risk patients.

CHAPTER 6

1. *Answer: C*
The coronary artery that supplies the PDA determines coronary "dominance." Most people (approximately 70% of the population) have a "right dominant" system, which means that the right coronary supplies these arteries. 10% of people have a "left dominant" system, which means that the left circumflex supplies these arteries. Approximately 20% of the population has a "codominant" system, meaning both the right coronary artery and left circumflex artery feed the PDA.

2. *Answer: A*
The five terms that describe key physiological properties of the heart are
- Inotropy: the ability to contract
- Chronotropy: the ability to alter the heart rate
- Dromotropy: the ability to affect the conduction speed of an electrical impulse
- Bathmotropy: the ability to modify of the degree of excitability (threshold of excitation)
- Lusitropy: the ability of the myocardium to relax

3. *Answer: A*
SVR refers to the resistance to blood flow throughout *all* of the systemic vasculature, excluding the pulmonary vasculature. Mechanisms that cause vasoconstriction increase SVR, and those mechanisms that cause vasodilation decrease SVR. Although SVR is primarily determined by changes in blood vessel diameter, changes in blood viscosity also affect SVR. Normal SVR is 900 to 1,200 dyn-s/cm^5.

For this question, the MAP is calculated as the DBP + 1/3 (pulse pressure) = 55 + 1/3 × 30 = 65 mm Hg. The SVR is calculated as:

$$SVR = 80 \times (MAP - CVP)/CO = 80 \times (65-5)/10 = 480$$
$$dyn\text{-}s/cm^5$$

4. *Answer: B*
Sodium nitroprusside, when used in high doses or over a period of days, can produce toxic blood concentrations of cyanide. In most patients, cyanide release from sodium nitroprusside is slow enough that the body's innate detoxification mechanisms can eliminate the cyanide before it interferes with cellular respiration. However, patients with hepatic impairment, renal insufficiency, hypoalbuminemia, or patients undergoing hypothermic cardiopulmonary bypass procedures are at increased risk for developing symptoms, even with therapeutic dosing.

One of the early *signs* of cyanide accumulation is *nitroprusside* tachyphylaxis. Toxicity due to accumulation of cyanide ions should be suspected in any patient who develops resistance to the hypotensive effect of nitroprusside despite progressive adjustment of infusion rates to higher levels or in a previously responsive patient who becomes unresponsive to the hypotensive action despite increasing dose.

A severe anion gap metabolic acidosis, combined with a reduced arterial–venous oxygen gradient (less than 10 mm Hg due to venous hyperoxia), suggests the diagnosis of cyanide toxicity. Vomiting, bradycardia, hypotension, shallow respirations and seizures are other signs of cyanide toxicity. The treatment of cyanide poisoning is empiric because laboratory confirmation can take hours or days. Treatment includes administration of both sodium thiosulfate and hydroxocobalamin.

5. *Answer: D*
pH-stat and alpha-stat refer to the acid–base management strategies employed during CPB. *With pH-stat acid–base management, the patient's pH is maintained at a constant level by managing pH at the patient's temperature.* In order to maintain normal pH, either the gas flow is reduced or the CO_2 is added to the CPB circuit, that is, the pH is corrected to 7.4 and Pa_{CO_2} at 40 mm Hg according to patient's body temperature. Consequently, pH-stat leads to higher pCO_2 *(respiratory acidosis)*, and *increased cerebral blood flow.*

In contrast, alpha-stat pH management is *not* temperature-corrected—as the patient's temperature falls, the partial pressure of CO_2 decreases (and solubility increases); thus a hypothermic patient with a pH of 7.40 and a pCO_2 of 40 (measured at 37°C) will, in reality, have a lower pCO_2 (because partial pressure of CO_2 is lower), and this will manifest as a relative *respiratory alkalosis* coupled with *decreased cerebral blood flow.*

There is evidence to suggest that the best acid–base management strategy to follow for patients undergoing deep hypothermic circulatory arrest during cardiac surgery is dependent upon the age of the patient with better results using pH-stat in the pediatric patient and alpha-stat in the adult patient.

CHAPTER 7

1. *Answer: D*
The superior laryngeal nerve provides sensory innervation to the posterior epiglottis, arytenoids, and vocal cords.

2. *Answer: B*
Injury to the recurrent laryngeal nerve explains the stridor and upper airway obstruction. Some surgeons routinely do recurrent laryngeal nerve monitoring during thyroidectomies in an effort to prevent this injury. The recurrent laryngeal innervates the posterior cricoarytenoid muscle, which opens the vocal cords. As a result, the cords will not be in an open position. However, because the cricothyroid muscle is innervated from the superior laryngeal nerve, there is still tension on the cords. As a result, the cords will be in an intermediate, or partially open, position.

3. *Answer: D*
During one-lung ventilation, shunt fraction increases substantially. The body compensates through pulmonary hypoxic vasoconstriction to decrease blood flow to the operative side. Vasodilators, especially nitroglycerin and nitroprusside, can worsen hypoxic pulmonary vasoconstriction.

4. *Answer: B*
The equation for oxygen content is $1.34 \times Hb \times$ saturation $+ 0.003 \times Pa_{O_2}$. On the basis of this patient's vitals and labs:

$$1.34 \times 10 \times 0.95 + 0.003 \times 70 = 13.2 + 0.2 = 13.4 \text{ mL/dL}$$

5. *Answer: B*
Tracheomalacia is classified as a variable extrathoracic lesion, which is why B is the answer. With tracheomalacia, the airway collapses during inspiration due to the negative pressure. Expiration is unaffected. A is normal, C is an intrathoracic lesion, and D is a large fixed obstruction.

CHAPTER 8

1. *Answer: C*
Carbon dioxide (CO_2) has a profound and reversible effect on cerebral blood flow, such that hypercapnia causes marked dilation of cerebral arteries and arterioles and increased blood flow, whereas hypocapnia causes constriction and decreased blood flow. Although several mechanisms involved in hypercapnic vasodilation have been proposed, the major mechanism appears to be related to a direct effect of extracellular H^+ on vascular smooth muscle. Cerebral blood flow increases linearly by 1 to 2 cc/100 g/min for 1 mm Hg increase in Pa_{CO_2}. Cerebral blood flow decreases by 1 to 2 cc/100 g/min for each 1 mm Hg decrease in Pa_{CO_2}. Under normal conditions, cerebral blood flow is 50 cc/100 g/min, so a 5-mm Hg increase in Pa_{CO_2} would bring the CBF to 50 + (5 to 10) cc/100 g/min = 55 to 60 cc/100 g/min.

2. *Answer: A*
Spinal cord ischemia resulting in postoperative paraplegia is a devastating complication of thoracoabdominal aortic aneurysm repair, and has been attributed to many causes. To prevent spinal cord compartment syndrome, CSF drainage has been used as an adjunct to thoracoabdominal aortic aneurysm repair, with procedure-related complications generally occurring infrequently. Subdural hematoma is a reported complication of thoracoabdominal repair with CSF drainage, which may result from the stretching and tearing of the bridging vein between the dura and cerebral hemispheres in cases of excessive CSF drainage. To prevent this complication, it has been recommended that CSF drainage not exceed hourly production, that is, 0.3 to 0.4 cc/min.

3. *Answer: B*
The Glasgow Coma Scale (GCS) is based on a 15-point scale for estimating and categorizing the initial severity of brain injury. The GCS is scored between 3 and 15, 3 being the worst, and 15 the best. It is composed of three parameters: best eye response, best verbal response, and best motor response, as given below:

I. **Motor response**
   6: obeys commands fully
   5: localizes to noxious stimuli
   4: withdraws from noxious stimuli
   3: abnormal flexion, i.e., decorticate posturing
   2: extensor response, i.e., decerebrate posturing
   1: no response
II. **Verbal response**
   5: alert and oriented
   4: confused, yet coherent, speech
   3: inappropriate words and jumbled phrases consisting of words
   2: incomprehensible sounds
   1: no sounds
III. **Eye opening**
   4: spontaneous eye opening

3: eyes open to speech

2: eyes open to pain

1: no eye opening

The patient in the question receives 3 points for opening eyes to speech, 3 points for incoherent speech, and 4 points for withdrawal from noxious stimuli for a total score of 10 points.

4. *Answer: B*

5. *Answer: A*

Rationale for questions 4 and 5

Central neurogenic DI, SIADH are syndromes affecting both sodium and water balance; however, they have differences in pathophysiology, diagnosis, and treatment. Differentiating between hypernatremia (central neurogenic DI) and the two hyponatremia syndromes (syndrome of inappropriate secretion of antidiuretic hormone, and cerebral salt-wasting syndrome) is critical for preventing worsening neurological outcomes. DI is a syndrome of fluid imbalance due to decreased secretion of ADH in the posterior lobe of the pituitary gland (central DI) or to renal unresponsiveness (nephrogenic DI) to the release of ADH. SIADH results from increased production of ADH, resulting in water intoxication and a volume-expanded state, and cerebral salt-wasting results from renal loss of sodium leading to true hyponatremia and a volume-contracted state in which the kidneys do not reabsorb sodium. Assessment of volume status and measurements of serum and urine sodium, osmolarity, and specific gravity are helpful in distinguishing between these three syndromes.

	Diabetes insipidus	Syndrome of inappropriate secretion of antidiuretic hormone	Cerebral salt wasting
Serum Na level	Na > 145	Na < 135	Na < 135
Serum osmolarity	>295 (high)	<275 (low)	<275 (low)
Urine osmolarity	Decreased (<200)	Elevated (>100)	Elevated (>100)
Urinary Na level	Within normal reference range or decreased	Within normal reference range or elevated (>25)	Elevated (>25)
Urine output	Increased	Decreased	Decreased
Urinary pecific gravity	<1.005 (dilute)	>1.010 (concentrated)	>1.010 (concentrated)
Volume status	Decreased	Increased	Decreased
Treatment	Fluid replacement (0.45% saline), desmopressin acetate or aqueous vasopressin	Fluid restriction (800–1,000 mL/24 hr) Slow sodium replacement with normal saline or hypertonic saline	Replacement of fluid volume and sodium. Slow sodium replacement with hypertonic (3%) saline

CHAPTER 9

1. *Answer: A*

IOP can be influenced by a change in volume of the contents of the orbit or by external pressure. Blinking, forceful eye closure, and direct compression are extrinsic factors that increase IOP. Hyperventilation, head elevation, diuretic administration, and anesthetics all decrease IOP by reducing the intraocular volume.

2. *Answer: B*

The OCR is triggered by traction on the extraocular muscles (especially medial rectus), direct pressure on the globe, ocular manipulation, or ocular pain. The pressure associated with local infiltration, which occurs during a retrobulbar block, by ocular trauma, or manipulation of tissue in the orbital apex after enucleation of the globe can also trigger it. The reflex is mediated by nerve connections between the ophthalmic branch of the trigeminal cranial nerve via the ciliary ganglion, and the vagus nerve. The reflex can be prevented peribulbar or retrobulbar blocks prior to stimulation, or with administration with atropine or glycopyrrolate. If bradycardia resulting from the OCR does occur, removal of the stimulus is immediately indicated. The OCR fatigues with repeated stimulation.

3. *Answer: C*

IOP is the fluid pressure inside the globe of the eye. Tonometry is the method used to determine this. Normal IOP is between 10 and 20 mm Hg. Ocular hypertension is defined by IOP being higher than normal, in the absence of optic nerve damage or visual field loss. Ocular hypotony, is typically defined as IOP equal to or less than 5 mm Hg. Such low IOP could indicate fluid leakage and deflation of the eyeball.

4. *Answer: B*

Management of airway fires includes early recognition, halting the surgical procedure, extinguishing the fire, and delivering post airway fire care to the patient. If an airway fire is identified, the flow of all airway gases should be stopped immediately and the endotracheal tube should be removed. Saline should be poured into the patient's airway to extinguish any residual embers and cool the tissues. Once the airway fire is extinguished, ventilation should be reestablished by mask, avoiding supplemental oxygen and nitrous oxide, if possible. Bronchoscopy (preferably rigid) may be beneficial to assess injury, and remove residual debris.

5. *Answer: B*
Understanding the innervation of the airway is essential airway management of the awake patient. Innervation of the airway can be divided into three regions based on the cranial nerves involved (figure). If nasal intubation is required, the maxillary branches from the trigeminal nerve must be anesthetized. For airway management that involves the pharynx and posterior third of the tongue, blockade of the glossopharyngeal nerve is required. Structures more distal in the airway to the epiglottis require block of vagal branches.

The larynx receives both sensory and motor innervation from the superior and recurrent laryngeal nerves, which are branches of the vagus nerve. The superior laryngeal nerve further divides into internal and external branches: the internal branch provides sensory innervation to the larynx above the level of the vocal folds while the external branch provides motor innervation to the cricothyroid muscles only. The recurrent laryngeal nerve provides motor innervation to all of the intrinsic muscles of the larynx except for the cricothyroids. It provides sensory innervation to the larynx below the level of the vocal cords as well as a small portion of the upper trachea.

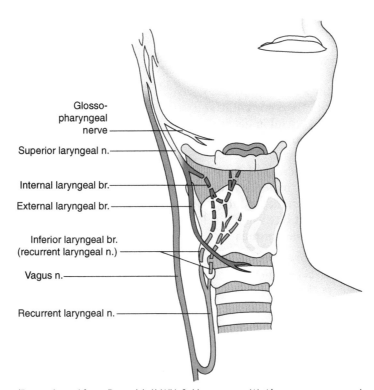

Glosso-
pharyngeal
nerve

Superior laryngeal n.

Internal laryngeal br.

External laryngeal br.

Inferior laryngeal br.
(recurrent laryngeal n.)

Vagus n.

Recurrent laryngeal n.

(Reproduced from Rosenblatt WH, Sukhupragarn W. Airway management. In: Barash PG, Cullen BF, Stoelting RK, et al., eds. *Clinical Anesthesia*. 7th ed. Philadelphia, PA: Wolters Kluwer; 2013:790.)

CHAPTER 10

1. *Answer: A*
Postoperative hemorrhage is a well-known complication following thyroid surgery that can rapidly lead to life-threatening, acute airway obstruction. Hematomas may be either superficial (directly below the platysma) or deep (inferior to the deep cervical fascia), with superficial hematomas generally appearing more impressive in terms of neck swelling. Deeper hematomas are more dangerous as they are less easily detected and require less blood accumulation to cause symptoms. If there is evidence of respiratory compromise, the neck wound should be opened immediately and the hematoma should be evacuated to relieve the mass compressing the

airway. Intubation may be difficult and should be performed by an experienced anesthesiologist. In case of inability to intubate, a surgical airway should be performed early.

2. *Answer: C*

The STOP-Bang questionnaire is a commonly used method to screen presurgical patients for sleep apnea. It consists of eight yes or no questions, which include the presence of snoring, tiredness/sleepiness, observed apneas, hypertension, BMI > 35 kg/m², age >50 years, neck circumference >40 cm, and male gender. A composite score of 5–8, 3–4, and 0–2 indicate high, moderate, and low risk of sleep apnea, respectively. For the patient in the question, the composite score is 1 (snore) + 1 (observed apnea) + 1 (hypertension) = 3. Thus, one could confidently exclude the possibility of at least severe OSA; however, the test is less reliable in excluding mild sleep apnea.

3. *Answer: D*

MELD is a scoring system for assessing the severity of chronic liver disease. It was initially developed to predict mortality within 3 months of surgery in patients who had undergone a transjugular intra-hepatic portosystemic shunt (TIPS) procedure and was subsequently found to be useful in determining prognosis and prioritizing for receipt of a liver transplant.

It has largely replaced the older Child–Pugh score (see table). MELD uses the patient's values for serum bilirubin, serum creatinine, and the INR for prothrombin time to predict survival. It is calculated according to the following formula

MELD = 3.78 × ln[serum bilirubin (mg/dL)] + 11.2 × ln[INR] + 9.57 × ln[serum creatinine (mg/dL)] + 6.43 × etiology (0: cholestatic or alcoholic, 1: otherwise)

Patients awaiting a liver transplant undergo periodic testing to update their MELD score and status on the liver transplant list, as scores may increase or decrease, depending on the severity of liver disease.

A comparison of the MELD and Child–Pugh scores are provided in the table below

Score	MELD	Child-Pugh
Components	INR, bilirubin, and creatinine	INR, bilirubin, albumin, ascites, hepatic encephalopathy
Scoring	Numerical	A through C (C is the worst)
Correlation with mortality	3-month mortality	1- and 2-year mortality

4. *Answer: A*

(IAP is the steady state pressure within the abdominal cavity. For most patients, an IAP of 5 to 7 mm Hg is usually considered normal but is not applicable for all patients. For example, morbidly obese and pregnant individuals can have chronically elevated intra-abdominal pressure (as high as 10 to 15 mm Hg) without adverse sequelae. Abdominal compartment syndrome is defined as a sustained IAP > 20 mm Hg, that is associated with organ dysfunction. Signs and symptoms of acute coronary syndrome (ACS) are often subtle and include decreases in venous return and cardiac output, elevated airway pressures, and decreased urine output.

The treatment of patients with ACS is urgent decompressive laparotomy, which provides rapid relief of intra-abdominal hypertension. The peritoneal cavity is usually left open postoperatively and closure is performed when the swelling subsides.

While the patient in this question has elevated IAP, there is no evidence of associated organ dysfunction. The borderline low blood pressure, low central venous pressure (CVP), and urine output are consistent with hypovolemia and a fluid bolus should be administered.

5. *Answer: C*

TURP syndrome is a clinical constellation of symptoms and signs associated with excessive absorption of irrigating fluid into the circulation. It comprises acute changes in intravascular volume, plasma solute concentrations, and osmolality, as well as specific effects resulting from the type of irrigation fluid used. While initially described with prostatic resection, other types of endoscopic surgery that use irrigation solution, for example, hysteroscopy, may also give rise to TURP syndrome. http://ceaccp.oxfordjournals.org/content/9/3/92. full - ref-3.

If TURP syndrome is suspected, surgery should be discontinued as soon as possible and IV fluids stopped. The rapid absorption of a large volume of irrigation fluid can cause hypertension with reflex bradycardia and can precipitate acute cardiac failure and pulmonary edema. Correction of bradycardia and hypotension should be treated with atropine, adrenergic drugs, and IV calcium. Intubation and positive pressure ventilation may be necessary if pulmonary edema has developed. Diuretic therapy is effective for treating acute pulmonary edema caused by the hypervolemia. However, furosemide can worsen hyponatremia due to its natriuretic effect. Mannitol causes less sodium loss than loop diuretics. Acute changes in plasma sodium concentration and osmolality predominantly affect the central nervous system (CNS). Acute hyponatremia produced by the dilutional effect of the large volume of absorbed irrigation may cause headache, altered level of consciousness, nausea and vomiting, and seizures. Hypertonic saline is indicated to correct severe hyponatremia, (serum sodium <120 mmol L or if symptoms develop). Raising the sodium at a rate of 1 mmol/L/hr is considered safe. Anticonvulsants (e.g., lorazepam) should be used to control seizures.

CHAPTER 11

1. *Answer: B*

Acute kidney injury (AKI), formerly called acute renal failure (ARF), was historically defined as an abrupt decline in renal function, clinically manifesting as an increase in BUN and serum Cr levels—over the course of hours to weeks. The vague nature of this definition made it difficult to compare between patient populations in studies of prevention or treatment of AKI. In 2002, the Acute Dialysis Quality Initiative (ADQI) was created for the purpose of developing evidence-based guidelines for the treatment and prevention of AKI. The *RIFLE criteria*, proposed by the ADQI group, aid in the staging of patients with AKI:

Risk: 1.5-fold increase in the Cr, or glomerular filtration rate (GFR) decrease by 25%, or urine output <0.5 mL/kg per hour for 6 hours.

Injury: Twofold increase in the Cr, or GFR decrease by 50%, or urine output <0.5 mL/kg per hour for 12 hours

Failure: Threefold increase in the Cr, or GFR decrease by 75%, or urine output of <0.3 mL/kg per hour for 24 hours, or anuria for 12 hours

Loss: Complete loss of kidney function (e.g., need for renal replacement therapy) for >4 weeks

End-stage renal disease: Complete loss of kidney function (e.g., need for renal replacement therapy) for >3 months

2. *Answer: A*

The Stewart approach is an alternative to the Henderson–Hasselbalch approach to acid–base physiology. An important component of the Stewart approach is the strong ion difference, which is the difference between the strong cations and strong ions:

$$[SID] = [Na^+] + [K^+] + [Ca^{2+}] + [Mg^{2+}] - [Cl^-] - [Other\ Strong\ Anions].$$

With normal protein levels, SID is about 40 mEq/L. Processes that increase the strong ion difference increase blood pH, whereas processes that reduce it decrease pH. As the patient's acidosis improves, the SID will increase.

3. *Answer: D*

Hypercalcemia may produce ECG abnormalities related to altered transmembrane potentials that affect conduction time. QT interval shortening is common, and, in some cases, the PR interval is prolonged. At very high levels, the QRS interval may lengthen, T waves may flatten or invert, and a variable degree of heart block may develop. Hypercalcemia has also been known to cause Osborn waves a positive deflection occurring at the junction between the QRS complex and the ST segment (indicated by the arrow in the figure). Osborn waves are also associated with severe hypothermia.

4. *Answer: A*

Contrast-induced nephropathy (CIN) is defined as either a 25% increase in serum creatinine from

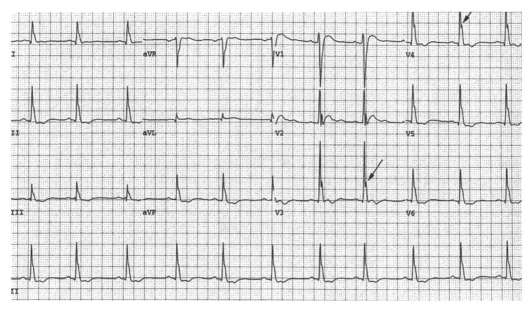

baseline or 0.5 mg/dL increase in absolute value, within 48 to 72 hours of intravenous contrast administration. Hydration therapy is the cornerstone of CIN prevention. Intravascular volume expansion maintains renal blood flow, preserves nitric oxide production, prevents medullary hypoxemia, and enhances contrast elimination. A number of other therapies for CIN have been investigated, without clear benefit. These include the use of statins, bicarbonate, *N*-acetylcysteine (NAC), ascorbic acid, theophylline and aminophylline, vasodilators, forced diuresis, and renal replacement therapy.

5. *Answer: C*

Acute tubular necrosis (ATN) is the most common cause of AKI in the renal category. It is important to exclude prerenal and postrenal causes of AKI since they are quickly reversible with appropriate therapy. There is no single test that can always distinguish prerenal azotemia from ATN. The proper approach is to rely on all available clinical information and lab tests.

Urinalysis and urine electrolytes may be helpful to differentiate ATN from prerenal azotemia. The urinalysis is typically normal in prerenal azotemia, with the only common finding being the presence of hyaline casts. In ATN, by comparison, the urine characteristically contains many muddy-brown granular casts with free renal tubular epithelial cells and epithelial cell casts. In patients with prerenal azotemia, FENa tends to be less than 1% and greater than 1% with ATN. A urinary osmolality (Uosm) greater than 500 mOsm/kg is highly suggestive of prerenal azotemia. In ATN there is damage in the loop of Henle, impairing the ability of the kidney to generate a high interstitial osmolality. Typically, the Uosm in ATN is approximately 300 to 350 mOsm/kg, a value that is similar to the plasma osmolality (Posm).

CHAPTER 12

1. *Answer: E*

Heparin-induced thrombocytopenia (HIT) is a prothrombotic adverse drug reaction caused by heparin. The "4 Ts" clinical scoring system is useful for estimating the pretest probability of HIT based on its characteristic features (**T**hrombocytopenia, **T**iming, **T**hrombosis) and the absence of other explanation(s) which are present in the patient in this case. If HIT is strongly suspected, all heparin should be stopped and further heparin avoided. Bivalirudin, a parenteral direct thrombin inhibitor and hirudin analog, has been successfully used in patients with HIT. Dose should be reduced and safely used in patients with renal failure, and in patients with combined hepatic and renal failure, its effect is monitored by the aPTT. Warfarin predisposes to microvascular thrombosis in patients with acute HIT. Fondaparinux is recommended for prophylaxis in patients with HIT but not for treatment

2. *Answer: B*

Thromboelastography (TEG) is a method of testing the efficiency of blood coagulation. More common tests of blood coagulation include prothrombin time (PT/INR) and partial thromboplastin time (aPTT), which measure coagulation factor function, but TEG also can assess platelet function, clot strength, and fibrinolysis, which these other tests cannot. Four values that represent clot formation are determined by this test: the reaction time (*R* value), the *K* value, the angle, and the maximum amplitude (MA). The *R* value represents the time until the first evidence of a clot is detected. The *K* value is the time from the end of *R* until the clot reaches 20 mm and this represents the speed of clot formation. The angle is the tangent of the curve made as the *K* is reached and offers similar information to *K*. The MA is a reflection of clot strength. TEG also measures clot lysis, which is reported as both the estimated percent lysis (EPL) and the percentage of clot, which has actually lysed after 30 minutes (LY 30, %). DIC is suggested by increased clot formation and clot lysis.

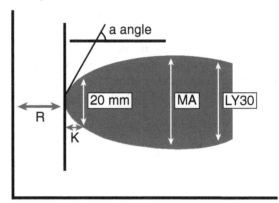

3. *Answer: D*

Bacterial contamination of transfusion products is a problem that has been improved through modern phlebotomy practices, refrigeration of red cells, freezing of plasma, and improved materials for transfusion product storage. Bacterial contamination of platelet products is the most frequent infectious risk from transfusion occurring in approximately 1 of 2,000 to 3,000 whole blood–derived random donor platelets and apheresis-derived single donor platelets.

4. *Answer: B*

Transfusion-related pulmonary edema is an under-recognized and potentially serious complication, which can result from adverse immune reactions and circulatory overload. TRALI results from neutrophil-mediated damage to the pulmonary microvasculature. The current proposed model is a "two-hit hypothesis," wherein a primary stimulus (e.g., surgery, hypoxia, infection, trauma, malignancy) is thought to activate the vascular endothelium and ultimately result in pulmonary neutrophil priming. The second hit is the transfusion of blood products containing lipids, antibodies, or cytokines that "activate" previously primed neutrophils. These activated neutrophils damage the endothelial layer such that fluid and protein leaks into the alveolar space.

In contrast to TRALI is TACO, which is the development of hydrostatic pulmonary edema, resulting from blood transfusion. Distinguishing between hydrostatic (TACO) and permeability (TRALI) pulmonary edema after transfusion is difficult, in part because the two conditions may coexist. Both TRALI and TACO are clinical diagnoses, and clinical features can sometimes distinguish between them. With both, patients present with respiratory distress due to acute onset pulmonary edema. With TRALI, patients also often have hypotension and fever, and can have transient leukopenia. With TACO, one would typically expect hypertension and a lack of fever and leukopenia. Features sometimes seen with TACO that would not be expected in TRALI include jugular venous distention, an S3 heard on cardiac auscultation, and peripheral edema.

5. *Answer: B*

Sickle-cell disease (SCD) is an inherited disorder of Hb associated with significant morbidity and mortality. It arises from a mutation in chromosome 11, where valine is substituted for glutamic acid, producing an abnormal β-globin chain. Under adverse conditions, these chains undergo polymerization, leading to deformation of red cells, which result in hemolysis, vaso-occlusion, and subsequent sickling crises. Perioperative conditions including suboptimal hydration, poor oxygenation, and acidemia can lead to SCD-related complications such as acute chest syndrome, painful vaso-occlusive episodes, and infections. The transfusion alternatives preoperatively in SCD (TAPS) trial randomized 70 children and adults with SCD to no preoperative transfusion or preoperative transfusion with a target Hb level of 10 g/dL. The median Hb at entry was 7.7 to 8.0 g/dL, and most patients underwent intermediate-risk surgery. The study was terminated early due to an increased incidence of serious adverse events in the no-transfusion arm. On the basis of these findings, exchange transfusion is generally recommended before major surgical interventions to minimize sickling and reduce the circulating HbS concentration below 30%. Use of erythropoietin may be considered in sickle-cell disease patients with renal failure but its effects in increasing the hematocrit are gradual and unpredictable.

CHAPTER 13

1. *Answer: D*

Corticosteroids and their synthetic derivatives differ in their metabolic (glucocorticoid) and electrolyte-regulating (mineralocorticoid) activities. These agents are employed at physiological doses for replacement therapy when endogenous production is impaired. It is important for anesthesiologists to be aware of the need for corticosteroid replacement as well as the relative potencies of available agents.

Name	Gluco-corticoid potency	Mineralo-corticoid potency	Duration of action ($t_{1/2}$ hours)
Cortisol (hydrocortisone)	1	1	8
Prednisone	3.5–5	0.8	16–36
Prednisolone	4	0.8	16–36
Methylprednisolone	5–7.5	0.5	18–40
Dexamethasone	25–80	0	36–54
Fludrocortisone	15	200	24

2. *Answer: A*

Pheochromocytoma is a rare catecholamine-secreting tumor arising commonly from adrenal medulla. The presence of a pheochromocytoma may be associated with unpredictable and fluctuating clinical course during anesthesia and surgical intervention. Hypertensive crises associated with pheochromocytoma may be managed with $MgSO_4$, which can be titrated to achieve the hemodynamic control. Magnesium decreases catecholamine release and is also a highly effective α-adrenergic antagonist and antiarrhythmic. Furthermore, magnesium reduces peripheral vascular resistance with minimal effects on venous return. Phenoxybenzamine is a long-acting, irreversible, alpha-adrenoceptor antagonist commonly used for preoperative blockade in patients with pheochromocytoma. It is usually administered orally and is not readily titratable, which limits its use for acute hypertensive crises. β-blockers should not be considered as a first option for management of a pheochromocytoma despite the presence of excessive tachycardia as unopposed alpha stimulation could worsen the hypertensive crisis.

Ketamine should be avoided due to its sympathomimetic properties.

3. *Answer: D*

Carcinoid tumors are uncommon, slow-growing neuroendocrine tumors of enterochromaffin cells. These tumors secrete hormones, including serotonin, bradykinin, histamine, and other vasoactive peptides that are metabolized quickly by the liver after being released into the portal circulation. Tumors of the small intestine are most likely to metastasize to the liver, allowing the hormones to escape hepatic metabolism and be released into the systemic circulation. Carcinoid crisis is a life-threatening event involving cardiac instability that results from the release of biologically active compounds from the tumor that may be triggered by tumor manipulation (biopsy or surgery) or by anesthesia.

Octreotide is a somatostatin analog that acts both to block the release of hormones and to stabilize blood pressure directly. For carcinoid crises, octreotide is typically administered in bolus doses or hourly infusion rates of 100 to 500 μg IV. Much higher doses are sometimes used for patients with complicated conditions in urgent situations.

The response to vasopressor agents is unpredictable and, in general, drugs such as norepinephrine and epinephrine can be hazardous in carcinoid patients. Any pharmacological stimulation of the autonomic nervous system has the potential to provoke further problems with vasoactive hormone release. Norepinephrine has been shown to activate kallikrein in the tumor and can even lead to the synthesis and release of bradykinin, resulting paradoxically in further vasodilatation and worsening hypotension, although exaggerated hypertensive responses may be seen. In practice, cautious administration of small doses of phenylephrine may be helpful in some patients.

4. *Answer: A*

Thyroid storm is an acute, life-threatening, hypermetabolic state induced by excessive release of thyroid hormones in individuals with thyrotoxicosis. The clinical presentation includes fever, tachycardia, hypertension, and neurological and GI abnormalities. Hypertension may be followed by congestive heart failure that is associated with hypotension and shock. Thyroid storm is often brought on by illness, usually an infection or by surgery. Thyrotoxic crisis associated with surgery

can manifest intraoperatively but more likely occurs 6 to 12 hours postoperatively. Management is supportive with cooling and fluids, alongside measures taken to reduce thyroid hormone synthesis, prevent hormone release, and inhibit the peripheral effects of excessive thyroid hormone. In addition, the management of thyroid storm should not disregard the search and appropriate treatment of any precipitating factors. For treating thyroid storm, the "five B'" are a useful memory aid for recalling the treatment of thyroid storm: **B**lock synthesis (i.e., antithyroid drugs); **B**lock release (i.e., iodine); **B**lock T_4 into T_3 conversion (i.e., high-dose propylthiouracil [PTU], propranolol, corticosteroid and, rarely, amiodarone); β-blocker; and **B**lock enterohepatic circulation (i.e., cholestyramine). Surgery (total or partial thyroidectomy) is typically reserved for patients who are intolerant of antithyroid medications or radioactive iodine. Radioactive iodine is contraindicated during pregnancy or when breast-feeding.

5. *Answer: A*

Sheehan syndrome, or necrosis of the pituitary gland, is a rare complication of postpartum hemorrhage. The pituitary gland is physiologically enlarged in pregnancy and is therefore very sensitive to the decreased blood flow caused by massive hemorrhage and hypovolemic shock. Women with Sheehan syndrome have varying degrees of hypopituitarism, ranging from panhypopituitarism to only selective pituitary deficiencies. The anterior pituitary is more susceptible to damage than the posterior pituitary.

The diagnosis of Sheehan syndrome is based on clinical evidence of hypopituitarism in a woman with a history of a postpartum hemorrhage. Deficiencies of specific anterior pituitary hormones will cause varied symptoms. Corticotropin deficiency can cause weakness, fatigue, hypoglycemia, or dizziness. Gonadotropin deficiency will often cause amenorrhea, oligomenorrhea, hot flashes, or decreased libido. Growth hormone deficiency causes many vague symptoms including fatigue, decreased quality of life, and decreased muscle mass. Patients with hypothyroidism caused by hypopituitarism have low T_3 and T_4 levels with normal or even inappropriately low TSH levels. Diagnosis of panhypopituitarism is straightforward, but partial deficiencies are often difficult to elicit. A woman with panhypopituitarism will have low levels of pituitary hormones (luteinizing hormone, corticotropin, and thyrotropin) as well as the target hormones (cortisol and thyroxine). Stimulation tests (insulin-induced hypoglycemia or metyrapone stimulation test) are often necessary for diagnosis in the acute phase or in situations where a partial deficiency is suspected.

Treatment of young women with hypopituitarism includes replacement of hydrocortisone first and then replacement of thyroid hormone and estrogen with or without progesterone depending on whether she has a uterus. Hydrocortisone is replaced first because thyroxine therapy can exacerbate glucocorticoid deficiency and theoretically induce an adrenal crisis.

CHAPTER 14

1. *Answer: A*
Hyperkalemic periodic paralysis is an autosomal dominant disease characterized by episodes of flaccid paralysis. The paralysis is associated with increased serum potassium concentrations and precipitated by cold, hunger, and stress. Respiratory muscles are usually spared. Dysrhythmias may occur. Any drugs that cause potassium release from cells should be avoided, including depolarizing neuromuscular blocking agents as well as potassium-containing fluids. Calcium should be available for the emergency treatment of hyperkalemic-induced weakness. Fasting should be minimized and glucose-containing fluids infused during fasting periods. Hypothermia should be avoided. The use of volatile agents and nondepolarizing neuromuscular blocking agents is thought to be safe.

2. *Answer: A*
Myasthenia gravis is an autoimmune disease in which antibodies are produced against the nicotinic acetylcholine receptors within the neuromuscular junction. The autoantibodies lead to destruction of the receptors. Symptoms include fatigable weakness, which can be localized to specific muscle groups (ocular, bulbar, and respiratory) or become widespread. The thymus gland is abnormal in up to 75% of cases, and thought to be the site of the abnormal antibody production. In contrast to most other neuromuscular disorders, myasthenia gravis patients exhibit a relative resistance to depolarizing neuromuscular blocking agents and the dose used may need to be increased. Conversely, patients show an increased sensitivity to nondepolarizing neuromuscular blocking agents, often requiring only 10% of normal dose. Cholinesterase inhibitors should be avoided, as they can not only prolong the duration of a depolarizing neuromuscular blocking agents block, but also precipitate a cholinergic crisis. Drugs that interfere with neuromuscular transmission should be avoided.

3. *Answer: D*
Guillain–Barré syndrome is an immune-mediated polyneuropathy that often follows a viral or bacterial illness within the preceding 4 weeks. The weakness typically ascends from the legs and is symmetrical. Sensory and autonomic dysfunction can also occur. Ascending weakness can lead to respiratory compromise requiring prolonged ventilatory support. Patients with Guillain–Barré syndrome require close monitoring of their respiratory function using either forced vital capacity (FVC; by far the most common approach) and/or arterial blood gases. An FVC of less than 15 mL/kg (less than 30% of FVC predicted) or a rising $Paco_2$ are indications for mechanical ventilation.

4. *Answer: C*
MS is an autoimmune disease of inflammation, demyelination, and axonal damage to the central nervous system. This damage can result in a wide range of neurological signs and symptoms, including physical, mental, and sometimes psychiatric problems. The disease progression may be subacute with relapses and remissions or chronic and progressive. Although exacerbations can be triggered by physical and emotional stress, exacerbations and remissions often occur unpredictably.

Preoperative evaluation of the patient with MS should consist of a thorough baseline neurologic history and examination. Patients receiving corticosteroid therapy should continue therapy and may require stress dosing. General anesthesia is most often used in patients with MS although both spinal and epidural anesthesia have been successfully employed in parturients with MS. In some studies, spinal anesthesia has been implicated in postop exacerbations whereas epidural and peripheral nerves blocks have not.

Nondepolarizing neuromuscular blockers are safe to use although patients with MS may have altered sensitivity to these drugs in the setting of baseline weakness and reduced "physiologic reserve" (neurologic and respiratory) and be less able to tolerate stressors such as a mild degree of postoperative residual muscle relaxant. Succinylcholine should be used with caution as demyelination and denervation may increase the risk of succinylcholine-induced hyperkalemia in these patients

In patients with MS, temperature should be monitored closely and efforts taken to minimize increases above baseline as even slight increases in body temperature may precipitate a decline in neurologic function postoperatively.

5. Answer: C

Acute compartment syndrome is a complication following fractures, soft tissue trauma, and reperfusion injury after acute arterial obstruction. It is caused by bleeding or edema in a closed, nonelastic muscle compartment surrounded by fascia and bone. The diagnosis is based on clinical examination and intracompartmental pressure measurement. Pain out of proportion to injury and increasing analgesic requirements should raise the suspicion of a developing compartment syndrome. Further, paresthesias may occur as an early symptom in acute compartment syndrome, representing a potentially reversible state because peripheral nerves are more sensitive to ischemia than muscle. Pallor, pulselessness, and poikilothermia are late findings and when observed, ischemic changes may be irreversible.

Perfusion within a compartment is only present when the diastolic blood pressure exceeds the intracompartmental pressure. During vasoconstriction or hypertension, perfusion ceases at even lower pressures. Although it is unclear at which pressure tissue damage occurs, clinical studies suggest a difference between diastolic and intracompartmental pressure of less than 30 mm Hg as an indication for fasciotomy.

A fasciotomy should be performed when the difference between compartment pressure and diastolic blood pressure is less than 30 mm Hg or when clinical symptoms are obvious. Once the diagnosis is made, immediate fasciotomy of all compartments is required.

CHAPTER 15

1. Answer: B

Compared to adults, infants have very little hemodynamic derangement with spinal anesthetics. This is due to a smaller peripheral blood pool, immature sympathetic autonomic system, and compensatory reduction in vagal efferent activity. Hence, preloading before SA is not a routine in children. From age 6 onward children can exhibit signs of a sympathectomy similar to that of adults, with older children (teenagers) having cardiovascular responses almost identical to that of adults. Children require higher dose of local anesthetic (LA) drug due to higher total CSF (neonates 10 mL/kg, infants and toddlers 4 mL/kg, adults 2 mL/kg) and spinal CSF volumes (50% in children vs. 33% in adults). Highly vascular pia mater and high cardiac output lead to rapid reabsorption of LA and shorter duration of block in children.

2. Answer: B

Appropriate fluid resuscitation is one of the cornerstones of modern burn treatment. Burn injuries of less than 15% are associated with minimal fluid shifts and can generally be resuscitated with oral hydration, except in cases of facial, hand and genital burns, as well as burns in children and the elderly.

For patients with burns of 15% total body surface area (TBSA) or less, the following are indicated

- Patients with burns 5% to 10% TBSA who are taking oral fluids well—Oral fluids only
- Patients with burns 5% to 10% TBSA who are not taking oral fluids well—maintenance fluids
- Patients with burns 10% to 15% TBSA—1.5 × maintenance fluids

This patient has suffered 12% TBSA burns, so maintenance would be (4 mL/kg) 40 mL/hr and 1.5× maintenance is 60 mL/hr.

When the TBSA involved in the burn exceeds 15%, the systemic inflammatory response syndrome is initiated and massive fluid shifts, which result in burn edema and burn shock, can be expected. Current recommendations are to initiate formal intravascular fluid resuscitation when the surface area burned is greater than 15%. Several burn resuscitation formulas can be used in pediatric burn care; however, the modified Parkland formula is most commonly used. Ringer lactate solution is initially used in pediatric patients at 3 to 4 mL/kg for each percent of the body surface area burned for the first 24 hours. One half of the calculated fluid needs are administered in the first 8 hours after the burn occurs, and the remaining half are administered over the following 16 hours. Rates of fluid administration should be altered based on the patient's response, which can be assessed by measuring urine output, monitoring sensorium, peripheral circulation, and lactate concentration.

3. Answer: D

The development of postoperative apnea is a major concern with surgery in the neonate. Risk factors for postoperative apnea include prematurity (less than 46 to 60 weeks), the presence of congenital anomalies, a history of apnea and bradycardia, and chronic lung disease. The etiology of postoperative apnea is likely multifactorial. Anesthetic agents may potentiate decreased ventilatory control and hyporesponsiveness to hypoxia and hypercarbia. Hypothermia, anemia, and respiratory muscle fatigue may also play a role. Anemia (hematocrit < 30%) has been determined to be independent of post-conceptual age for risk in the development of postoperative apnea. Infants at high risk for development of postoperative apnea may benefit from a regional anesthetic as opposed to a general anesthetic. If supplemental sedation is used, the advantage is lost.

An important issue regarding postoperative apnea in infants is who should be admitted and monitored (and for how long) after outpatient surgery. The incidence of significant apnea and bradycardia is highest in the first 4 to 6 hours after surgery but has been reported up to 12 hours after surgery. **A widely accepted guideline is to monitor all infants younger than 50 weeks post-conceptual age for at least 12 hours after surgery.** In addition, outpatient or elective/nonurgent surgery may be delayed in infants younger than 50 weeks post-conceptual age if possible. **Caffeine and theophylline have been used as respiratory stimulants** to prevent and/or treat postoperative apneic episodes. Blood transfusion in anemic infants is not clearly beneficial in preventing postoperative apnea. Instead, it is recommended that anemic children get iron supplementation and the surgery be postponed (if possible) until the anemia resolves.

4. *Answer: D*
Propofol-related infusion syndrome (PRIS) is a rare and potentially lethal side effect of patients receiving propofol infusions for sedation. The physiopathology of PRIS mechanism remains unclear; however, a direct mitochondrial respiratory chain inhibition or impaired mitochondrial fatty acid metabolism mediated by propofol has been implicated. Clinical features consist of arrhythmias, metabolic acidosis, lipemia, rhabdomyolysis, and myoglobinuria. PRIS has been classically described in children and adults undergoing a long-term infusion with propofol (more than 48 hours) at doses higher than 4 mg/kg/hr. However, it can be observed with lower doses and after shorter duration of sedation. Predisposing factors include young age, severe critical illness of central nervous system or respiratory origin, administration of steroids, vasopressors, and low carbohydrate intake.

5. *Answer: A*
Tetralogy of Fallot consists of right ventricular outflow obstruction, right ventricular hypertrophy, and a VSD with an overriding aorta. The right ventricular outflow obstruction is usually secondary to hypertrophy of the subpulmonic muscle. Up to 25% of patients also have pulmonic stenosis. The infundibular obstruction is dynamic and can be increased secondary to sympathetic tone"; this obstruction is responsible for "tet spells" or the hypercyanotic spells seen in young patients. The primary physiologic goal when managing a tetralogy spell (cyanosis following a sudden increase in PVR) is reducing the right-to-left shunt (through the VSD), that is, by redirecting blood through the lungs. Pharmacologic management of tetralogy spells includes alpha-agonism (increases both PVR and SVR; however, if PVR is already elevated, this does not have an additional effect), β-blockade (may help to relieve infundibular spasm), bicarbonate (acidosis can increase PVR), and morphine. PHENYLEPHRINE is the correct answer here because it was specified that the cyanosis occurred after induction of general anesthesia. Oxygen and morphine are first-line treatments, followed by beta blockade, then alpha agonism if the question did not apply to treatment following induction.

CHAPTER 16

1. *Answer: D*
Post-dural puncture headaches rarely begin less than 1 day after a neuraxial procedure. A severe headache 1 hour after a neuraxial is more likely pneumocephalus.

2. *Answer: B*
An epidural that is slowly dosed allows the least change in hemodynamic fluctuations. Epidurals also have the option for an opioid-only anesthetic with the avoidance of local anesthetic.

3. *Answer: E*
Pregnancy is associated with a decrease in systemic vascular resistance.

4. *Answer: A*
An elevated PTT is an artifact of laboratory testing of antiphospholipid syndrome. Patients with antiphospholipid syndrome are procoagulant.

5. *Answer: C*
Acceptable antihypertensive drugs during pregnancy include methyldopa, labetolol, nifedipine, and hydralazine.

CHAPTER 17

1. *Answer: C*
Notalgia paresthetica (NP) is a sensory neuropathic syndrome of the mid-back skin, the classic location of which is the unilateral infrascapular area. The etiology is neuropathy from degenerative cervicothoracic disk disease or direct nerve impingement. NP patients classically present with the hallmark symptom of localized pruritus of the unilateral infrascapula. However, there are many atypical presentations of NP, including localized pruritus of the upper back, neck, scalp, and shoulder. *Cheiralgia*

paraesthetica is a neuropathy of the hand generally caused by compression or trauma to the superficial branch of the radial nerve. *Meralgia paraesthetica* is a neurological condition caused by nerve entrapment of the lateral cutaneous nerve of the thigh.

Analgia paresthetica is not a diagnostic entity.

2. *Answer: D*
The World Health Organization (WHO) created a practical pain ladder diagram in 1986 to help guide clinicians treating cancer pain throughout the world. The pain ladder was designed intentionally to be extremely simple: there are three rungs to the ladder: (1) anti-inflammatory agents, (2) weak opioids, and (3) strong opioids corresponding to increasing pain intensity. The clinician prescribes medications as pain worsens, moving from one rung to the next. Recently, a fourth rung was added to the pain ladder to account for nerve blocks (e.g., epidural), neurolysis, brain and nerve stimulators.

3. *Answer: B*
Gabapentin binds and inhibits α2-δ voltage-gated calcium channels in the central nervous system. Baclofen is agonist at GABA$_B$ channels commonly used to treat spasticity. Tricyclic antidepressants act by inhibition of reuptake of norepinephrine and serotonin. Ketamine is an NMDA receptor antagonist, but it also acts at numerous other sites (including opioid receptors and monoamine transporters). Lidocaine acts by blockade of voltage-gated sodium channels leading to inhibition of neuronal depolarization.

4. *Answer: D*
PLP is a painful sensation following limb amputation that missing limb is still present. The time of onset is 60% to 85% in the first week of limb loss, but pain can occur years later. Pain typically fades with time, but rarely disappears. PLP can be reactivated by epidural/spinal anesthetics.

5. *Answer: D*
Complex regional pain syndrome (CRPS) is a chronic pain condition most often affecting one of the limbs (arms, legs, hands, or feet), usually after an injury or trauma to that limb. CRPS is believed to be caused by damage to, or malfunction of, the peripheral and central nervous systems. There are two similar forms: individuals without confirmed nerve injury are classified as having CRPS-I (previously called reflex sympathetic dystrophy syndrome) and CRPS-II (previously called causalgia) is the term used for patients with confirmed nerve injuries. CRPS is characterized by prolonged or excessive pain and mild or dramatic changes in skin color, temperature, and/or swelling in the affected area. Complex Regional Pain Syndromeis

associated with nondermatomal patterns of pain, allodynia (pain due to a stimulus that does not usually provoke pain), and unusual movement disorders such as tremors. CRPS symptoms vary in severity and duration. Studies of the incidence and prevalence of the disease show that most cases are mild and individuals recover gradually with time. In more severe cases, individuals may not recover and may have long-term disability.

CHAPTER 18

1. *Answer: C*
Interscalene blocks and catheters are used for intraoperative as well as postoperative pain control in patients undergoing surgery of the shoulder, elbow, and upper arm. The triad "ptosis, miosis, and anhidrosis" characterizes Horner syndrome. It is a common complication of interscalene nerve blocks/catheters secondary to the local anesthetic spreading proximally and therefore blocking the sympathetic fibers of the cervicothoraco ganglion. This complication is generally benign in nature and the patient should not expect to suffer any long-term consequences as a result. The ipsilateral phrenic nerve is almost always blocked, resulting in an elevated hemidiaphragm and reduced pulmonary function. This procedure should possibly be avoided in patients who have limited pulmonary reserve secondary to underlying respiratory disease. The recurrent laryngeal nerve can also be blocked and is therefore contraindicated in patients with known preexisting vocal cord paralysis. Inadvertent vascular injection of local anesthetic or placement of a catheter can result in systemic local anesthetic toxicity.

2. *Answer: B*
Axillary nerve blocks provide anesthesia for surgical procedures involving the elbow, forearm, and hand. This block encompasses the terminal nerves of the brachial plexus. The median nerve originates from the medial and lateral cords, the radial nerve is the terminal branch from the posterior cord, and the ulnar nerve is the terminal branch of the medial cord. These three nerves surround the axillary artery in the following manner: the median nerve is superior, the radial nerve is posterior, and the ulnar nerve is inferior. The injection of local anesthetic around the axillary artery should anesthetize all three nerves, as they are located in the neurovascular sheath. One should note when performing this procedure, the musculocutaneous nerve will require a separate block.

3. *Answer: B*
Some of the earliest signs of local anesthetic toxicity are secondary to blockade of normal inhibitory

pathways of the cerebral cortex. In general, (with bupivacaine being the possible exception), systemic local anesthetic toxicity is more likely to affect the central nervous system vs. the cardiovascular system. Early symptoms that suggest local anesthetic toxicity include dizziness, lightheadedness, tinnitus, circumoral numbness, shivering, tremors, and seizures. Later symptoms are central nervous system depression. Cardiovascular complications include dysrhythmias, decreased myocardial contractility, and decreased cardiac output. Profound vasodilatation can also occur. The maximum dose of lidocaine that should be administered in patients is 7 mg/kg (max 500 mg) with epinephrine and 4.5 mg/kg (max 300 mg) without epinephrine.

4. *Answer: C*

Celiac plexus blocks are useful in treating the pain of pancreatic cancer, as well as abdominal pain secondary to issues involving the stomach, liver, gallbladder, spleen, and pancreas. The celiac plexus consists of sympathetic nerve fibers from the greater and lesser splanchnic nerves. The parasympathetic supply of the abdominal organs is from the anterior and posterior vagal trunks. Orthostatic hypotension is one of the most common complications secondary to venous pooling; this can be avoided, or at least attenuated, by adequate pre-procedural hydration with IV fluids. Diarrhea is also a common complication secondary

to blockade of the sympathetic nerve fibers. Far less common complications include hemorrhage (due to needle puncture of the aorta or inferior vena cava), abdominal organ/viscera damage (due to needle puncture), intravascular injection/local anesthetic toxicity, paraplegia (from injection of phenol or alcohol into the spinal arteries/artery of Adamkiewicz), and pneumothorax (can occur if the needle is angled too cephalad). It should be noted that this block should be performed when the patient has a limited life span, as the nerves will regenerate, which can cause increased pain. Both alcohol and phenol have similar efficacies with regard to destruction of nerve tissues.

5. *Answer: A*

An ankle block will provide anesthesia for surgery or procedures involving the feet and/or toes by blocking the five nerves that supply the foot, namely, the superficial peroneal, deep peroneal, posterior tibial, sural, and saphenous. The three "superficial" nerves are the superficial peroneal, sural, and saphenous nerves, which only provide sensory innervation; the "deep" nerves are the deep peroneal and posterior tibial nerves, which provide both sensory and motor innervation. The superficial peroneal, deep peroneal, posterior tibial, and sural nerves are the four terminal branches of the sciatic nerve, whereas the saphenous nerve is a cutaneous branch of the femoral nerve.

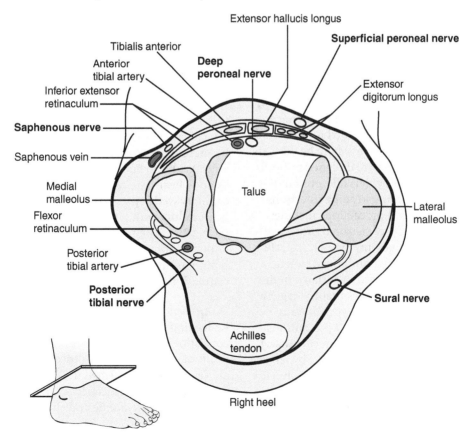

CHAPTER 19

1. *Answer: C*

Classes of hemorrhage have been defined, based on the percentage of blood volume loss. Treatment should be aggressive and directed by both the initial classification and the response to therapy. In patients without other injuries or fluid losses, 30% to 40% is the smallest amount of blood loss that consistently causes a decrease in systolic BP (Class 3 hemorrhage).

- Class I hemorrhage (loss of 0% to 15%): usually, no changes in BP, pulse pressure, or respiratory rate occur. A delay in capillary refill of longer than 3 seconds corresponds to a volume loss of ~10%.
- Class II hemorrhage (loss of 15% to 30%): clinical symptoms include tachycardia, tachypnea, decreased pulse pressure, cool clammy skin, delayed capillary refill, and slight anxiety.
- Class III hemorrhage (loss of 30% to 40%): patients usually have marked tachypnea and tachycardia, decreased systolic BP, oliguria, and significant changes in mental status, such as confusion or agitation.
- Class IV hemorrhage (loss of >40%): symptoms include marked tachycardia, decreased systolic BP, narrowed pulse pressure (or immeasurable diastolic pressure), markedly decreased (or no) urinary output, depressed mental status (or loss of consciousness), and cold and pale skin.

2. *Answer: A*

Standard precautions are the minimum infection prevention practices that apply to all patient care, regardless of suspected or confirmed infection status of the patient, in any setting where health-care is delivered. These practices are designed to both protect the health-care providers and prevent the health-care providers from spreading infections among patients. Standard precautions include: (1) hand hygiene, (2) use of personal protective equipment (e.g., gloves, gowns, masks), (3) safe injection practices, (4) safe handling of potentially contaminated equipment or surfaces in the patient environment, and (5) respiratory hygiene/cough etiquette. There are three types of transmission-based precautions: contact precautions (for diseases spread by direct or indirect contact), droplet precautions (for diseases spread by large particles in the air), and airborne precautions (for diseases spread by small particles in the air). Each type of precautions has some unique prevention steps that should be taken, but **all** have standard precautions as their foundation.

3. *Answer: D*

In 1994 the American–European Consensus Conference laid the foundations for the definition of ARDS, including the following clinical criteria: the recent onset of symptoms after a known risk factor, severe hypoxemia defined by a PaO_2/FIO_2 ratio less than 200 mm Hg, bilateral infiltrates on chest radiograph, and absence of cardiogenic pulmonary edema. While commonly used in practice, this definition has a number of limitations including: the acute nature of symptoms was not specified, level of positive end-expiratory pressure was not taken into account in oxygenation criteria, and cardiogenic pulmonary edema was defined as an increase in pulmonary artery wedge pressure, whereas recent studies found that high pressures could coexist with ARDS. The Berlin definition of ARDS was developed to address these limitations.

The new Berlin definition categorize ARDS as being mild, moderate, or severe based on degree of hypoxemia: mild (200 mm Hg < PaO_2/FIO_2 ≤ 300 mm Hg), moderate (100 mm Hg < PaO_2/FIO_2 ≤ 200 mm Hg), and severe (PaO_2/FIO_2 ≤ 100 mm Hg) and four ancillary variables for severe ARDS: radiographic severity, respiratory system compliance (≤40 mL/cm H_2O), positive end-expiratory pressure (≥10 cm H_2O), and corrected expired volume per minute (≥10 L/min). Under the Berlin definition, the entity of "acute lung injury" no longer exists as patients with PaO_2/FIO_2 of 200 to 300 are classified as having "mild ARDS." Onset of ARDS (diagnosis) must be acute, as defined as within 7 days of some defined event, which may be sepsis, pneumonia, or simply a patient's recognition of worsening respiratory symptoms. Bilateral opacities consistent with pulmonary edema must be present but may be detected on CT or chest x-ray. With the Berlin definition there is no need to exclude heart failure; patients with high pulmonary capillary wedge pressures, or known congestive heart failure with left atrial hypertension can still have ARDS. The new criterion is that respiratory failure simply be "not fully explained by cardiac failure or fluid overload," in the physician's best estimation using available information.

4. *Answer: B*

Re-feeding syndrome is a potentially fatal syndrome consisting of metabolic disturbances that occur as a result of reinstitution of nutrition to patients who are severely malnourished. It is characterized by hypophosphatemia associated with fluid and electrolyte shifts and metabolic and clinical complications.

Patients at high risk include chronically under-nourished patients and those who have had little or no nutritional intake for more than 1 week. For patients at high risk of developing re-feeding syndrome, nutritional repletion of energy should be started slowly and plasma electrolytes (especially phosphate, sodium, potassium, and magnesium) and glucose should be measured at baseline before feeding and any deficiencies corrected during feeding with close monitoring. Vitamin supplementation should also be started immediately and circulatory volume should also be restored.

5. *Answer: A*
The systemic inflammatory response syndrome (SIRS) is defined as the presence of two or more of the following variables:
- Fever of more than 38°C or less than 36°C
- HR > 90 beats/minute
- Respiratory rate > 20 breaths/minute or $Pa_{CO_2} < 32$ mm Hg
- White blood cell count >12,000/μL or <4,000/μL or >10% immature [band] forms

Sepsis is defined as a systemic inflammatory response to infection. The term "severe sepsis" is used to describe instances in which sepsis is complicated by acute organ dysfunction, and "septic shock" is sepsis complicated by either hypotension that is refractory to fluid resuscitation or by hyperlactatemia. Signs of a systemic inflammatory response, such as tachycardia or an elevated white cell count, may also occur in noninfectious conditions (i.e., after surgery) and therefore is not specific for the presence of infection.

CHAPTER 20

1. *Answer: A*
The compulsive use of a drug despite harmful consequences is referred to as addiction. It is characterized by an inability to stop using a drug, failure to meet work, social, or family obligations, and sometimes (depending on the drug) tolerance and withdrawal. Physical dependence occurs when the body adapts to the drug, requiring more of it to achieve a certain effect (tolerance) and eliciting drug-specific physical or mental symptoms if drug use is abruptly ceased (withdrawal). Physical dependence in and of itself does not constitute addiction, but it often accompanies addiction.

2. *Answer: C*
Substance abuse is a serious public health problem and physicians are susceptible. Anesthesiologists

have drawn special attention because of their ready access drugs such as intravenous opioids; however, only indirect evidence exists that substance abuse is more common in anesthesiologists than in other physicians' specialties. The most consistent early sign of substance abuse problems in physicians is increasing isolation manifested by changes in personal relationships and withdrawal from community activities. The addicted anesthesiologist usually becomes extraordinarily attentive at work as maintaining proximity to the source of drugs becomes more important than other aspects of the physician's personal life. Spending more time at the hospital, even when off duty, refusing relief for breaks, and signing out increasing amounts of narcotics or quantities inappropriate for the given case are other signs that should raise concern for a substance abuse problem. Changes in behavior are common with periods of irritability, anger, depression, and euphoria. Neglect of physical appearance with weight loss and pale skin may be other indicators. Impaired job performance is often the last sign of a substance abuse problem. Early identification of the affected individual is essential as it can often prevent harm, both to the impaired physician and to his or her patients.

3. *Answer: D*
Alcohol withdrawal is the clinical syndrome that occurs when people who are physically dependent upon alcohol stop drinking or reduce their alcohol consumption. Minor withdrawal symptoms such as tremor, anxiety, nausea, vomiting, and insomnia typically occur within 6 to 24 hours following the patient's last drink. Major withdrawal symptoms usually occur within 10 to 72 hours after the last drink and are manifested by visual and tactile hallucinations, whole-body tremor, diaphoresis, and hypertension. Alcohol withdrawal seizures occur within 6 to 48 hours of alcohol cessation; they are major motor seizures that take place during withdrawal in patients who normally have no seizure history. They usually occur only once or recur only once or twice, and they generally resolve spontaneously. DT is the most severe form of ethanol withdrawal. It occurs 3 to 10 days following the last drink. Clinical manifestations include global confusion, hallucinations, fever, hypertension, diaphoresis, and autonomic hyperactivity. If untreated, DT can progress to cardiovascular collapse.

4. *Answer: A*
Pseudocholinesterase is the major enzyme for detoxification of cocaine and is important for metabolizing succinylcholine. With both succinylcholine and cocaine acting as substrates for

pseudocholinesterase, a prolonged neuromuscular block can occur in a cocaine-abusing patient. Although prolonged blockade is a potential risk, succinylcholine in standard doses has been used when cocaine-abusing parturients required a rapid sequence induction.

5. *Answer: A*
Anthrax is caused by *Bacillus anthracis*, a spore-forming, gram-positive bacillus. The disease can be manifested in three ways: pulmonary, cutaneous, and gastrointestinal. Pulmonary anthrax begins with nonspecific flu-like symptoms. Chest x-ray reveals a widened mediastinum, and gram-positive bacilli can be seen on blood culture after 2 to 3 days. Two to four days later, there is an abrupt onset of respiratory failure and shock. Death generally occurs within 24 to 48 hours after shock develops.

Botulism is a potentially life-threatening paralytic illness resulting from a neurotoxin produced by *Clostridium botulinum*. Though mainly a foodborne intoxication, botulism can also be caused by intestinal infection in infants, wound infections, and by inhalation. Early symptoms include fatigue, weakness, and vertigo usually followed by blurred vision, and difficulty in swallowing and speaking. The disease can then progress to weakness of the respiratory muscles, which can result in respiratory failure. There is no fever and no loss of consciousness. Treatment consists of administration of antitoxin and intensive respiratory care.

Smallpox is a contagious, and often deadly disease caused by the variola virus. It was one of the world's most devastating diseases but was declared eradicated in 1980 following a global immunization campaign. Smallpox was transmitted from person to person via infective droplets during close contact with infected symptomatic people. Vaccine administered up to 4 days after exposure provided protective immunity and was effective in preventing infection.

Bubonic plague is one of three types of infection caused by the bacterium *Yersinia pestis*. The other two types of plague are septicemic plague and pneumonic plague. With bubonic plague, flu-like symptoms develop 3 to 7 days after exposure to the bacteria. Swollen and painful lymph nodes (buboes) occur in the area closest to where the bacteria entered the skin. Left untreated, bubonic plague bacteria can quickly multiply in the bloodstream, causing septicemic plague, or even progress to the lungs, causing pneumonic plague. Antibiotics are (streptomycin, gentamicin, or doxycycline) effective for treatment. Without treatment, bubonic plague results in the death of 30% to 90% of those infected.

CHAPTER 21

1. *Answer: D*
The paired *t*-test compares one set of measurements with a second set from the same sample of subjects. It is often used to compare "before" and "after" scores in experiments to determine whether significant change has occurred. The null hypothesis is that the mean difference between *paired* observations is zero. When the mean difference is zero, the means of the two groups must also be equal. The unpaired *t*-test is used to compare means from data, which is collected from two different and independent groups of subjects or patients. The size between the two samples may be equal or not. *Regression analysis* is a statistical method for modeling and analyzing the relationship between a dependent variable and one or more independent variables. Analysis of variance (ANOVA) provides a statistical test of whether or not the means of several groups (≥ 2) are equal, and therefore generalizes the *t* test to more than two groups.

2. *Answer: D*
The standard error of the mean (SEM) is the standard deviation (SD) of the sample mean's estimate of a population mean. SEM is estimated by the sample estimate of the population SD (sample SD) divided by the square root of the sample size:

$$\text{SEM} = \text{SD}/\sqrt{n} = 100 \text{ minutes}/10 = 10 \text{ minutes}$$

3. *Answer: C*
Positive predictive value (PPV) represents the probability that a person has a disease or condition given a positive test result. That is, it is the proportion of individuals with positive test results who are correctly identified or diagnosed. It is important because it reflects the accuracy with which a test can identify a disease or condition. In a population, it can be defined as the number of true positives divided by the *sum* of true positives and false positives. The sensitivity refers to the true positive rate for people with a disease or condition having a positive test result, and the specificity refers to the true negative rate for healthy people having a negative test result. The negative predictive values is the probability that an individual is not affected with the condition when a negative test result is observed.

4. *Answer: A*

The chi-square test is used to determine if there is a significant relationship between two categorical variables. The frequency of one categorical variable is compared with different values of the second categorical variable. The data can be displayed in an R $\times$ C contingency table, where R is the row and C is the column. The null hypothesis is that there is no relationship between anesthetic type and patient satisfaction. If the null hypothesis is rejected then it can be concluded that that there is a relationship between anesthetic type and patient satisfaction.

5. *Answer: A*

While sample size calculations can become extremely complicated, there are just a few factors that influence the calculations:

- The effect size, that is, how large a difference you want to be able to detect
- The variability in the variable of interest
- The alpha level (α)
- The statistical power

Increasing the effect size or the alpha level reduces the sample size, while increasing the variability or the statistical power increase the sample size.

CHAPTER 22

1. *Answer: D*

The ACGME core competencies are comprised of

- Patient care
- Medical knowledge
- Practice-based learning and improvement
- Systems-based practice
- Interpersonal skills and communication

These six indicators serve to help evaluate resident and fellow progression and improvement in these areas.

2. *Answer: B*

The patient is expressing the ethical tenet of "autonomy"; namely, the right to make her own medical decisions. She has metastatic cancer and wishes to spend time with her family. Whether or not you personally agree with your patient's decision, it is their right to express their wishes and the care team should always make the best effort possible to respect the patient's wishes. A family meeting, including the patient, their family, health-care providers, social workers, and so on, is always in the best interest of the patient and helping to provide them the best possible care, even if the "care" is no longer "medical or curative" and the goal is now "comfort." At times, a psychiatry or ethical consult

can be appropriate if the patient is not competent or specific procedures are not in the best interest of the patient.

3. *Answer: C*

The patient was clear with her wishes prior to surgery and she stated that she did not want any blood products. This is consistent with "informed refusal" and she has a right to refuse treatment if she is of capacity and the physician caring for her has explained the possible consequences of refusing specific therapies and/or treatment. The physician should ask in detail about the acceptance of other products besides red cells; IE: albumin, cell saver, and so on, as there are some patients who may have selective acceptance to specific products.

4. *Answer: A*

Brain death is defined as "the irreversible loss of all clinical functions of the brain, including the brainstem." Coma, absence of brainstem reflexes, and apnea are the three essential components that must be present before a patient is declared "brain dead." In addition, other potential variables must be ruled out, including hypothermia (core temperature must be greater than 36.5°C), normal metabolic profile/absence of metabolic disarray and electrolyte disturbances, absence of residual neuromuscular blockade, and absence of intoxication with drugs or other poisoning agents. The diagnosis of "brain death" is primarily clinical; however, there are ancillary tests that can support or possibly abandon the clinical conclusion. These include electroencephalogram, angiography, and transcranial Doppler.

5. *Answer: A*

There are many reasons patients file malpractice claims against physicians; however, the most common cause is "negligence", namely, that the physician did not provide what is known as the "standard of care" and there was resulting harm to the patient. "Medical errors," such as delayed or misdiagnosis, incorrect drug administration, and so on should be revealed to the patient if harm did indeed occur as a result of the mistake. (The physician can always consult the hospital lawyer or their malpractice insurance company if they have questions with regard to this). When physicians disclose an error to the patient, in a kind and empathetic manner, this may reduce the risk of a claim against them; maintaining patient–physician communication is imperative, even in difficult times. Lack of informed consent can be claimed when the patient feels as though they were not provided adequate information with regard to risks and complications and/or they were given incorrect information. The patient would likely need to prove that an injury occurred secondary to lack of informed consent; battery/assault can fall under this category; however, physical harm does not necessarily occur in this situation, the "intention" to provide care or perform a procedure without appropriate consent comprises the damage. Vicarious liability imposes responsibility of the failure of one person onto another. One can file a claim under vicarious liability if they feel that harm was inflicted as a result of inadequate supervision by the attending of record.

Note: Page numbers followed by *f* and *t* indicate figures and tables.

Abciximab, 244*t*
Abdominal aortic aneurysms (AAA),
    112–114
    DeBakey classification, 112, 113*f*
    paralysis, 113–114
    Stanford classification, 112, 113*f*
Abdominal blocks, 279–280
Abdominal compartment syndrome,
    161–162, 162*f*
Abdominal organ transplantation, 164–165
Abdominal trauma, 290
Abortion, spontaneous, 248
Accreditation Council for Graduate Medical
    Education (ACGME), 307
Accreta, 252
ACE inhibitors, for takotsubo
    cardiomyopathy, 90
Acetaminophen, 260
    for migraines, 267
    for pain, 258
    for tension, 267
Acetazolamide, for ophthalmic surgery, 151
Acetylcholine, for ophthalmic surgery, 151
Achondroplasia, 230
Acid–base disorders, in renal
    acidosis, 175
    alkalosis, 175–176
    buffering systems, 174
    framework for understanding, 174
Acidosis, 192
    lactic, 176–177
    metabolic, 175, 176
    respiratory, 175, 176
Acromegaly, 200
Activated clotting time (ACT), 188, 189*f*
    cardiac bypass and, 107
Acupuncture, 267
    for postoperative nausea and vomiting,
        76
Acute chest syndrome, with sickle-cell
    disease, 182
Acute normovolemic hemodilution, 196
Acute respiratory distress syndrome
    (ARDS)
    characteristics of, 291
    pathophysiology of, 291
    treatment for, 291–292
Acyclovir, 285
Addiction, definition of, 295
Adenoidectomy, 231
Adenosine, 246
    for arrhythmia, 99
    for hepatic dysfunction, 159
Adrenals
    anatomy and function of, 199–200
    disorders of, 204–205
Adrenocorticotrophic hormone (ACTH),
    199
Adults
    anxiolysis and analgesia, 57

noncardiac surgery and chronic disease
    in, 226–227
    vs. infant airway, 216
    vs. newborn airway, 221
Advanced Cardiovascular Life Support
    (ACLS), 254
Advanced directives, 309–310
Adverse event, definition of, 310
Air embolism, 247
Air gas cylinders, 7
Airway. *See also* Respiratory system
    altered anatomy, 229–230
    assessment, general anesthesia and
        endotracheal tubes, 59–60
        induction, 59
        preoxygenation, 59
        supraglottic airways, 59
    complications
        airway injuries, 72
        intraoperative complications, 72
    edema, 73
    infections, 229
    innervation, 118
    nerve injuries, 118
    obstruction, 229
    and oral surgery, 154–155
    and respiratory anatomy, 117
    and respiratory muscles, 117–118
    surgical, 60–61
Albendazole, 285
Albumin, 65, 186
Albuterol, for hypokalemia, 178
Alcohol abuse, 296
Aldosterone antagonists, 172
Aldosterone receptor blocker (ARB), 87
Alfentanil, 37
Alkalosis
    metabolic, 175–176
    respiratory, 176
Allergic reactions
    anaphylactoid, 71
    anaphylaxis, 70
    drugs for, 71
    of local anesthetics, 272
Allodynia, definitions of, 257
α_2-agonists, 261
α-agonists, 84
Alveolar uptake, 46, 47*f*
    gas concentration effect, 47–48, 48*f*
American Board of Anesthesiology (ABA),
    307
American College of Cardiology/American
    Heart Association (ACC/AHA), 55–56,
    55*f*
American Heart Association 2007, 94
American Society of Anesthesiologist
    (ASA), 53
    2006 Task Force Practice Guidelines
        for Perioperative Blood Transfusion,
        189

preoperative testing recommendations,
    54
    standard monitors, 17
Amiloride, for conn, 204
Aminocaproic acid, for platelet function,
    187
Aminoglycosides, 41, 285
Amiodarone
    for arrhythmia, 99–100
    for ventricular tachycardia, 98
Amniocentesis, 240
Amniotic fluid
    embolism, 247
    pregnancy and, 240
Amphotericin B, 285
Amyotrophic lateral sclerosis, 210
Anaerobes, for infection control, 285
Analysis of variance (ANOVA), 302–303
Anaphylactoid, 71
Anemia, 181
Anesthesia. *See also* Anesthetics
    and analgesia, 267
    changes with, 26
    closed claims project, 308
    for craniotomies, 145–146
    definition of, 54
    for electroconvulsive therapy, 146–147
    epidural. *See* Epidural anesthesia
    general. *See* General anesthesia
    machine. *See* Anesthesia machine
    maintenance of, 246
    neuraxial. *See* Neuraxial anesthesia
    ophthalmic, 151–153
    pediatric. *See* Pediatrics, anesthesia
    pollution, 8
    regional. *See* Regional anesthesia
    remote, 233
    for specific neurosurgical procedures,
        146
    spinal. *See* Spinal anesthesia
    stages of, 217–218
    topical, 153
Anesthesia dolorosa, definitions of, 257
Anesthesia information management system
    (AIMS), 14
Anesthesia machine, 4*f*
    basic components for fresh gas delivery,
        3–5
        flow meters, 4
        gas analyzers, 4
        gas cylinders/pipeline source, 3, 4*f*
        inspiratory and expiratory limbs, 3
        power source and bellows, 4–5
        pressure regulators, 3
        pressure relief valves, 3–4
        reservoir bag, 5
    CO_2 elimination, 5
    heat and moisture exchangers, 5
    safety devices, 8
    sterilization, 8

Anesthetic breathing circuits
    bag valve mask, 2–3
    circle breathing system, 1–2, 3f
    classification of, 1
    definition of, 1
    Mapleson breathing circuits, 1, 2f
Anesthetic depth monitoring
    bispectral index, 24–25
    expired gas analysis, 24
Anesthetic gas
    calculating output, 7
    pollution, 8
    vapor pressures, 7
Anesthetic Gas to Reduce Explicit Recall
    (BAG-RECALL) trial, 46
Anesthetics. See also Anesthesia
    and cerebral blood flow, 132
    cerebral blood flow and, 130
    epidural anesthesia, 62–63
    general anesthesia, 58–61
    inhaled, 45–51, 132
    issues for specific surgeries, 231–233
    neuraxial anesthesia, 61
    neurologic disorders and, 143–144
    planning, 233
    regional anesthesia, 63
    in renal failure, 174
    spinal anesthesia, 61–62
    types of, 57–64
    unique considerations, 73
    volatile. See Volatile anesthetics
Angiotensin-converting enzyme (ACE)
    inhibitors, 56, 87
Ankle block, 279
Ankylosing spondylitis, 212–213
Antepartum testing, pregnancy and, 240
Anterior cord syndrome, 142
Anterior tibial nerve injury, 281
Anthrax, 297
Antibiotics
    and allergic reactions, 71
    for infection control, 285
        classification, 285–286
Anticholinergics
    for bronchospasm, 72
    for electroconvulsive therapy, 147
Anticoagulation, 192–193, 244
    cardiac bypass and, 105
    for surgery, 56
    for takotsubo cardiomyopathy, 90
Anticonvulsants, for herpes zoster, 265
Antidiuretic hormone (ADH), 169, 199
    defects in secretion, 200
Antiepileptics
    for pain, 258
    for seizures, 144
Antifungal agents, for infection control, 285
Antihistamines, for anaphylaxis, 71
Antihypertensives
    for electroconvulsive therapy, 147
    for surgery, 56
Antimicrobials, for infection control, 285
Antiparasitics, for infection control, 285
Antiphospholipid disease, 251
Antiplatelets, 193
    for surgery, 56
Antispasmodics, 261
Antivirals, for infection control, 285
Anxiolysis, 267
    and analgesia, 57
    for headache, 267
Aorta, coarctation of, 226
Aortic dissections, 114
Aortic insufficiency (AI), 92–93
Aortic sinuses, 80

Aortic stenosis, 91–92
Aortic valve, 80
Aortic valve replacement (AVR), 92
Aortocaval compression, 247
APGAR neonatal score, 240, 241t
Aplastic crisis, with sickle-cell disease, 182
Apnea
    obstructive sleep. See Obstructive sleep
        apnea (OSA)
    of prematurity, 218–219
Apnea–Hypopnea index (AHI), 158
Aprotinin (bovine), for platelet function,
    188
Argatroban, 244t
Arrhythmia, 40, 249
    classification of, 95
    and electrical disorders, 95–98
    implications of, 95
    treatment options, 98–100
Aspiration, 72–73, 247
    precautions, 157–158
Aspirin, 56, 193
    intoxication, 177
    for myocardial infarction, 89
Asthma, 123
Atlanto-occipital dislocation, 289
Atracurium, 40
    metabolism of, 41
Atrial fibrillation, 95–96
Atrial flutter, 96
Atrioventricular cardiac cycle, 81
Atropine, 246
    for arrhythmia, 99
    for fetal heart rate, 239
    for heart rate, 97
    for ophthalmic surgery, 151
Auscultation, 17–18
Autoimmune disorders, pregnancy and,
    250–251
Autologous blood, 187
Automated external defibrillator (AED),
    11, 114
Autonomic hyperreflexia, 142–143
Autonomic nervous system, 135–136,
    135f
Awake intubation, 155
Awake tracheostomy, 155
Axillary block, 276
Azoles, 285
Aztreonam, 285

Back pain
    evaluation of, 262–263
    procedures for, 263–264
    types of, 263
Baclofen, 261
Bacterial meningitis, 245
Bag valve mask, 2–3
Barbiturates
    for CBF and CMR, 132
    for fetal heart rate, 239
    hypercapnia and, 122
    mechanism of, 33
    metabolism/excretion of, 33
    organ system effects by, 33
    pharmacodynamics and kinetics of, 33
    for porphyrias, 183
    side effects of, 33
    somatosensory evoked potentials and, 25
    uses of, 33
Bariatric surgery
    anesthetic management, 163
    pharmacologic considerations for, 163
    preoperative patient risk factors, 162

Baroreceptors, 83
    for nervous systems, 136
Basal ganglia, 129–130
Bathmotropy, 82
Becker muscular dystrophy, 210
Beckwith–Wiedemann syndrome, 229
Benzodiazepines, 33, 86, 246, 273
    for CBF and CMR, 132
    for C-section, 245
    for electroconvulsive therapy, 147
    for fetal heart rate, 239
    hypercapnia and, 122
    for liver disease, 161
    mechanism of, 34
    metabolism/excretion of, 34
    organ system effects by, 34
    pharmacodynamics and kinetics of, 34
    for seizures, 144
    side effects of, 34
    uses of, 34
β-agonists, 84
    for bronchospasm, 72
β-blockers, 56, 85
    for arrhythmia, 98
    for heart rate, 97
    for myocardial infarction, 89
    for ophthalmic surgery, 151
    for pheochromocytoma, 205
β-lactams, 285
Betamethasone, 223, 253
Bezold–Jarish reflex, 247
Bicarbonate, 174
    for hypokalemia, 178
Bier block, 276–277
Bifasicular block, 96–97
Binary statistical analysis, 301–302
Biophysical profile, pregnancy and, 240
Bispectral index, 24–25
Bisphosphonates, for hypercalcemia, 179
Bivalirudin, 244t
Blood disorders
    hematological disorders and anesthetic
        implications, 182–183
    red blood cell. See Red blood cell (RBC)
        disorders
Blood filters, during transfusions, 186
Blood flow, autoregulation of, 84
Blood pressure (BP)
    modulation, 83
    monitoring, 17–19
        invasive, 18–19
        noninvasive, 17–18
Blood product
    allergic reaction, 190
    complications, 191–192
    hemolytic reactions, 190–191
    nonhemolytic febrile reaction, 190
Blood urea nitrogen (BUN), 172
Blunt injury, 290
Bohr effect, 121
Bosentan, for pulmonary hypertension,
    103
Botulism, 297–298
Boyle law, 45
Brachial plexus
    anatomy of, 275, 275f
    blocks, 275–277
    injury, 281
    neuropathy, 68
Bradycardia, 35
Brain death, organ donation after, 77, 310
Brain relaxation, anesthesia for, 145
Brain stem auditory potentials, 25
Brain tumors, 231
Breathing, work of, 119–120

Broken heart syndrome. *See* Takotsubo cardiomyopathy
Bronchial blockers, 125
Bronchiectasis, 123
Bronchodilators, for bronchospasm, 72
Bronchopleural fistula, 126
Bronchopulmonary dysplasia, 223
Bronchospasm, 72
Brown–Sequard syndrome, 142
Brugada syndrome, 97
Bupivacaine, 243, 246, 273
Buprenorphine, 37
Burn surgery, anesthetics for, 232
Butylcholinesterase, 39–40

CABG
    complications and considerations of, 106
    off-pump, 106
Caffeine, 245
    for apnea of prematurity, 219
    for electroconvulsive therapy, 147
    for migraines, 267
Calcium
    balance, in renal, 178–179
    for labor, 242
    for parathyroid disorders, 202
Calcium-channel blockers, 85–86
    for arrhythmia, 98
        for labor, 242
Cannabis abuse, 296
Cannulation, cardiac bypass and, 105
Capnography, 20–21, 21*f*
Capsaicin, 262, 265
Carbamazepine (tegretol), 41
    for seizures, 144
    for trigeminal neuralgia, 265
Carbapenems, 285
Carbon dioxide gas cylinders, 7–8
Carbonic anhydrase inhibitor, 172
Carbon monoxide, 124
Carboprost tromethamine (Hemabate), 242
Carboxyhemoglobin, 124
Carboxyhemoglobinemia, 196–197
Carcinoid syndrome, 206
Carcinoid tumor, 205–206
Cardiac arrest, in neonatal/pediatrics, 234
Cardiac bypass. *See also* Cardiopulmonary bypass
    anesthetic events for, 105–106
    components of, 103–105, 104*f*
    monitoring during, 107
    purpose of, 103
    unique surgeries, 106–107
Cardiac death, organ donation after, 77, 310
Cardiac disorders, pregnancy and, 249–250
Cardiac output
    alveolar uptake and, 47
    assessment and calculation, 24
Cardiac surgery, pediatrics, 226
Cardiac system, sepsis and, 283
Cardiac tamponade, 100–101
Cardiac work, 83
Cardiogenic shock, 284–285
Cardiomyocytes, 81
    stretching of, 82
Cardiopulmonary bypass. *See also* Cardiac bypass
    initiation of, 105–106
    preparation for weaning from, 106
Cardiopulmonary resuscitation (CPR), 114
Cardiovascular system
    barbiturates and, 33
    benzodiazepines and, 34
    blood pressure and flow, 83–84

cardiac mechanical support, 107–108
changes during labor, 237
coronary artery disease and heart failure, 88–91
development in neonates, 221
dexmedetomidine and, 35
etomidate and, 32–33
hemodynamic drugs for, 84–87
ketamine and, 31–32
local anesthetics and, 273
nitrous oxide and, 51
physiology of, 81–83
postoperative issues in, 74
propofol and, 30
structure and mechanisms of, 79–81
volatile anesthetics on, 48–49
Carotid endarterectomy (CEA)
    anesthetics for, 110–111
    indications for surgery, 110
    pathophysiology of, 110
    procedure of, 110
    surgical considerations, 111–112
Case-control studies, for statistical analysis, 301
Catheter ablation, for arrhythmia, 100
Cauda equine, 263
Celiac plexus block, 280
Central anticholinergic syndrome, 75
Central chemoreceptors, 121
Central cord syndrome, 142
Central diabetes insipidus (DI), 200
Central line–associated bloodstream infections, 286
Central nerves system (CNS), 272
    changes during labor, 237
    demyelinating disease of, 43
    local anesthetics and, 273
    volatile anesthetics on, 48–49
Central processing unit, 14
Central venous catheterization, 21–22
Central venous pressure (CVP), 22, 22*f*
Cephalosporins, 285
Cerebellum, 129
Cerebral autoregulation, 130
Cerebral blood flow (CBF), 130
    anesthetics and, 132
    critical levels of, 131
    factors altering or uncoupling, 130
Cerebral cortex, 129
Cerebral metabolic rate (CMR), 130
Cerebral oximetry, 26
Cerebral palsy, 230
Cerebral perfusion pressure (CPP), 130
Cerebral system
    anatomy and physiology, 129–132
        cerebral blood flow, 130–131
        cerebral organization, 129–130
        cerebrospinal fluid, 131–132, 131*f*
    barbiturates and, 33
    benzodiazepines and, 34
    dexmedetomidine and, 35
    etomidate and, 32
    ketamine and, 31
    nitrous oxide and, 51
    propofol and, 30
Cerebrospinal fluid (CSF), 131–132, 131*f*
Certification, for anesthesiologists, 307
Cervical incompetence, 248
Cervical plexus, blocks and landmarks, 274
Charcot-Marie-Tooth disease, 209–210
Charles law, 45
Cheiralgia paresthetica, definitions of, 257
Chemical burning injury, 290–291
Chemoreceptors, for Nervous systems, 136

Chest X-ray (CXR), for preoperative testing, 54
Child–Pugh score, 164
Chi-square test, 303
Chloramphenicol, for plague, 297
Chloroprocaine, 246
Chorioamnionitis, 253
Chronic hypertension, pregnancy and, 249
Chronic obstructive pulmonary disease (COPD), 123
Chronotropy, 82
Cidofovir, for smallpox, 297
Ciprofloxacin, for anthrax, 297
Circle breathing system, 1–2, 3*f*
Circumcision, 232
Cisatracurium, 41, 292
Citrate toxicity, 191–192
Cleft lip/palate, 231
Clindamycin, 285
Clonidine, 56, 261
    for emergence delirium, 219
Clopidogrel, 56, 244*t*
    for myocardial infarction, 89
Cluster headaches, 267
Coagulation
    disorders
        disseminated intravascular coagulation, 184
        hemophilia, 184
        von Willebrand Disease (vWD), 183–184
    pregnancy and, 238
Cocaine abuse, 296
Codeine, 37
    for pain, 258
Cohort studies, for statistical analysis, 301–302
Colloid, for perioperative management, 65
Combined spinal-epidural (CSE), 243
Common peroneal nerve injury, 69, 69*f*, 247
Compartment syndrome, 213
Complex regional pain syndrome (CRPS), 264
Computed tomography (CT), for C-spine injuries, 288–289
Congenital diaphragmatic hernia, 227
Congenital heart disease, 224, 249–250
    classifications of, 224–225
    coarctation of aorta, 226
    hypoplastic left heart, 226
    pediatric cardiac surgery, 226
    tetralogy of fallot, 225, 225*f*
    transposition of the great vessels, 226
    tricuspid atresia, 226
    truncus arteriosus, 225–226
Congenital hip dysplasia, 232
Congenital long QT syndrome, 97
Congenital muscular dystrophy, 210–211
Conn, 204
Constrictive pericarditis, 101
Context-sensitive half-time, 29, 29*f*
Continuous renal replacement therapy, 173
Contraction stress test, pregnancy and, 240
Contrast nephropathy, definition of, 173
Controlled hypotension, 73
Controlled hypothermia, 73
Corneal abrasions, 67
Coronary artery, 81
    disease, 88
Coronary changes, with age, 88
Coronary perfusion, 88
Coronary vessels, 80–81, 80*f*
Corticosteroids

for preterm labor, 253
for traumatic brain injury, 138
Corticotrophin-releasing hormone
(CRH), 199
Coumadin, 56
COX-1, 260
COX-2, 260
CPDA-1, 186
Cranial nerves, 136
Craniosynostosis, 231
Craniotomies, 231
anesthesia for, 145–146
Creatinine, 172
Cricothyroidotomy, 61
Critical care myopathy, 293
Critical pressure, 45
Critical temperature, 45
Cross-sectional studies, for statistical
analysis, 301
Croup (laryngotracheobronchitis), 229
Crouzon syndrome, 230
Cryoprecipitate, 190
C-section
epidural and spinal anesthesia for,
243–245
general anesthesia, 245–246
regional anesthesia for, 245
risks, 246–247
C-spine injuries, 288–289
types and management of, 289
Cushing disease, 204
Cyanide abuse, 298
Cyclobenzaprine, 261
Cyclosporine, for kidney transplantation,
166
Cystic fibrosis, 123

Dabigatran, 244t
Dampening, arterial Line, 19, 19f
Dantrolene, for malignant hyperthermia, 67
Daptomycin, 285
DDAVP
for isovolemic hypernatremia, 177
for von Willebrand Disease, 184
Deep brain stimulator, 146
Deep cervical plexus block, 110, 274
Deep vein thrombosis (DVT) prophylaxis,
57
Defibrillation, for arrhythmia, 100
Defibrillators
cardioversion of, 12
function of, 11
types of, 11–12
Dehydration, signs of, 222
Delirium, 75
Delirium tremens (DT), 296
Delta gap (DG), 176
Demeclocycline, for isovolemic
hyponatremia, 178
Dependence, definition of, 295
Depolarizing muscle relaxant
metabolism of, 40–41
pharmacokinetics and
pharmacodynamics of, 40
side effects of, 40
Depth of anesthesia. See Anesthetic depth
monitoring
Dermatome, 243
Desflurane, 46, 47
for CBF and CMR, 132
metabolism of, 48
and unique properties, 49–50
Desmopressin, for platelet function, 187
Developmental disorders, in pediatrics, 230

Dexamethasone, 200
for brain relaxation, 145
for hyperthyroidism, 201
for postoperative nausea and vomiting,
76
Dexmedetomidine, 261
for emergence delirium, 219
mechanism of, 35
metabolism/excretion of, 35
organ system effects by, 35
pharmacodynamics and kinetics of, 35
side effects of, 35
uses of, 34–35
Dextran, 65, 112, 190
Diabetes
anesthetic considerations, 203–204
classification of, 202
emergent conditions, 202–203
Diabetes insipidus, 140
central, 200
Diabetic ketoacidosis (DKA), 202–203
Dialysis, hemofiltration and, 173
Diastolic dysfunction, 89
Diazepam, 34
Diffusion hypoxia, 51
Digoxin, for arrhythmia, 98–99
Dihydropyridines, 86
Dipyridamole, 193
Direct laryngoscopy, 60
Direct thrombin inhibitors, 193
Discogenic pain, 263
Disodium edentate, 30
Disseminated intravascular coagulation
(DIC), 184, 247
Diuretics, 170–172
for kidney transplantation, 166
for negative-pressure pulmonary edema,
72
sites of action, 172f
for takotsubo cardiomyopathy, 90
Dobutamine, 84
sepsis and, 284
Donor blood, release of, 187
Dopamine, 85, 200
sepsis and, 284
Dopexamine, 84
Doppler effect, 9
Doppler ultrasound, 18
for cardiac output, 24
for fetal heart rate monitoring, 239
Double-lumen tube (DLT), 125
Downers, 85

Down Syndrome. See Trisomy 21
Doxycycline, for plague, 297
Dromotropy, 82
Droperidol, for postoperative nausea and
vomiting, 76
Drowning, 291
Duchenne muscular dystrophy, 43, 210
Dutch Echocardiographic Cardiac
Risk Evaluation Applying Stress
Echocardiography (DECREASE), 56
Dye dilution, for cardiac output, 24
Dysesthesia, definitions of, 257
Dystrophies, muscular. See Muscular
dystrophies

Ear surgery, anesthetic considerations for,
155
Ebola, 298
ECG monitoring, 17, 18f
Echinocandins, 285
Echothiophate, 40

for ophthalmic surgery, 151
Ectopic pregnancy, 247
Edrophonium, 42
Electrical burning injury, 290
Electrical cardioversion, for arrhythmia,
96, 100
Electrical disorders, arrhythmia and, 95–98
Electrical stimulation, for back pain,
263–264
Electricity
defibrillators, 11–12
in operating room, 12
pacemakers, 10–11
Electrocardiogram (ECG)
for preoperative testing, 54
Electrocautery, in operating room, 12
Electroconvulsive therapy (ECT), anesthesia
for, 146–147
Electroencephalography (EEG)
for depth of anesthesia, 24–25
for nervous system, 25–26
for vascular surgery, 111
Electrolyte disorders, in renal, 177–179
hypercalcemia, 179
hyperkalemia, 178
hypernatremia, 177
hypocalcemia, 179
hypokalemia, 178
hyponatremia, 177–178
osmolality, 178
Electromyography (EMG), for nervous
system, 26
Emergence delirium, in pediatrics, 219
Endobronchial intubation, 124
Endocarditis prophylaxis, 94–95
Endocrine system
anatomy and function of, 199–200
disorders
adrenal, 204–205
neuroendocrine tumors, 205–206
pancreatic, 202–204
pituitary, 200
pregnancy and, 250
thyroid and parathyroid, 201–202
sepsis and, 283
Endotracheal tube (ETT), 216–217
exchangers, 60
placement, 60
types of, 59–60
End-stage liver disease (ESLD), 164
Enflurane, 46
metabolism of, 48
and unique properties, 50
Enoxaparin, 244t
Ephedrine, 84
for heart rate, 97
for hypotension, 247
Epicardial pacemaker, 10
Epidural analgesia, delivery mechanisms,
259–260
Epidural anesthesia, 62–63
for flail chest, 290
for labor/C-section, 242–245
temperature regulation and, 243–244
Epidural hematoma, 138
Epidural steroid injection, 263
Epiglottitis, 229
Epinephrine, 84–85, 200
for anaphylaxis, 71
for heart rate, 97, 108
liposuction and, 163–164
to local anesthetics, 272
protamine and, 193
sepsis and, 284
for takotsubo cardiomyopathy, 90

Epoprostenol, for pulmonary hypertension, 103
Eptifibatide, 244*t*
Error, definition of, 310
Erythropoietin, 187
Esmolol, 246
Esophageal detector device, 21
Essential hypertension, 87
Estrogen, 200
EtCO₂, 20–21
Etomidate
    for CBF and CMR, 132
    for electroconvulsive therapy, 147
    mechanism of, 32
    metabolism/excretion of, 32
    organ system effects by, 32–33
    pharmacodynamics and kinetics of, 32
    for porphyrias, 183
    side effects of, 33
    somatosensory evoked potentials and, 25
    uses of, 32
Evoked potentials, 25
Expiratory muscles, 117–118
Eye, anatomy of, 149*f*

Facet joint pain, 263
Facet medial branch blocks, 263
Facial ulcerations, 72
Failed back surgery syndrome, 263
Fat emboli, 213
Femoral block, 278
Femoral nerve injury, 69, 247, 281
Fenoldopam, 87
Fentanyl, 36, 243
    for myringotomy, 231
    for pain, 258, 259
Fetal heart rate (FHR), 239–240
Fetal malposition, 253
Fetal nonstress test, pregnancy and, 240
Fetal pulse oximetry, 240
Fetal scalp blood gas, 240
Fiber-optic catheter, 26
Fiberoptic intubation, 60
Fibromyalgia, 266
Fick principle, for cardiac output, 24
Fire, operating room and, 12–13
Flail chest, 290
Flumazenil, 34
    for hypoventilation, 74
Fluoroquinolones, 285
Focused assessment with sonography for trauma (FAST), 287–288, 288*f*
Follicle-stimulating hormone (FSH), 199
Fondaparinux, 244*t*
Fospropofol, 30
Frank–Starling relationship, 82–83, 82*f*
Free water, for perioperative management, 65
Fresh frozen plasma (FFP), 186
    transfusion, 188–189
Furosemide, 191
    for brain relaxation, 145
    for hypercalcemia, 179
    for intracranial hypertension, 139

Gabapentin, 261, 265
Gas cylinders, 7–8
Gastric reflux medication, for surgery, 56–57
Gastroesophageal reflux disease, 157–158
Gastrointestinal system, 36
    changes during labor, 238
    ulcers and bleeding, 260
Gastroschisis, 228
Gay-Lussac law, 45

General anesthesia, 151
    airway assessment and, 58–61
    complications of, 218
    for C-section, 245–256
    effects of, 26
    nitrous oxide for, 51
    for ophthalmic surgery, 151
    for pediatrics, 217
    for vascular surgery, 110–111
    vs. local anesthesia, 111
Generic Propofol, 71
Genitofemoral block, 281
Genitourinary system
    abdominal organ transplantation, 164–165
    bariatric surgery, 162–163
    general surgery considerations
        abdominal compartment syndrome, 161–162
        aspiration precautions, 157–158
        hepatic dysfunction, 159–161
        obesity, 158–159
    intestinal obstruction, 163
    laparoscopy, 157
    liposuction, 163–164
    lithotripsy, 166–167
    transurethral resection of prostate, 166
Gentamicin, for plague, 297
Gestational diabetes, 250
Gestational hypertension, pregnancy and, 249
Glasgow Coma Score, 137–138
Glomerular filtration rate (GFR), 172
Glossopharyngeal nerve, 118
Glucagon, 200
    for heart rate, 108
Glucocorticoids, 200
Glucose
    control in intensive care unit, 293
    management in diabetes, 203
    in pediatrics, 222
    requirements for perioperative management, 65
Glucose-6-phosphate deficiency (G6PD), 197
Glycoprotein IIb/IIIa inhibitors, 193
Glycopyrrolate, for heart rate, 97
Goldenhar syndrome, 230
Gonadotropin-releasing hormone (GRH), 199
Gray matter, 129
Great vessels, transposition of, 226
Growth hormone (GH), 199
Growth hormone–releasing hormone (GHRH), 199
Guillain–Barré syndrome, 209

H2-blockers, 57
    for postoperative nausea and vomiting, 76
Haldane effect, 121
Haloperidol, for postoperative nausea and vomiting, 76
Halo placement, 231–232
Halothane, 46, 49
    metabolism of, 48
    and unique properties, 50
Headaches, 267. *See also specific Headaches*
    postdural puncture, 244
Head and neck blocks, 274
Health Insurance Portability and Accountability Act (HIPPA), 310
Heart
    block, 96

disease
    interventions, 90–91
    medical management, 91
    risk factors and stratification, 90
failure
    causes of, 89
    classification of, 90
    definition of, 89
function, definitions of, 82
newborn, 221
position of, 79, 79*f*
rate, 222
transplantation, 108–110
HEENT system
    ophthalmic anatomy and physiology, 149–151
    ophthalmic anesthesia for, 151–153
    otolaryngology surgery, 154–155
    preoperative ophthalmic assessment, 151
    specific ophthalmic situations, 153
Helium gas cylinders, 7
Hematologic system
    anticoagulants, 192–193
    antiplatelets, 193
    blood disorders. *See* Blood disorders
    changes during labor, 238
    coagulation disorders, 183–184
    infectious disorders, 194–196
    non-RBC transfusion medicine, 188–190
    platelet disorders, 184–185
    reactions and complications, 190–192
    transfusion medicine, 185–188
Hemodialysis, 173
Hemodynamic drugs
    for C-section, 246
    for heart disease, 84–87
Hemodynamic effects, on kidney, 174
Hemofiltration, and dialysis, 173
Hemoglobin (Hb), 174
    in pediatrics, 222
Hemophilia A, 184
Hemophilia B, 184
Hemorrhage, intra-axial and extra-axial, 138
Hemothorax, 289–290
Heparin, 192–193, 244*t*
    cardiac bypass and, 105
Heparin-induced thrombocytopenia (HIT), 185
Hepatic system
    anatomy, 159
    changes during labor, 238–239
    dysfunction, 159–161
    liver function and, 159–160, 159*f*
    sepsis and, 283
Hepatitis B, 195–196
Hepatitis C, 196
Hepatopulmonary syndrome, 160
Hepatorenal syndrome, 160–161
Hepatotoxicity, 49
Herbals, for surgery, 57
Hereditary angioneurotic edema, 143
Hereditary hemorrhagic telangiectasia. *See* Osler–Weber–Rendu syndrome
Hereditary spastic paraplegia, 210
Herpes zoster, 265
Hetastarch, 65
Hiatal hernia, 158
Highly active antiretroviral therapy (HAART), 252
Hippocampus, 129
Histamine, 37
HIV/AIDS, 194–195
    blood product and, 191
    pregnancy and, 252
Horner syndrome, 245

Humate-P, 184
Humidity, 45
Huntington chorea, 43
Hurler syndrome, 230
Hydralazine, 87
  for hypertension, 249
Hydrocephalus, 231
Hydrocortisone, 200
Hydromorphone, 36
  for pain, 258
Hyperalgesia, definitions of, 257
Hyperbaric oxygen, 73
Hypercalcemia, 98, 179
Hypercapnia, effects of, 122
Hyperesthesia, definitions of, 257
Hyperexcitable ion channel myopathies, 211
Hyperglycemia, 206, 293
Hyperglycemic hyperosmolar syndrome
  (HHS), 203
Hyperkalemia, 40, 98, 178, 192
Hyperkalemic periodic paralysis, 211–212
Hyperoxia, 121
Hyperparathyroid, 202
Hyperpathia, definitions of, 257
Hypertension (HTN)
  anesthetic considerations, 88
  chronic, pregnancy and, 249
  essential, 87
  gestational, 249
  intracranial. See Intracranial hypertension
  morbidity, 88
  portopulmonary, 161
  pregnancy and, 248–249
  preoperative evaluation, 88
  pulmonary, 124
  types of, 87–88
Hyperthyroidism, 201, 250
Hypertonic saline
  for brain relaxation, 145
  for intracranial hypertension, 139
  for subarachnoid hemorrhage, 142
Hypertriglyceridemia, 31
Hypertrophic cardiomyopathy, 94
Hyperventilation
  for brain relaxation, 145
  for cardiovascular system, 273
  for intracranial hypertension, 139–140
Hypervolemic hypernatremia, 177
Hypervolemic hyponatremia, 178
Hypnosis, 267
Hypnotics, for induction of anesthesia,
  29–35
Hypoalgesia, definitions of, 257
Hypocalcemia, 179, 222–223
Hypoesthesia, definitions of, 257
Hypogastric plexus block, 280
Hypoglycemia, 293
Hypokalemia, 98, 178
Hypokalemic periodic paralysis, 212
Hypoparathyroid, 202
Hypophosphatemia, 202
Hypoplastic left heart, 226
Hypotension, 35, 74, 246–247
  controlled, 73
Hypothalamus, anatomy and function of, 199
Hypothermia, 75–76, 192
  consequences of, 66
  controlled, 73
Hypothyroidism, 201, 250
Hypoventilation, 74
Hypovolemia, 74
  response to, 169
Hypovolemic hypernatremia, 177
Hypovolemic hyponatremia, 177
Hypovolemic shock, 284

Hypoxemia, 73–74
Hypoxia, 121
Hypoxic pulmonary vasoconstriction, 121

Idiopathic thrombocytopenia purpura
  (ITP), 185
Ilioinguinal block, 280–281
Iloprost, for pulmonary hypertension, 103
Immunoglobulin A (IgA), 191
Impedance, for cardiac output, 24
Increta, 252
Indomethacin, 242
Induction, 59
Induction drugs
  hypnotics, 29–35
  muscle relaxants, 38–43
  opiates/opioids, 35–38
  pharmacokinetics and
    pharmacodynamics, 29
Infant airway, 216
  vs. adult airway, 216f, 221
Infection control, in intensive care unit
  antibiotics and, 285
  antimicrobial resistance, 285–286
  central line infections, 286
  precautions for, 286
Infectious disorders, pregnancy and,
  251–252
Informed consent, 309
Informed refusal, 309
Infraclavicular block, 276
Infrared absorption, for depth of anesthesia,
  24
Inhalational induction, 217
Inhalational injury, 233
Inotropy, 82
Inspiratory muscles, 117
Insulin, 200
Insulinoma, 204
Intercostal block, 279
Internal capsule, 130
Interscalene block, 275
Intestinal obstruction, 163
Intra-aortic balloon pump (IABP), 93, 107,
  108f
Intracranial aneurysms, 146
Intracranial hypertension, 138
  clinical signs of intracranial pressure, 139
  intracranial pressure monitoring, 139
  treatment for, 139–140
Intracranial pressure (ICP). See Intracranial
  hypertension
Intraoperative autotransfusion, 187
Intrapulmonary hemorrhage, 126
Intravenous anesthetic induction, 217
Intravenous fluid selection, for perioperative
  management, 64–65
Intraventricular hemorrhage, 223
Intubation
  awake, 155
  endobronchial, 124
  fiberoptic, 60
  retrograde, 60
Intussusception, 232
Ion channel myopathies, 211
Ischemic optic neuropathy, 67
Isoflurane, 46, 47
  for CBF and CMR, 132
  metabolism of, 48
  and unique properties, 49
Isoproterenol, 84
  for heart rate, 97, 108
Isovolemic hypernatremia, 177
Isovolemic hyponatremia, 177–178

Jehovah Witnesses, 187–188
Jugular venous bulb oxygen saturation, 26
Junctional escape rhythms, 97
Juvenile rheumatoid arthritis, 230

Ketamine, 217
  for CBF and CMR, 132
  complications of, 218
  in C-section, 245–246
  for intraocular pressure, 150
  for liver disease, 161
  mechanism of, 31
  metabolism of, 31
  for noncardiac surgery and chronic
    disease, 227
  organ system effects by, 31–32
  pharmacodynamics and kinetics of, 31
  for porphyrias, 183
  side effects of, 32
  somatosensory evoked potentials and, 25
  uses of, 31
Kidney
  hemodynamic effects on, 174
  structure of, 171f
  transplantation, 165–166
Kleihauer–Betke test, 253
Klippel–Feil syndrome, 230
Korotkoff, 18

Labetalol, 246
  for hypertension, 249
Labor. See also Pregnancy
  and C-section risks, 246–247
  drugs for, 241–242
  epidural and spinals, 242–245
  physiology of, 237–239
  preterm, 254
  progress of, 244
  stages of, 241
Lactated ringers (LR), 64
Lactic acidosis, 176–177
Lambert–Eaton syndrome, 212
Laryngeal mask airway (LMA), 59
Laryngospasm, 72, 218
Lasers, in operating room, 12
Lateral femoral cutaneous block, 278
Lateral femoral cutaneous nerve, 69–70
Laudanosine, 41
Left atrial pressure, 23
Left atrium (LA), 79–80
Left bundle branch block (LBBB), 96
Left ventricle (LV), 80
Left ventricular assist device (LVAD), 108, 109f
Left ventricular end-diastolic pressure, 23
Lepirudin, 244t
Levodopa, for Parkinson disease, 144
Lidocaine, 217, 276
  for arrhythmia, 99
  for Bier block, 276
  for C-section, 246
  for labor/C-section, 243
  liposuction and, 163–164
Lighted stylet, 60
Limb-girdle muscular dystrophy, 210
Limbic system, 129
Lincosamines, 41
Line-isolation monitor, in operating room, 12
Linezolid, 285
Liposuction, 163–164
Lithotripsy, 166–167
Liver
  anatomy and function of, 199
  anesthetic management in disease, 161

development in neonates, 222
disease markers, 160
failure, acetaminophen and, 260
function, 159–160, 159*f*
transplantation, 164–165
Lobectomy/pneumonectomy, for lungs, 125
Local anesthetics
additives to, 272
and allergic reactions, 71
allergic reactions of, 272
cervical plexus blocks and landmarks, 274
classification of, 271
for C-section, 246
head and neck blocks, 274
for herpes zoster, 265
for labor or C-section, 243
lower extremity blocks and landmarks, 277–279
mechanism of, 271–272, 271*f*
nerve injuries and, 281
qualities of, 272
systemic absorption, 272
systemic toxicity of, 272–273
thoracic, abdominal, and pelvic blocks and, 279–281
upper extremity blocks and landmarks, 275–277
Long thoracic nerve injury, 68–69
Loop diuretics, 171–172
for hypervolemic hyponatremia, 178
for isovolemic hyponatremia, 178
Lorazepam, 34
Lower extremity
blocks and landmarks, 277–279
nerve injuries, 69–70
Lumbar epidural, 242–243
Lumbar plexus
anatomy of, 277, 277*f*
blocks, 277–278
Lumbar sympathetic block, for labor or C-section, 246
Lumbosacral trunk, 247
Lungs. *See also* Respiratory system
flow–volume loops, 122–123, 122*f*
nonrespiratory functions of, 120
obstructive disorders, 123–124
one-lung ventilation, 124–125
pulmonary hypertension, 124
smoking cessation, 124
thoracic surgery, 125–126
transplantation, 110, 126
volumes, 118–119
zones, 118, 119*f*
Lupus, 213, 250–251
Lusitropy, 82
Luteinizing hormone (LH), 199

Magnesium
for eclampsia, 249
for labor, 241–242
for ventricular tachycardia, 98
Magnetic resonance imaging (MRI), 13–14
for C-spine injuries, 289
Mainstem bronchus, right and left, 117, 118*t*
Malignant hyperthermia, 66–67
Mallampati classification, 58–59, 58*f*
Malnourishment, 292
Malpractice, medical, 307–308
Mannitol, 191
for brain relaxation, 145
for intracranial hypertension, 139
for subarachnoid hemorrhage, 142
Mapleson breathing circuits, 1, 2*f*, 215

Marfan syndrome, 230, 251
Mass spectrometry, for depth of anesthesia, 24
Maternal ultrasound, pregnancy and, 240
MAZE procedure, for arrhythmia, 100
Mebendazole, 285
Meconium, 240–241
Median nerve injury, 281
Mediastinal mass, 124, 232
Mediastinoscopy, for lungs, 125
Medical informatics, 14
Medical malpractice, 307–308
Medulla oblongata, 130
Megaloblastic anemia, 51
Mendelson syndrome, 157
Meninges, 134
Meningomyelocele, 143
Meperidine, 37, 243
Meralgia paresthetica, definitions of, 257
Meta-analysis, 302
Metabolic acidosis, 175, 176
Metabolic alkalosis, 175–176
Metabolic equivalent of task (MET), 54, 83
Metabolic syndrome, 158–159
Metabolism/excretion
acetaminophen and, 260
barbiturates and, 33
benzodiazepines and, 34
dexmedetomidine and, 35
etomidate and, 32
ketamine and, 31
propofol and, 30
Metformin, for type 2 diabetics, 203
Methadone, 37–38
Methemoglobinemia, 196
Methohexital, 33, 217
for electroconvulsive therapy, 147
for sedation, 64
Methyldopa, for hypertension, 249
Methylergometrine, 242, 245
Methyl methacrylate, 213
Methylparaben, 272
Metoclopramide, 57
for postoperative nausea and vomiting, 76
Metronidazole, 285
Midazolam, 34, 217
for emergence delirium, 219
somatosensory evoked potentials and, 25
Migraines, 267
Milrinone, 85
for pulmonary hypertension, 103
Mineralocorticoids, 200
Minimum alveolar concentration (MAC), 217
application of, 46
for common anesthetics, 46
definition of, 45
factors affecting, 45–46
in pediatrics, 218
Misoprostol, 242
for labor, 241
Mitochondrial myopathies, 211
Mitral insufficiency, 93–94
Mitral stenosis, 93
Mitral valve replacement (MVR), 93
Mitral valves, 80
Mixed venous saturation, 23
Model for End-Stage Liver Disease (MELD), 164
Molar pregnancy, 248
Monitored Anesthesia Care (MAC), 57–58
Monro–Kellie hypothesis, 138–139
Morphine, 36–37, 243
for C-section, 245
for pain, 258, 259

Motor evoked potentials (MEP), 25
Multifocal atrial tachycardia, 96
Multiple sclerosis (MS), 43, 209, 251
Muscle relaxants
and allergic reactions, 71
conditions affecting use, 42–43
depolarizing. *See* Depolarizing muscle relaxant
enhancers of, 41
for induction of anesthesia, 38–43
interference of, 39
mechanism of action, 38–39
neuromuscular blockade monitoring, 41–42
neuromuscular junction, 38, 38*f*
nondepolarizing. *See* Nondepolarizing muscle relaxants
shorteners of, 41
Muscle rigidity, 36
Muscular dystrophies
definition of, 210
perioperative implications, 211
types of, 210–211
Musculoskeletal disorders, in pediatrics, 230
Myalgias, 40
Myasthenia gravis, 42–43, 212, 251
Myasthenic syndrome, 43
Myelomeningocele, 228–229
Myocardial infarction (MI)
antianginal treatment, 89
complications of, 89
coronary artery and, 89
diagnosis of, 88–89
Myofascial pain syndrome, 263, 266
Myopathies, 211–212. *See also specific myopathies*
Myotonia congenital, 211
Myotonic dystrophy, 43
Myotonic muscular dystrophy, 211
Myringotomy, 231
Myxedema coma, 201

N-acetylcysteine, 173, 260
Naloxone
for hypoventilation, 74
reversal, 38
Naltrexone, reversal, 38
Nasal surgery, Anesthetic considerations for, 155
National Fire Protection Association (NFPA), 12
National practitioner data bank, 308
Neck blocks, 274
Necrotizing enterocolitis (NEC), 224
Needlestick injury, 196
Negative-pressure pulmonary edema, 72
Negligence, requirements, 307
Neonatal lobar emphysema, 228
Neonatal/pediatric codes, 234
Neonatal respiratory distress syndrome, 223
Neonates
anatomy and physiology, 221–223
body distribution, 222
conditions and anesthetic considerations, 227–228
neonatal vitals and laboratory values, 222–223
organ system development, 221–222
pulmonary system development in, 221
temperature regulation, 222
in utero development, 221
Neostigmine, 42
Nerve injuries, 281

Nervous system, 25–26
    autonomic nervous system, 135–136,
        135f
    cerebral oxygenation and blood flow, 26
    chemoreceptors and baroreceptors, 136
    and communication, 136–137
    cranial nerves, 136
    electroencephalography and, 25–26
    electromyography and, 26
    evoked potentials, 25
    intracranial pressure, 26
Nesiritide, 87
Neuraxial anesthesia
    caudal, 220–221, 220f
    epidural, 220
    for postoperative pain, 259
    spinal, 219–220
    use of, 61
Neuroblastomas, 232
Neuroendocrine tumors, 205–206
Neurologic disorders
    and anesthetic implications, 143–144
    hereditary angioneurotic edema, 143
    parkinson disease, 144
    polio, 144
    pregnancy and, 251
    pseudotumor cerebri, 144
    seizures, 144
    spina bifida occulta, 143
    stroke, 143–144
Neurologic system
    anesthetics and cerebral blood flow, 132
    cerebral anatomy and physiology,
        129–132
    disorders associated with intracranial
        pathology, 138–141
    nervous systems, 135–136
    neurologic disorders and anesthetic
        implications, 143–145
    neuromuscular synapses and
        communication, 136–137
    postoperative issues in, 75
    spinal cord anatomy, 132–135
    spinal pathology, 142–143
    subarachnoid hemorrhage, 141–142
    traumatic brain injury, 137–138
Neurolytic blocks, 279–280
Neuromuscular blockade
    sequence of, 41
    somatosensory evoked potentials and, 25
    train of four monitoring, 41–42, 43f
Neuromuscular junction, 38, 38f
Neuromuscular synapses, and
    communication, 137f
    action potential, 136–137
    structure of, 136
Neuromuscular system
    and musculoskeletal system
        muscular dystrophies, 210–211
        myopathies, 211–212
        neuropathic diseases, 209–210
        orthopedic conditions, 213
        rheumatoid conditions, 212–213
    volatile anesthetics on, 48–49
Neuromyotonia, 211
Neuropathic diseases
    amyotrophic lateral sclerosis, 210
    Charcot–Marie–Tooth disease, 209–210
    Guillain–Barré syndrome, 209
    hereditary spastic paraplegia, 210
    multiple sclerosis, 209
    spinobulbar muscular atrophy, 210
Neuropathic pain, 257
Neurosurgery, anesthetics for, 231
Newborn

distress, 234
    heart, 221
    transient tachypnea of, 223
    vs. adults airway, 221
New York Heart Association (NYHA), 90
Nicardipine, 86
Nifedipine, 86, 242, 249
Nimodipine, 86, 141
Nitric oxide, for pulmonary hypertension,
    103
Nitroglycerin, 87, 89
Nitrous oxide (N_2O), 46, 51, 151
    for CBF and CMR, 132
    gas cylinders, 7
Nociceptive pain, 257
Nondepolarizing muscle relaxants
    for bariatric surgery, 163
    classes of, 40
    metabolism of, 41
    pharmacodynamics and kinetics, 40–41
Nonopioid analgesics, and adjuvants,
    260–262
Nonsteroidal anti-inflammatory drugs
    (NSAIDs), 260–261
    for labor, 242
    for migraines, 267
    for pain, 258
    for tension, 267
Norepinephrine, 84, 200
    for heart rate, 108
    reuptake inhibitors, 265
    sepsis and, 284
Normal saline (NS), 64–65, 145
Normoglycemia in the Intensive Care-
    Evaluation (NICE-SUGAR) trial, 293
Notalgia paresthetica (NP), definitions of,
    257
Null hypothesis, 302
Nutrition, 292–293
    caloric needs, in intensive care unit, 292
    methods of support, 292–293
    re-feeding syndrome, 293

Obesity, 158–159
    obstetrical risks and, 250
Obesity hypoventilation syndrome, 158
Obstetrics. See Labor; C-section
Obstructive disorders
    anesthetic management, 123
    asthma, 123
    bronchiectasis, 123
    chronic obstructive pulmonary disease,
        123
    constrictive pericarditis, 101
    cystic fibrosis, 123
    mediastinal masses, 124
    obstructive sleep apnea, 123
    pericardial effusion and cardiac
        tamponade, 100–101
    pulmonary embolism, 101–102
Obstructive sleep apnea (OSA), 123
    obesity and, 158
Obturator block, 278
Obturator nerve injury, 69, 281
Octreotide, for carcinoid tumor, 206
Oculocardiac reflex (OCR), 150
Oligohydramnios, 240
Omphalocele, 228
Ondansetron, for postoperative nausea and
    vomiting, 76
One-lung ventilation, 124–125
Open-eye injury, 153
Operating room
    and airway fires, 12–13

costs, 309
    interests, 308
    scheduling, 308
    setup, 215–217
Ophthalmic anesthesia, 151–153
Opiates/opioids, for induction of
    anesthesia, 36t
    mode of delivery, 35
    non-analgesic effects by, 35–36
    properties of, 36–38
    receptors and their functions, 35
    reversal, 38
Opioids
    analgesics, for pain, 258–260
    for bariatric surgery, 163
    for CBF and CMR, 132
    for cerebral palsy, 230
    for C-section, 245
    for emergence delirium, 219
    for fetal heart rate, 239
    hypercapnia and, 122
    for labor or C-section, 243
    for liver disease, 161
    for myocardial infarction, 89
    for obstructive sleep apnea, 158
    somatosensory evoked potentials and, 25
Organ donation
    after brain death, 77, 310
    after cardiac death, 77, 310
Organophosphates abuse, 298
Organ transplantation
    abdominal, 164–165
    heart, 108–110
    kidney, 165–166
    liver, 164–165
    lungs, 110, 126
    pancreas, 166
Orthopedic surgery, anesthetics for, 232
Oscillometry, 18
Oseltamivir, 285
Osler–Weber–Rendu syndrome, 183
Osmolality, 178
Osmotic diuretics, 172
Osteogenesis imperfect, 230
Otolaryngology, anesthetics for, 231
Oxycodone, for pain, 258
Oxygen analyzer, 19–20
    inspired oxygen, 19–20
    pulse oximetry, 20
Oxygen gas cylinders, 7
Oxyhemoglobin dissociation curve, 120–
    121, 120f
Oxytocin, 199, 242
    for labor, 241

Pacemakers
    interrogation of, 10–11
    intraoperative considerations, 11
    nomenclature, 10
    postoperative considerations, 11
    preoperative considerations, 11
    risk of, 11
    types of, 10
Packed red blood cells (PRBCs), 185–186
PACU discharge, 76–77
Pain
    back. See Back pain
    definitions of, 257
    fibers, 257–258
    headache, 267
    nonopioid analgesics and adjuvants,
        260–262
    opiods and delivery options, 258–260
    pathways, 258

syndromes and conditions, 264–266
types of, 257
World Health Organization analgesic
ladder, 258
Pancreas
anatomy and function of, 200
disorders, 202–204
transplantation, 166
Pancreatitis, 31
Para-aminobenzoic acid metabolite, 272
Paracervical block, for labor or C-section,
246
Paralysis, abdominal aortic aneurysms and,
113–114
Parasympathetic nervous system (PNS), 136
Parathyroid
anatomy and function of, 199
disorders, 202
Paravertebral block, 279, 280f
Paresthesia, definitions of, 257
Parkinson disease, 144
Patient-controlled analgesia (PCA), 259
Patient safety, 310
Pectus excavatum, 232
Pediatrics
anesthesia
operating room, 215–217
setup and type, 215–221
anxiolysis and analgesia, 57
diseases and conditions, 229–230
sedation, 233
Pelvic blocks, 280–281
Pelvic instability, 290
Pelvic trauma, 290
Percreta, 252
Peribulbar blocks, 152–153, 152f
Pericardial effusion, 100–101
Periodic paralysis, 211
Peripartum cardiomyopathy, 250
Peripheral chemoreceptors, 122
Peripheral neuropathy, 264–265
Peritoneal dialysis, 173
Peritonsillar abscess, 229
Permanent pacemaker, 10
Peroneal nerve injury, 281
Phantom limb pain (PLP), 265–266
Phenothiazines, for postoperative nausea
and vomiting, 76
Phenoxybenzamine, for
pheochromocytoma, 205
Phentolamine
for autonomic hyperreflexia, 143
for pheochromocytoma, 205
Phenylalkylamine, 86
Phenylephrine, 84
for hypotension, 247
for ophthalmic surgery, 151
Phenytoin, 41
for arrhythmia, 99
for seizures, 144
Pheochromocytoma, 205
Phosgene abuse, 298–299
Phosphate, for parathyroid disorders, 202
Pickwickian syndrome. See Obesity
hypoventilation syndrome
Pierre Robin syndrome, 229
Pilocarpine, for ophthalmic surgery, 151
Piperacillin/tazobactam, 285
Pituitary
anatomy and function of, 199
disorders, 200
Placental abruption, 252
Placental attachment, disorders of, 252
Placental previa, 252
Placental transfer, 246

Placenta, retained, 253
Plague, 297
Platelets
disorders
heparin-induced thrombocytopenia,
185
idiopathic thrombocytopenia purpura,
185
thrombocytopenia, 184–185
thrombotic thrombocytopenia
purpura, 185
pregnancy and, 238
storage, 186
transfusion, 189–190
Polio, 144
Polycythemias, 182
Polyhydramnios, 240
Popliteal block, 278
Porphyrias, 183
Portopulmonary hypertension, 161
Posterior cord syndrome, 142
Postoperative cognitive dysfunction, 75
Postoperative nausea and vomiting
(PONV), 76, 267
Potassium balance, in real, 178
Potassium-wasting diuretics, for
hypokalemia, 178
Power analysis, 304
Prednisone, 200
Preeclampsia/eclampsia
anesthetic implications, 249
diagnosis of, 248
management and treatment, 249
morbidity and mortality, 248–249
pathophysiology of, 248
risk factors of, 248
Pregnancy. See also Labor
complicated/high-risk, 247–252
delivery complications, 252–254
drug safety in, 254t
ectopic, 247
molar, 248
myasthenia gravis and, 212
Prematurity, disorders of, 223–224
Preoperative medications
management of chronic medications,
56–57
management of herbals, 57
Preoxygenation, 59
Pressure transducer, 19
Preterm labor, 253
Prilocaine, 217, 276
Primary certification, 307
Procainamide, 41
for arrhythmia, 100
Professional liability insurance, 308
Progesterone, 200
Propofol, 217, 227
and allergic reactions, 71
for bariatric surgery, 163
for CBF and CMR, 132
for C-section, 245
for electroconvulsive therapy, 147
for emergence delirium, 219
for liver disease, 161
mechanism of, 29–30
metabolism of, 30
organ system effects by, 30
pharmacodynamics and kinetics of, 30
for porphyrias, 183
for sedation, 64
for seizures, 144
side effects of, 30–31
uses of, 29
Propofol infusion syndrome, 31

Propofol-related infusion syndrome (PRIS),
219
Propranolol, for hyperthyroidism, 201
Propylthiouracil, for hyperthyroidism, 201
Prostaglandin E_1, 218
Protamine, 106, 193
Prothrombin complex concentrates (PCC),
190
Proton pump inhibitors, for postoperative
nausea and vomiting, 76
Pruritis, 36
Pseudocholinesterase. See
Butylcholinesterase
Pseudotumor cerebri, 144
Psoas block, 277–278
Psychogenic pain, 257
Pudendal block, 281
for labor or C-section, 246
Pulmonary artery (PA)
catheterization, 22–23, 23f
occlusion pressure, 23
pressure, 23
Pulmonary contusion, 290
Pulmonary embolism, 101–102
Pulmonary function testing, 119
Pulmonary hypertension, 102–103, 124
Pulmonary system
development in neonates, 221
nitrous oxide and, 51
sepsis and, 283
volatile anesthetics on, 48–49
Pulmonary vascular resistance (PVR), 84
Pulmonic valve, 80
Pulse oximetry, 20
Pulse wave analysis, for cardiac output, 24
Purkinje system, 81
Pyloric stenosis, 228
Pyridostigmine, 42

QTC prolongation, 97–98
Quinidine, 41

Radial nerve injury, 281
Radiation, 299
in anesthetic locations, 13
Radiofrequency ablation, for back pain, 263
Raman Scatter analysis, for depth of
anesthesia, 24
Randomized control trial, 302
Rebreathing, 1
circle system with, 215
Recurrent laryngeal nerve (RLN) palsy, 155
Red blood cells (RBCs)
disorders
anemia, 181
packed, 185–186
polycythemias, 182
transfusion, 186
pregnancy and, 238
Re-feeding syndrome, 293
Regional anesthesia, 63
local. See Local anesthetics
for multiple sclerosis, 209
principles, 273–274
for vascular surgery, 110
Remifentanil, 37
Renal system
abdominal aortic aneurysms and, 114
acid–base disorders, 174–177
anatomy and physiology, 169–172
anesthetic considerations in failure, 174
changes during labor, 238
development in neonates, 221–222

Renal system (*continued*)
    disorders, 172–173
    electrolyte disorders, 177–179
    failure, nonsteroidal anti-inflammatory
        drugs and, 260–261
    postoperative issues in, 74–75
    sepsis and, 283
    volatile anesthetics on, 48–49
Renin–angiotensin–aldosterone (RAA)
    system, 83, 169, 170*f*
Reproductive organs, anatomy and function
    of, 200
Respiratory acidosis, 175, 176
Respiratory alkalosis, 176
Respiratory depression, 35
Respiratory system. *See also* Lungs
    anatomy and innervation, 117–118
    barbiturates and, 33
    benzodiazepines and, 34
    changes during labor, 237–238
    dexmedetomidine and, 35
    etomidate and, 33
    infections, in pediatrics, 230
    ketamine and, 32
    mechanics, 118–119
    oxygen exchange, 120–121
    physiology, 119–120
    postoperative issues in, 73–74
    propofol and, 30
    ventilation control, 121–122
Reticular activating system, 130
Retinal vessel occlusion, 67
Retinopathy of prematurity (ROP), 223–224
Retrobulbar block, 151–152, 151*f*
Retrograde intubation, 60
Revised cardiac risk index (RCRI), 53
Rheumatoid arthritis, 213
Right atrium (RA), 79
Right bundle branch block (RBBB), 96
Right ventricle (RV), 79
Risk assessment, 303–304
Robin Hood syndrome, 138
Robotic-assisted cardiac surgery, 106–107
Rocuronium, 40
    metabolism of, 41
Romano–Ward syndrome, 97–98
Ropivacaine, 273, 276

Sacral plexus
    anatomy of, 277, 277*f*
    blocks, 278–279
Sacroiliac joint
    block, 263
    pain, 263
Sciatic nerve
    block, 278
    injury, 69, 281
Scoliosis, 232
Scopolamine, 151
    for postoperative nausea and vomiting, 76
Secondary hypertension, 87–88
Sedation
    definition of, 54
    for nonanesthesiologists, 63–64
    pediatrics, 233
Seizures, 144
Sentinel event, definition of, 310
Sepsis
    definitions of, 283
    pathophysiology of, 283
    severe, 283
    treatment for, 284
Septal rupture, myocardial infarction
    and, 89

Septic shock, 283
Serotonin, 265
    and norepinephrine reuptake inhibitors,
        262
Serum ascites albumin gradient (SAAG),
    160
Severe sepsis, 283
Sevoflurane, 46, 47
    for CBF and CMR, 132
    metabolism of, 48
    and unique properties, 49
Shivering, postoperative, 75–76
Shock
    cardiogenic, 284–285
    hypovolemic, 284
    septic, 283
    severe, 283
Shoulder dystocia, 253
Sickle-cell disease, 182
Sildenafil, for pulmonary hypertension, 103
Single shot spinal (SSS) anesthetic, 243
Sinoatrial cardiac cycle, 81
Sitting craniotomy, 145
Skin burning, 232–233
Smallpox, 297
Smoking cessation, 124
Sodium balance, in renal, 177–178
Sodium bicarbonate, 262, 272
Sodium citrate, 57
    for postoperative nausea and vomiting,
        76
Sodium iodine, for hyperthyroidism, 201
Sodium nitroprusside (SNP), 86–87
Sodium polystyrene sulfonate, for
    hypokalemia, 178
Somatosensory evoked potentials (SSEP),
    25
Somatostatin, for carcinoid tumor, 206
Spina bifida occulta, 143
Spinal anesthesia, 61–62
    for labor/C-section, 242–245
    for multiple sclerosis, 209
Spinal cord
    anatomy, 132–135
    injury, 142, 251
    stimulator, 263–264
    structure, 133, 134*f*
Spinal stenosis, 142, 263
Spinal tumors, 142
Spinobulbar muscular atrophy, 210
Spironolactone, for conn, 204
Stellate ganglion, 274
Stereotactic surgery, 146
Steroids
    for anaphylaxis, 71
    for brain relaxation, 145
    for bronchospasm, 72
    injections, for back pain, 263
    for intracranial hypertension, 140
    for subarachnoid hemorrhage, 142
Stewart model, 174
Strabismus, 153
Streptomycin, for plague, 297
Stress testing, heart disease and, 91
Stroke, 143–144
Subarachnoid analgesia, 260
Subarachnoid hematoma, 138
Subarachnoid hemorrhage, 141–142, 251
Subarachnoid space, 135
Subdural hematoma, 138
Substance abuse, 295–296
    in anesthesiologist, 296–297
    causes of increased, 296
    poisons and weapons, 297–299
    rates of, 296

risk factors for, 296
signs of, 296
treatment for, 296–297
Sub-tenon block, 153, 153*f*
Succinylcholine, 39, 150, 217
    for bariatric surgery, 163
    for cerebral palsy, 230
    for electroconvulsive therapy, 147
Sufentanil, 37
Sulfites, and allergic reactions, 71
Sulfonylureas, for type 2 diabetics, 203
Sumatriptan, 245
Superficial cervical plexus block, 110, 111*f*,
    274
Superior laryngeal nerve (SLN) palsy, 155
Supraclavicular block, 275–276
Suprascapular nerve injury, 68–69
Supraventricular tachycardias, 249
Sympathetic nervous system (SNS), 83,
    135–136
Sympathetic surge, 140–141
Syndrome of inappropriate ADH (SIADH)
    secretion, 140, 200
Systemic inflammatory response syndrome
    (SIRS), 283
Systemic vascular resistance (SVR), 84
Systolic dysfunction, 89

Takotsubo cardiomyopathy, 90
Temperature monitoring, 21
Temperature regulation, for perioperative
    management, 65–67
Tension, 267
Tension pneumothorax, 289
Terbutaline, for labor, 241
Testosterone, 200
Tetanus, 298
Tethered cord, 231
Tetracycline, for plague, 297
Tetralogy of fallot, 225, 225*f*
Thalamus, 129
Thalassemias, 182–183
Thermal burning injury, 290
Thermodilution, for cardiac output, 24
Thiazide, 170
    for hypertension, 249
Thienopyridine, 193
Thiopental, 33
Thoracic and abdominal aortic
    reconstruction–112–114
Thoracic blocks, 279
Thoracic injuries, 289–290
Thoracic surgery
    anesthetics for, 232
    for lungs, 125–126
Thrombocytopenia, 184–185
Thromboelastography, for coagulation, 194,
    194*f*, 195*f*
Thrombotic thrombocytopenia purpura
    (TTP), 185
Thyroid
    anatomy and function of, 199
    disorders, 201–202, 250
    storm, 201
Thyroidectomy, 164
    postoperative complications of, 201–202
Thyroid-stimulating hormone (TSH), 199
Thyrotropin-releasing hormone (TRH), 199
Ticlopidine, 244*t*
Tirofiban, 244*t*
Tizanidine, 261
Tocolysis, 241
Tolerance, definition of, 295
Tonsillectomy, 154–155, 231

Toradol, for emergence delirium, 219
Total IV anesthetic (TIVA), 25
Tourniquet, for sickle-cell disease, 182
Tracheal injury, 72
Tracheoesophageal fistula/esophageal
    atresia, 227–228
Tracheostomy, 60–61
Tramadol, 37
    for pain, 258
Transcranial Doppler, 26
Transcutaneous electrical nerve stimulation,
    263
Transcutaneous pacemaker, 10
Transesophageal echocardiogram, 10
Transexamic acid, for platelet function,
    187
Transfusion associated circulatory overload
    (TACO), 192
Transfusion-related acute lung injury
    (TRALI), 192
Transient tachypnea, of newborn, 223
Transsphenoidal resection, 146
Transthoracic echocardiogram, 9–10
Transurethral resection of the prostate
    (TURP), 166
Transvenous pacemaker, 10
Trauma
    obstetric resuscitation and, 253–254
    specific injuries, in intensive care unit,
        289–291. *See also specific injuries*
    surveys, in intensive care unit
        primary, 287
        purpose of, 287
        radiological evaluation of, 287–289
        secondary, 287
Traumatic brain injury (TBI), 137–138, 289
Treacher Collins syndrome, 230
Trial of labor after C-section (TOLAC). *See*
    Vaginal birth after C-section (VBAC)
Triamterene, for conn, 204
Tricuspid atresia, 226
Tricuspid regurgitation, 94
Tricuspid stenosis, 94
Tricuspid valve, 80
Tricyclic antidepressants (TCAs), 261–262
    for herpes zoster, 265
    peripheral neuropathy and, 265
    for tension, 267
Trigeminal nerve block, 274
Trigeminal neuralgia, 265
Trigeminal rhizotomy, 265
Triggers, 150–151
Trimethaphan, for autonomic hyperreflexia,
    143

Triptans
    for cluster headaches, 267
    for migraines, 267
Trisomy 21, 230
Trivalent botulinum antitoxin, for botulism,
    298
Truncus arteriosus, 225–226
t test, 302
Tumors, brain, 231
12-lead ECG testing, heart disease and, 90
2, 6-diisopropylphenol, 30
2-chloroprocaine, 243
Type 1 diabetics, 203
Type 2 diabetics, 203

Ulnar nerve injury, 281
Ulnar neuropathy, 68, 68f
Ultrasound imaging
    applications of, 9–10
    in central venous catheterization, 22
    frequency and image quality, 8–9, 9f
    image acquisition, 9
    for nervous system, 26
Umbilical cord prolapse, 253
Unifasicular block, 96
Upper extremity
    blocks and landmarks, 275–277
    injuries, 68–69
Upper respiratory tract infection, in
    pediatrics, 229
Uterine atony, treatment of, 242
Uterine blood flow (UBF), 239
Uterine rupture, 252

Vaginal birth after C-section (VBAC),
    252–253
Vagus nerve, 118
Valvular disease
    aortic insufficiency, 92–93
    aortic stenosis, 91–92
    endocarditis prophylaxis, 94–95
    hypertrophic cardiomyopathy, 94
    mitral insufficiency, 93–94
    mitral stenosis, 93
    tricuspid regurgitation, 94
    tricuspid stenosis, 94
Vancomycin, 285
Vaporizers, 6–7
    variable-bypass, 6f
Vasa previa, 252
Vascular malformations, 231
Vascular resistance, 83–84
Vascular surgery, 110–114

carotid endarterectomy, 110–112
    thoracic and abdominal aortic
        reconstruction–112–114
Vasodilators, for autonomic hyperreflexia,
    143
Vasopressin, 83, 85
    for diabetes insipidus, 140
    for isovolemic hypernatremia, 177
    for kidney transplantation, 165
    sepsis and, 284
Vasopressors, for electroconvulsive therapy,
    147
Vecuronium, 40
    metabolism of, 41
Venous air embolism, 145
Ventilation, one-lung, 124–125
Ventilatory system, 174
Ventricular fibrillation, 98
Ventricular tachycardia, 98
Ventricular tachycardias, 249
Ventriculostomy, 146
Verapamil, 86
Vertebrae, anatomy of, 132–133, 133f
Video-assisted laryngoscopy, 60
Visual evoked potentials, 25
Visual injuries, 67–68
Volatile anesthetics
    for CBF and CMR, 132
    elimination of, 48
    for fetal heart rate, 239
    fluoride concentration of, 50f
    hypercapnia and, 122
    mechanism of, 45
    minimum alveolar concentration, 45–46
    motor evoked potentials and, 25
    nitrous oxide, 51
    organ-specific effects of, 48–49
    somatosensory evoked potentials and, 25
    for subarachnoid hemorrhage, 142
    and unique properties, 49–51
    uptake, 46–48
        factors associated with, 46–47
von Willebrand Disease (vWD), 183–184

White blood cells (WBC), pregnancy and,
    238
White matter, 129
Wilms tumor, 232
Wolff–Parkinson–White syndrome, 95f, 97
World Health Organization (WHO),
    recommended pain medications, 258

Ziconotide, 262
Zoster vaccine, 265